T0184850

"I have had the pleasure of being a contributing author to one of Professor Wickramasinghe's previous books on digital health. Once again, she and her co-editors have assembled a roster of domain experts that cover currently relevant topics in the rapidly changing field of digital health. I appreciate how this book weaves in the areas of technical, management, clinical, and human factor considerations into the delivery of healthcare today. As a practicing clinician, I understand how analytic and AI technologies will play an increasingly critical role in effecting value-based care outcomes that are more precise and bespoke to the individual patient. I recommend this book as a critical read to all stakeholders who seek a greater understanding of just how technology plays an increasingly pertinent role in the delivery of care now and into the future."
Duane F. Wisk, *DO, MPH, FACOEM, Managing Partner, GlobalMed Physicians*

"AI is the tool that promises to change everything—with good reason. But without the intelligent analytics discussed in this groundbreaking book, it could just be the source of confusion and error. The two dimensions are critical to realizing its promise."
Albert J. Weatherhead III, *Professorship of Management, Dean and Professor, Department of Banking and Finance, Weatherhead School of Management, USA*

"Using data driven approaches in providing highly reliable patient care is the right thing to do. As technologies have advanced, Wickramasinghe et al. provide a glimpse into the management, technical, clinical and human factors associated with the critically important topics of applying analytics, artificial intelligence and machine learning to healthcare. Developing patient centered and clinician derived approaches to improving care models using descriptive, diagnostic, predictive and prescriptive analytics is the right approach, and the authors are expertly leading the readers to expedite their journey to improving healthcare."
Jonathan Schaffer, *MD, MBA, Managing Director, eCleveland Clinic, Information Technology Division of Cleveland Clinic, USA*

Dimensions of Intelligent Analytics for Smart Digital Health Solutions

This title demystifies artificial intelligence (AI) and analytics, upskilling individuals (healthcare professionals, hospital managers, consultants, researchers, students, and the population at large) around analytics and AI as it applies to healthcare.

This book shows how the tools, techniques, technologies, and tactics around analytics and AI can be best leveraged and utilised to realise a healthcare value proposition of better quality, better access and high value for everyone every day, everywhere. The book presents a triumvirate approach including technical, business and medical aspects of data and analytics and by so doing takes a responsible approach to this key area.

This work serves to introduce the critical issues in AI and analytics for healthcare to students, practitioners, and researchers.

Analytics and AI for Healthcare

Artificial Intelligence (AI) and analytics are increasingly being applied to various healthcare settings. AI and analytics are salient to facilitate better understanding and identifying key insights from healthcare data in many areas of practice and enquiry including at the genomic, individual, hospital, community and/or population levels. The Chapman & Hall/CRC Press Analytics and AI in Healthcare series aims to help professionals upskill and leverage the techniques, tools, technologies and tactics of analytics and AI to achieve better healthcare delivery, access, and outcomes. The series covers all areas of analytics and AI as applied to healthcare. It will look at critical areas including prevention, prediction, diagnosis, treatment, monitoring, rehabilitation, and survivorship.

The Series Editor: Professor Nilmini Wickramasinghe is a Professor of Digital Health and the Deputy Director of the Iverson Health Innovation Research Institute at Swinburne University of Technology, Australia, and is the inaugural Professor and Director Health Informatics Management at Epworth HealthCare, Victoria, Australia. She also holds honorary research professor positions at the Peter MacCallum Cancer Centre, Murdoch Children's Research Institute and Northern Health. For over 20 years, Professor Wickramasinghe has been researching and teaching within the health informatics/digital health domain. She was awarded the prestigious Alexander von Humboldt award in recognition of her outstanding contribution to digital health.

Data Analysis in Medicine and Health Using R
Kamarul Imran Musa, Wan Nor Arifin Wan Mansor and Tengku Muhammad Hanis

Data-Driven Science for Clinically Actionable Knowledge in Diseases
Daniel R. Catchpoole, Simeon J. Simoff, Paul J. Kennedy and Quang Vinh Nguyen

Translational Application of Artificial Intelligence in Healthcare – A Textbook
Edited by Sandeep Reddy

Dimensions of Intelligent Analytics for Smart Digital Health Solutions
Edited by Nilmini Wickramasinghe, Freimut Bodendorf and Mathias Kraus

For more information about this series please visit: https://www.routledge.com/analytics-and-ai-for-healthcare/book-series/Aforhealth

Dimensions of Intelligent Analytics for Smart Digital Health Solutions

Edited by

Nilmini Wickramasinghe

Freimut Bodendorf

Mathias Kraus

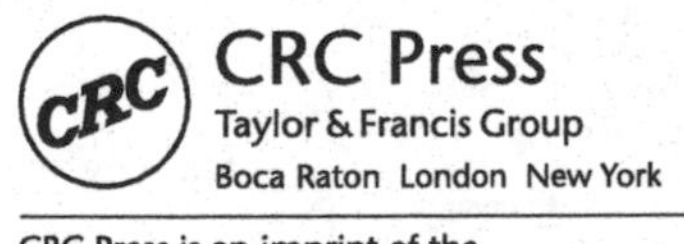

CRC Press is an imprint of the
Taylor & Francis Group, an **informa** business
A CHAPMAN & HALL BOOK

Designed cover image: Doctor Hands on Laptop in Abstract Scan with Futuristic Healthcare Wellness Analytics

First edition published 2024
by CRC Press
2385 NW Executive Center Drive, Suite 320, Boca Raton FL 33431

and by CRC Press
4 Park Square, Milton Park, Abingdon, Oxon, OX14 4RN

CRC Press is an imprint of Taylor & Francis Group, LLC

ISBN: 978-1-032-69973-8 (hbk)
ISBN: 978-1-032-69972-1 (pbk)
ISBN: 978-1-032-69974-5 (ebk)

DOI: 10.1201/9781032699745

Typeset in Minion
by MPS Limited, Dehradun

For our families for their support, our students for their thirst for knowledge, and all healthcare stakeholders who strive to realise superior, patient-centred healthcare delivery.

Contents

Editors

Nilmini Wickramasinghe is the Professor and Optus Chair of Digital Health at La Trobe University. In addition, she is the inaugural Professor and Director of Health Informatics Management at Epworth HealthCare. She also holds honorary research professor positions at the Peter MacCallum Cancer Centre, Murdoch Children's Research Institute (MCRI), and Northern Health. After completing five degrees at the University of Melbourne, she earned a PhD at Case Western Reserve University, Cleveland, Ohio, USA, and later completed the executive education at Harvard Business School, Harvard University, Cambridge, Massachusetts, USA, in value-based healthcare. For over 25 years, Professor Wickramasinghe has been actively researching and teaching within the health informatics/digital health domain in the United States, Germany and Australia, with a particular focus on designing, developing and deploying suitable models, strategies and techniques grounded in various management principles to facilitate the implementation and adoption of technology solutions to effect superior, value-based patient-centric care delivery. Professor Wickramasinghe collaborates with leading scholars at various premier healthcare organizations and universities throughout Australasia, the United States and Europe and is well published, with more than 400 referred scholarly articles, more than 15 books, numerous book chapters, an encyclopaedia and a well-established funded research track record securing over $25M in funding from grants in the United States, Australia, Germany and China as a chief investigator. She holds a patent around analytics solutions for managing healthcare data and is the editor-in-chief of the *International Journal of Networking and Virtual Organisations* (www.inderscience.com/ijnvo) as well as the editor of the Springer book series *Healthcare Delivery in the Information Age*. In 2020, she was awarded the prestigious

Alexander von Humboldt award for outstanding contribution to digital health, the first time this honour has been bestowed to someone in the discipline of digital health.

Freimut Bodendorf earned a degree in computer science at the School of Engineering, University of Erlangen-Nuremberg. He also earned a PhD in information systems. Subsequently, he was head of an IS Department at the University Hospital and Medical School at the University of Freiburg, Germany; professor at the Postgraduate School of Engineering in Nuremberg, Germany; and head of the Department of Computer Science and Information Systems at the University of Fribourg, Switzerland. He also is the head of the research group Management Intelligence Systems of the Institute of Information Systems at the University of Erlangen-Nuremberg. He is a faculty member of the School of Business and Economics as well as the School of Engineering and the School of Natural Sciences. Recently he was appointed to be a Research Fellow of the Fraunhofer Institute IIS, the largest institute in Germany. His scientific work focuses on business intelligence and digital health, including advanced data analytics, responsible artificial intelligence, intelligent assistance, data sharing and federated learning ecosystems. His research projects investigate and create solutions in the fields of digital transformation in healthcare and digital support of individual wellness.

Mathias Kraus is an Assistant Professor for Data Analytics at the Institute for Information Systems, FAU Erlangen-Nürnberg, where he also heads the White-Box AI research group. Prior to this appointment, he was a research assistant at ETH Zurich and the University of Freiburg. In his current role, he develops advances in data analytics with a focus on transparency and reliability in machine learning models. He has made several contributions to the scientific community through his work, which has been published in leading information systems and operations research journals and at prestigious computer science conferences.

Contributors

Dr. Belal Alsinglawi earned a PhD in computer science at Western Sydney University. He is currently a Senior Research Fellow at Swinburne University of Technology, Melbourne, Australia. His research interests span the areas of machine learning and medical computing, explainable AI, pervasive healthcare, and the Internet of Things.

Dr. Amir Eslami Andargoli is a Lecturer in Information Systems with research interests in digitalisation and innovation within healthcare. With a focus on the evolution of digital platforms, he explores how these technologies add value to organizations and individuals, aiming to contribute to more effective and efficient healthcare solutions.

Hanna Debus is a Researcher and Doctoral student at Siemens Healthineers, working at the intersection of machine learning and healthcare information systems. Her research focuses on predictive models for customer satisfaction. Her background is in biomedical engineering, which she studied at the University of Tübingen.

Dr. Isabella Eigner worked as a Research Assistant at the University Erlangen-Nuremberg in the area of healthcare analytics, particularly the prediction of high-risk patients for hospital readmissions. She is working in the industry as a Data Scientist in the area of market research and supply chain network design.

Dr. Andreas Hamper studied information systems at the Friedrich-Alexander University. He focused on digital health technologies at the Chair of Prof. Dr. Freimut Bodendorf.

Since 2021, Dr. Hamper is Head of the Business Transformation research group at the Fraunhofer Institute for Integrated Circuits IIS, focusing on digital and sustainable transformation.

Maximilian Harl studies Information Systems at the University Erlangen-Nuremberg and Interdisciplinary Brain Science at ETH Zurich, focusing on explainable predictive business process monitoring using graph-based neural networks.

Tobias Hatt recently completed his doctoral studies at ETH Zurich in the field of causal machine learning. During this time he spent a research stay at the University of Cambridge. His work has been published in leading computer science outlets such as KDD, ICML and AISTATS.

Prof. Prem Prakash Jayaraman is a Professor in Internet of Things and Distributed Systems and Director of Swinburne's Factory of the Future and Digital Innovation Lab. His research focus is in the areas of Internet of Things (IoT), and mobile and cloud computing. He has authored or coauthored 150+ journal, conference and book chapters in highly ranked venues of the above research areas.

Kevin Kohler recently completed his studies in Information Systems at FAU Erlangen-Nürnberg. During this time, he focused on explainable and interpretable machine learning with a focus on the healthcare domain.

Pavlina Kröckel is a Habilitation Candidate at the Institute for Information Systems at the University of Erlangen-Nuremberg in Germany. Her research interests are in the field of responsible AI in healthcare, specifically privacy and security in data sharing, responsible business models and ethics in the design and implementation of AI-based systems in healthcare.

Tong Lei Liu is a Critical Care Resident at Monash Health. He holds MD and MClinEpi degrees from Monash University and the University of Newcastle, respectively. Their research focuses on clinical applications of prediction modelling in perioperative care, with a particular emphasis on optimising postoperative pain and reducing complications.

Annika Lurz holds a data science position at Siemens Healthineers and is a collaborating researcher at the Institute of Information Systems at the University of Erlangen-Nuremberg in Germany. Her research interests include competitive intelligence in healthcare, particularly mergers and acquisitions prediction. She is an expert in graph neural networks and natural language processing methods.

Wendy D. Lynch As a research scientist working in the business world, Dr. Wendy D. Lynch is a sense-maker and translator. A consultant to numerous Fortune 100 companies, startups and academic institutions, her current work focuses on applying big data analytics in business. Founder of analytic-translator.com, Dr. Lynch also trains analytic translators.

Dr. Daniel Neumann worked as a Data Scientist and Industrial Engineer in the field of collaborative planning of changeable systems for complex products at TU Chemnitz and subsequently in the field of IT-supported healthcare. He is now researching the creation and analysis of process models for patient journeys, particularly for the development and operation of collaborative decision support systems at the University of Leipzig.

Mark Nevin has held executive positions in international healthcare organisations involving leading strategy, policy development, regulation, and advocacy. He has wide-ranging experience in health workforce and the adoption of new technologies. Mark was awarded a Fellowship of the Australasian Institute of Digital Health in 2020 in recognition of his expertise in telehealth and artificial intelligence.

Gurdeep Sarai is a PhD student in the Faculty of Health Science at Swinburne University of Technology. His thesis focuses on the degree of fidelity with which a sailing simulator can reproduce the health benefits associated with real-life sailing. Her research is funded by Northern Health and VSail.

Muhammad Nadeem Shuakat, PhD, MS, BE, works at Epworth HealthCare and Swinburne University of Technology on various projects for technology integration for superior health. He is also involved in digital health education. His research interests include IT

Solutions, eTextiles, modelling, sensors and the use of technology for eHealth.

Josh Ting is a Medical Student at the University of Melbourne School of Medicine. His research interest focuses on healthcare service process improvement and healthcare technological innovation.

Oren Tirosh's expertise is in biomechanics, specifically in gait analysis and development of wearable sensors technology and applications for digital teleplatforms in sport and rehabilitation. Tirosh developed several digital health platforms used in hospitals and smartphone applications, allowing clinicians to remotely quantify their patients' gait and postural control.

Nalika Ulapane earned BSc (Hons) and PhD degrees in electrical and electronics engineering at the University of Peradeniya, Sri Lanka, and the University of Technology Sydney (UTS), Australia, respectively. He has gone on to serve research fellowships at UTS, the University of Melbourne, and Swinburne University of Technology. He works on mathematical modelling, machine learning, sensor technologies, robotics and digital health.

Eva van Weenen is a Doctoral Student in the field of wearable technology in diabetes at ETH Zurich. Prior to her doctoral studies, she graduated from the University of Leiden in astrophysics. She has published her work in leading medical journals, such as *Diabetes Care* and *Diabetes, Obesity and Metabolism*.

Dr. Stephen Vaughan conducts a part-time practice as a Locum Consultant Physician in haematology/medical oncology in various public and private clinics throughout Victoria and New South Wales. He has also worked as a Consultant to the Health Insurance Commission on high-cost drugs and for the Department of Health and Human Services on IT implementation. He was a part-time Director of the Grampians Integrated Cancer Service.

Doug Vogel is a Professor of Information Systems (IS) and an Association for Information Systems (AIS) Fellow as well as AIS Past President and, currently, Director of the eHealth Research Institute as a

State Specially Recruited Expert in the School of Management at the Harbin Institute of Technology in China. He is an Australian Institute of Digital Health Fellow and has published widely, received over 20,000 citations and has a presence in over 100 countries.

Adjunct Professor John Zelcer is a Healthcare Strategy Consultant, Clinician and Informatician whose career has included clinical and academic medicine, health informatics, executive management and management consulting in Australia and the United States, and board director roles in public, private and not-for-profit organisations in the healthcare sector.

Foreword

It's indeed my pleasure to write the foreword to this book by Nilmini Wickramasinghe, Mathias Kraus and Freimut Bodendorf. The title *Dimensions of Intelligent Analytics for Smart Digital Health Solutions* conveys the essence of the subject area and context. The sections of the book adequately address the many complex and intertwined topics associated with this important domain.

Technical considerations (Section I) lay the foundations for successful application. The rapid development and introduction of new technologies and associated data provide avenues for understanding and learning that, historically, could only be imagined. As we have moved from an era of big data to huge data, artificial intelligence in conjunction with analytics and machine learning has come to the rescue to provide insight and opportunity for personalization, albeit given correct interpretation. However, technical considerations are only part of the bigger picture as addressed in the remaining sections.

Management perspectives (Section II) deserve special attention as organizations seek to benefit from artificial intelligence, analytics and machine learning applications in healthcare contexts. Implementation in terms of getting systems and associated data used and useful is a perennial issue. Of special concern in healthcare are aspects of data privacy, ownership and governance. Breaches occur and mistrust can fester, which presents special challenges. New models and approaches for successful management are paramount to deal not only with these issues but also with the rapid rise of chronic conditions to meet the needs of the future in a sustainable and competitive fashion. The chapters in this section successfully explore the broad range of managerial issues and implications.

Clinical applications (Section III) demonstrate effectively how technical considerations and management perspectives come together to deliver robust solutions. It's important to have examples to draw upon and learn from to move forward to meet an ever-demanding future. Artificial intelligence, analytics, and machine learning play key roles in achieving success in the presence of barriers and challenges, especially in unexpected circumstances amidst desires for effective care with sensitivity to privacy and security. The chapters in this section deal with a wide range of possible clinical applications and their implications for delivering better patient-centric outcomes.

Human factors (Section IV) are often overlooked and can often lead to system demise over time from issues that could have been addressed, with implications that can be long-lasting. Artificial intelligence, analytics ,and machine learning have the potential for great success but also present issues that have not previously surfaced. Workforce considerations are paramount as well as more general patient issues. The concept of digital twins provides a novel opportunity for exploration and application. Developing shared meaning across a broad range of stakeholders is not easy but can lead to heightened degrees of trust and application success in the presence of ever-changing technical considerations and management challenges.

Overall, this book makes an important contribution and will, in my opinion, be well-received by a broad range of stakeholders and interested citizens. Many thanks go to Nilmini Wickramasinghe, Mathias Kraus and Freimut Bodendorf for their time and efforts which are, indeed, to be commended.

Doug Vogel
Association for Information Systems
Fellow and Past-President, Australasian Institute of
Digital Health Fellow, Professor and
eHealth Research Institute Director
Harbin Institute of Technology, P.R. China

Preface

In today's Information Age or Knowledge Economy, data has become a most indispensable raw material, in many ways as precious as gold or silver. This makes harnessing this most valuable asset and refining it into information and knowledge so it can be useful and useable to support decision-making not just a strategic necessity, but essential for all organisations to be effective, efficient and sustainable.

Over the last 10 years, the advances in technology and especially the Internet of Things have been tremendous and afforded us with a plethora of tools and techniques which can be utilised to enhance the value of the volumes of data we now find generated. In particular, the tools of analytics and artificial intelligence as well as the techniques of machine learning have been applied most successfully to revolutionise various industries and sectors, notably banking, finance, and manufacturing. To date, however, healthcare while very data rich, has been slow and cautious to embrace these tools and techniques.

Our book has been developed to highlight the benefits of applying analytics, artificial intelligence and machine learning to various healthcare contexts to enable the maximisation of critical data resources to enable superior healthcare delivery and the realisation of a healthcare value proposition of better access to care, better quality of care and high value of care. Recognising that healthcare is a complex area dealing with biological systems, we note this can be challenging and have identified key considerations; technical, managerial, clinical and human or people issues. Hence, we have structured the book to provide insights into the applications of analytics, artificial intelligence, and machine learning with respect to these considerations and perspectives as follows:

SECTION I: TECHNICAL CONSIDERATIONS

This section serves to highlight important and key technical considerations as follows:

Chapter 1: Medical Image Processing by Hanna Debus
Debus discusses the role of analytics, AI and ML in medical imaging. Given the advances in medical imaging and deeper reliance on images to inform clinical decision-making today, this is a significant area to apply these tools and techniques to enhance key data assets.

Chapter 2: Smart Wearables in Healthcare by Eva van Weenen
Weenen outlines key considerations around wearable devices, which are now so prevalent for supporting various aspects of self-monitoring. In particular, the role of analytics, artificial intelligence and machine learning serve to make these wearables at various levels of "smartness".

Chapter 3: Causal AI in Personalised Healthcare by Tobias Hatt
As Hatt outlines in this chapter, artificial intelligence can be used to make healthcare and healthcare decision-making more personalized. Personalization and patient centeredness are becoming essential aspects as we strive towards superior healthcare delivery.

Chapter 4: Interpretable AI in Healthcare by Kevin Kohler et al.
In order to maximise the benefits of artificial intelligence in healthcare, it is necessary for these solutions to be interpreted correctly. This forms the thesis of this chapter by Kohler et al.

SECTION II: MANAGEMENT PERSPECTIVES

This section focuses on managerial issues and implications with respect to artificial intelligence, analytics and machine learning applications in healthcare contexts.

Chapter 5: Data Ownership and Emerging Data Governance Models in Healthcare by Pavlina Kröckel
It is vital when managing healthcare data that issues of ownership and governance are well addressed. Kröckel unpacks these critical issues in this chapter.

Chapter 6: Privacy-Preserving Roadmap for Medical Data-Sharing Systems by Belal Alsinglawi et al.
Especially due to its high sensitivity, health data is vulnerable to breaches of privacy. Alsinglawi et al. discuss a roadmap for trying to preserve

privacy which utilises analytics, artificial intelligence and machine learning.

Chapter 7: A Comparative Review of Descriptive Process Models in Healthcare Operations Management and Analytics by Daniel Neumann et al.
As more and more models are emerging in healthcare, it becomes important to understand their respective strengths and weaknesses. This is the focus of the chapter by Neumann et al.

Chapter 8: AI Approaches for Managing Preventive Care in Digital Health Ecosystems by Andreas Hamper
In today's 21st century, we are plagued with a rapid rise in chronic conditions. Prevention is a vital aspect of good healthcare operations. This chapter by Hamper identifies how artificial intelligence can assist.

Chapter 9: Competitive Intelligence in Healthcare by Annika Lurz
Like all industries, healthcare needs to be sustainable and competitive. Lurz explores this in terms of competitive intelligence in this chapter.

SECTION III: CLINICAL APPLICATIONS

Possible clinical applications and their implications for delivering better patient-centred clinical outcomes, or not, are the focus of this section.

Chapter 10: Machine Learning for Healthcare Applications: Possibilities and Barriers by Nalika Ulapane et al.
In this chapter, Ulapane et al. unpack several machine learning applications and in doing so present key barriers and facilitators.

Chapter 11: Systematic Review of Prediction Models for Chronic Opioid Use Following Surgery by Tong Lei Liu et al.
Liu et al. present evidence from the literature which serves to highlight the impact of analytics, machine learning and/or artificial intelligence for identifying overuse and possible addiction to opioids.

Chapter 12: Addressing Challenges in the Emergency Department with Analytics and AI by Josh Ting et al.
One of the critical areas in hospitals is the emergency department. Ting et al. identify opportunities for analytics and artificial intelligence to support and facilitate effective and efficient deployment of essential care in this context.

Chapter 13: Using Simulators to Assist with Mental Health Issues: The Impact of a Sailing Simulator on People with ADHD, by Gurdeep Sarai et al.
Gurdeep Sarai et al. discuss the growing use of simulators, their advantages and the benefits of physical activity for people with attention deficit hyperactivity disorder (ADHD) offered by the VSail Sailing Simulator.

Chapter 14: A Possible Blockchain Architecture for Healthcare: Insights from Catena-X by Nalika Ulapane et al.
To address vital privacy and security concerns with sensitive data, Ulapane et al. present a private blockchain architecture model that is developed from outside of healthcare.

SECTION IV: HUMAN FACTORS

Ultimately healthcare is about people, so human factors while forming the last section of this book are definitely not the least important consideration.

Chapter 15: Implications and Considerations of AI for the Healthcare Workforce: A Theoretical Perspective by Mark Nevin
Nevin highlights the need for changes in the health workforce given the introduction of artificial intelligence, analytics and machine learning.

Chapter 16: Unplanned Readmission Risks for Comorbid Patients of Diabetes – An Action Design Research Paradigm Data-driven Decision Support by Nilmini Wickramasinghe
In this chapter, Wickramasinghe applies an action research methodology to highlight critical issues around unplanned readmission with diabetes comorbid patients.

Chapter 17: Establishing a Digital Twin Architecture for Superior Falls Risk Prediction by Nilmini Wickramasinghe
Wickramasinghe discusses how deriving a digital twin of a patient can be of assistance in preventing falls during an acute care visit.

Chapter 18: Facilitating a Shared Meaning of AI/ML Findings Amongst Key Healthcare Stakeholders: The Role of Analytic Translators by Wendy D. Lynch et al.
Lynch et al. highlight a current key void in healthcare given the introduction of analytics, artificial intelligence and machine learning; namely, the need for all healthcare stakeholders to be equally comfortable around terminology and far-reaching implications.

No single volume can capture all aspects of applying analytics, artificial intelligence and machine learning to healthcare, and this was definitely not our goal. Rather, we have set out to provide an indication of the possibilities and pitfalls that can be encountered as one traverses along this path under the four key areas of technical, management, clinical, and human. We hope that this miscellany of chapters serves to highlight key barriers, benefits and facilitators. Moreover, we trust it will encourage all healthcare stakeholders, researchers and individuals to embrace these techniques and move forward responsibly. We believe the future for healthcare delivery is indeed positive and that we can realise a vision of superior healthcare delivery if we embrace these tools and techniques to maximise critical healthcare data assets to support patient-centered high-quality clinical outcomes that are also high value. We trust you enjoy reading this book and working responsibly with healthcare data assets as you apply the tools and techniques of analytics, artificial intelligence, and machine learning in order to provide superior quality and high-value healthcare delivery.

Nilmini Wickramasinghe
Freimut Bodendorf
Mathias Kraus

Acknowledgements

This work would not be possible without the support and contributions of many people, too numerous to name individually. Moreover, as we have been coming out of COVID-19 during this time, it has been particularly challenging for us all; hence, we are doubly indebted to everyone who has, despite their own personal hardships, continued to support us in completing this project in a timely fashion. First and foremost, we thank all the authors who have contributed such thought-provoking chapters that fill the following pages. We are indebted to our respective institutions for affording us the time to work on this book project and our colleagues for their help. In addition, we are most grateful for the wonderful assistance provided by the team at CRC Routledge. Further, we acknowledge the Alexander von Humboldt Stiftung for awarding and funding Professor Nilmini Wickramasinghe to conduct research work at Friedrich Alexander University, Nuremberg, Germany with Professors Freimut Bodendorf and Mathias Kraus; this book being one of the outcomes of this collaboration. Finally, we thank our families for their ongoing encouragement and support.

Eva van Weenen acknowledges funding from the Swiss National Science Foundation (SNSF) as part of the Eccellenza grant 186932 on "Data-driven health management" for her Chapter 2, "Smart Wearables in Healthcare".

I

Technical Considerations

Nilmini Wickramasinghe, Freimut Bodendorf, and Mathias Kraus

The integration of artificial intelligence (AI) and analytics into healthcare has opened the door to numerous innovative applications that can drastically improve patient care and outcomes. As we enter a new era of healthcare, driven by technology and informed decision-making, it is essential to explore the various domains in which AI and analytics are making a significant impact. In this section, we delve into four key areas where technology is transforming healthcare: medical image processing, smart wearables, personalised healthcare, and interpretable AI. Each chapter offers insights into the challenges, opportunities, and best practices associated with these emerging technologies, providing a comprehensive overview of the current state of AI and analytics in healthcare.

Chapter 1: Medical Image Processing, by Hanna Debus, introduces the various types of imaging modalities as well as the use of machine learning and AI for medical image processing. Medical imaging plays a critical role in disease detection and diagnosis, and the use of AI and machine learning can significantly enhance the accuracy and speed of diagnosis.

Chapter 2: Smart Wearables in Healthcare, by Eva van Weenen, explores the use of smart wearables such as fitness trackers, smartwatches, and other connected devices in healthcare. These devices can provide

DOI: 10.1201/9781032699745-1

continuous monitoring of health data, enabling early detection of health issues and personalised treatment plans.

Chapter 3: Causal AI in Personalized Healthcare, by Tobias Hatt, focuses on the use of AI and machine learning to deliver personalised healthcare. Personalised healthcare takes into account the unique characteristics and needs of each patient, allowing for more precise diagnoses and treatment plans.

Chapter 4: Interpretable AI in Healthcare, by Kevin Kohler and Mathias Kraus, discusses the importance of interpretability in AI and machine learning models for healthcare. Interpretable AI can help clinicians understand how an AI model is making predictions, increasing transparency and trust in the decision-making process.

The chapters in this section offer a glimpse into the exciting possibilities that lie ahead for AI and analytics in healthcare. As we continue to innovate and push the boundaries of what is possible, it is crucial to maintain a focus on patient-centred care and to ensure that technology serves the best interests of patients and healthcare providers alike. By using the opportunities presented by AI and analytics while addressing the challenges they pose, we can create a healthcare system that is more efficient, effective, and personalised than ever before.

One of the key factors that will determine the success of AI and analytics in healthcare is the ability to integrate these technologies seamlessly into existing workflows and systems. This requires a collaborative approach, bringing together healthcare professionals, technologists, researchers, and policymakers to develop and implement effective solutions. By fostering a multidisciplinary dialogue, we can bridge the gap between cutting-edge research and real-world clinical practice, ensuring that technology serves the needs of both patients and healthcare providers.

CHAPTER 1

Medical Image Processing

Hanna Debus

INTRODUCTION

Medical imaging plays a critical role in modern medicine, allowing healthcare professionals to visualise the internal structures and functions of the human body (Bankman 2008). The availability of a wide range of imaging modalities, such as computed tomography (CT) (Kalender 2011; Kamalian, Lev, and Gupta 2016), magnetic resonance imaging (MRI) (Mazzoni et al. 2021; Y. Liu et al. 2021), and sonography (Sanders and Winter 2006), has revolutionised the way diagnoses are made and treatments are administered. With the help of these imaging techniques, healthcare professionals can obtain detailed insights into the human body, detect and diagnose various conditions, and plan appropriate interventions (Bankman 2008).

Medical image processing is a subfield of medical imaging that involves various steps involved in image formation, computation, and management. The process of image formation involves acquiring data from the imaging modalities and reconstructing it to form images. Image computation is a critical step that encompasses various techniques such as segmentation, enhancement of image features, and image analysis (Bankman 2008). Image management, on the other hand, involves tasks related to handling image data, including registration, storage, and other processes (Arenson et al. 1988).

One of the primary goals of medical image processing is to improve image quality. This involves reducing image noise, enhancing images to

DOI: 10.1201/9781032699745-2

highlight important features, and automating image analysis to increase efficiency and accuracy (Perumal and Velmurugan 2018). The availability of advanced image processing techniques and algorithms has enabled healthcare professionals to make more informed decisions and provide more effective treatments (Narin, Kaya, and Pamuk 2021; Jünger, Hoyer, and Schaufler 2021). Medical image processing also plays a crucial role in advancing medical research and development. For example, the use of advanced image processing algorithms has enabled researchers to analyse large datasets and uncover new insights into various medical conditions (Bankman 2008). The development of innovative imaging modalities, such as functional MRI (fMRI) and positron emission tomography (PET), has been enabled by advancements in medical image processing. Another important aspect of medical image processing is image registration, which involves aligning and merging multiple images of the same body region taken from different imaging modalities or at different time points (Kostelec and Periaswamy 2003). Image registration is essential in providing a comprehensive and holistic view of the human body and tracking changes over time. It also plays a critical role in radiation therapy planning, where images from multiple imaging modalities are used to define the treatment area and deliver radiation in a precise and effective manner. In addition to improving the quality of medical examinations and diagnoses, medical image processing has the potential to reduce healthcare costs (Srinivasan and Arunasalam 2013). By automating routine tasks, reducing the need for repeat examinations, and improving the accuracy of diagnoses, medical image processing can help reduce costs and increase efficiency. However, despite the many benefits of medical image processing, there are also challenges and limitations that must be addressed. For example, the quality of medical images can be affected by various factors such as patient motion, noise, and artifacts. Advanced image processing techniques can help reduce the impact of these factors, but they must be validated and standardised to ensure reliable and consistent results (Wiens et al. 2019).

Medical image processing is a critical aspect of modern medicine, playing a key role in improving the quality of medical examinations and diagnoses, advancing medical research and development, and reducing healthcare costs (Srinivasan and Arunasalam 2013). With the rapid pace of technological advancements and the growing availability of data, the field of medical image processing is expected to continue to evolve and make a significant impact on healthcare in the future.

The objective of this chapter is to give an introduction and overview of the field of medical image processing. We start by giving an introduction to conventional methods for image processing. Afterwards, we continue with more modern techniques for medical image processing, including machine learning and neural networks. To provide a more complete picture, we also briefly describe the underlying functionalities of the different imaging modalities. Finally, we discuss these techniques, highlight limitations, and link to current research.

CONVENTIONAL METHODS FOR IMAGE PROCESSING

Medical imaging plays a crucial role in modern medicine by providing physicians with a visual representation of the human body, enabling them to diagnose and treat various conditions (Bankman 2008). There are several imaging modalities available, including computed tomography, magnetic resonance imaging, positron emission tomography, and sonography, each of which provides unique insights into the body. To further analyse and extract meaningful information from the images produced by these modalities, a wide range of image processing techniques have been developed. These techniques can improve image quality, extract and enhance specific features, and support automated analysis. The choice of which techniques to use depends on various factors, including the type of image data, its contrast, grey-scale characteristics, and the imaging parameters used to produce it.

The following section provides an overview of some of the most commonly used image processing techniques for CT, MRI, PET, and sonography image data. However, due to the vast number of techniques available, only a selection of representative methods will be introduced. These techniques are important for improving the quality of medical examinations and diagnoses, and they are continually being developed and refined to meet the changing needs of modern medicine. The various imaging modalities and image processing techniques have been instrumental in advancing the field of medicine, and they continue to play a vital role in the diagnosis and treatment of various medical conditions. From reducing noise in images to targeted enhancement of specific features, the use of image processing has greatly improved the accuracy and speed of diagnoses, leading to better patient outcomes.

Windowing

As one of the first steps after image acquisition, windowing is the standard processing technique allowing for the extraction of useful information and contrast enhancement. For instance, sonographic images are greyscale images, whereby the brightness of each pixel can be mapped to grey values between 0 and 255. In CT, greyscale values are typically measured in the Hounsfield scale (HU values). They generally range between -1024 HU and 3071 HU but are usually transformed into grey values between 0 and 255 as that is the range visible to the human eye (Xue et al. 2012). As a result, the contrast between two adjacent image regions might not be high enough to differentiate these tissues properly.

As a remedy, the definition of a window with fixed HU values for centre c and width w ($w = HU_{max} - HU_{min}$) limits the used grey values and enables the accentuation of specific tissue types. Only HU numbers within the set width are distributed over the full range of the greyscale ($HU_{max} = 0 = black$, $HU_{min} = 255 = white$) (Xue et al. 2012). By setting the window width, the grey value representation of certain image regions can be changed, allowing for the regions of interest to be brought out. All parts of the image with HU numbers below the window's lower threshold are displayed in black, while all parts of the image with HU numbers above the window's upper threshold are displayed in white (Xue et al. 2012). This effectively eliminates parts of the image that are not within the range of HU values defined by the window, making the regions of interest more visible.

There are established window settings that are best suited for accentuating commonly examined tissue types, such as bone, brain, lung, or soft tissue. These established window settings make it easier for healthcare professionals to quickly and accurately visualise the regions of interest in an image. By changing the window settings, different tissue types can be accentuated and visualised, providing healthcare professionals with more information about the internal structures and functions of the human body.

In conclusion, window setting is an effective tool in medical image processing that helps to improve the quality of images and enables healthcare professionals to better visualise specific tissue types. By changing the window settings, different tissue types can be accentuated, providing healthcare professionals with a more comprehensive view of the human body and allowing them to make more informed decisions and provide more effective treatments.

Noise Reduction and Resolution Enhancement

Accurately imaging as many details as possible is the basis for exact medical statements and decisions. However, almost every image acquired by an imaging modality such as MRI, CT, or sonography contains some amount of noise. Image noise can be caused by different factors. The X-ray photons and certain properties of the detector lead to noise in CT imaging. In MRI, the static magnetic field, switching of the gradients, movement of the patient or metal parts in the body are just a few examples that cause noise in the resulting image. Hence, there are a variety of techniques for removing noise from the images.

Traditionally, these techniques involve so-called filters, where each of the available filters is optimised for a different type of noise. The existence of variations of the image signal leading to pixels of incorrect intensity or greyscale value is the general definition of noise (Perumal and Velmurugan 2018). Salt and pepper noise and Gaussian noise are the two most common types of noise in MR and sonographic imaging (Wahlang, Saha, and Maji 2020). Salt and pepper noise or speckle noise occurs as randomly occurring black and white pixels. Unavoidable external conditions lead to Gaussian noise. The image pixels vary from their actual value following the normal distribution (Perumal and Velmurugan 2018). Most filters follow the same functionality – eliminating noise by smoothing the image and enhancing the edges.

One of the most used filters is the average filter. This linear filter starts with the first image pixel and iterates through all pixels one by one. In this process, a quadratic convolution matrix (usually covering a window of $n \times m$ pixels, where $n = m$) is applied to a centre pixel and its neighbouring pixels. The filter calculates the average of all pixels and replaces the centre pixel with this value. By doing so, we obtain a blurred version of the image (Shedbalkar and Prabhushetty 2021). Equation 1.1 shows a 5×5 averaging convolution mask – to determine the new value for the centre pixel, all pixel values are added up and divided by the number of pixels.

$$C_{Average} = \frac{1}{25}[1\ 1\ 1\ 1\ 1\ 1\ 1\ 1\ 1\ 1\ 1\ 1\ 1\ 1\ 1\ 1\ 1\ 1\ 1\ 1\ 1\ 1\ 1\ 1\ 1] \quad (1.1)$$

For salt and pepper noise, the median filter is the most efficient filter. It works similarly to the average filter but determines the median of the pixels that are included in the convolution mask. However, the median filter is a non-linear filter coming with advantages over linear filters, since it protects the edges of the image from being changed (Shedbalkar and Prabhushetty 2021). To reduce Gaussian noise, a convolution matrix representing the Gaussian distribution (Equation 1.2) is applied to the image pixels. This convolution operation reduces the image contrast and has a blurring effect. Hence, the image is smoothed and noise is reduced, but at the same time image detail is lost (Shedbalkar and Prabhushetty 2021).

$$C_{Gaussian} = \frac{1}{256}[1\,4\,6\,4\,1\,4\,16\,24\,16\,4\,6\,24\,36\,24\,6\,4\,16\,24\,16\,4\,1\,4\,6\,4\,1]. \tag{1.2}$$

PET imaging is generally dealing with different types of noise. Noise in the image data can be caused by scattered or random coincidence events (Cho et al. 2010). In random coincidence events two gamma rays that do not belong together accidentally hit the detector at opposite locations. A scattered photon is a photon that collides with an electron in the tissue and deviates from its original path. As a result, it is possible that two scattered gamma rays are detected as a coincidence event. For both cases, the acquired PET data is incorrect, as the events do not result from a real annihilation event but are recorded as such. For correction of accidentally occurring events, the rate of the random events is calculated and subtracted from the recorded signal. However, the correction of scattered coincidence events is much more complicated. Scatter noise is therefore sometimes also ignored. However, this field is under active research and different methods for noise reduction are still being further developed (Chen and An 2017). By reducing as much image noise as possible, the resolution of the PET scan is enhanced.

Edge Detection and Threshold Segmentation

To automatically detect abnormal structures in the overall image or relevant changes in homogeneous regions of tissue, classical edge detection techniques are widely used.

Edges in images are defined as local contrasts, i.e., image parts with significant differences between two adjacent grey values (Sarkar and

Mandal 2015). Different filters and thresholds are used to reduce image noise and filter out some image details, thereby enhancing edges and borders between structures.

The difference in grey value between two image regions can be described as a gradient ∇G (Equation 1.3) (in both x-direction G_x and y-direction G_y for 2D-images), the gradient magnitude, therefore, describes the edge strength G (Equation 1.4) (Sarkar and Mandal 2015).

$$\nabla G = \begin{pmatrix} G_x \\ G_y \end{pmatrix} = \begin{pmatrix} \partial G/\partial x \\ \partial G/\partial y \end{pmatrix} \tag{1.3}$$

$$G = |\nabla G| = \sqrt{(G_x^2 + G_y^2)} = \sqrt{\left(\left(\frac{\partial G}{\partial x}\right)^2 + \left(\frac{\partial G}{\partial y}\right)^2\right)}. \tag{1.4}$$

The direction of the gradient (hence the direction of the largest change in grey value which is perpendicular to the imaged edge) can be determined using Equation 1.5.

$$\theta_G = \left(\frac{G_x}{G_y}\right). \tag{1.5}$$

One widely used example applicable to greyscale images is the *Canny Edge Detector* (Canny 1986).

As a first step, a Gaussian filter is applied to reduce and smooth out Gaussian noise (random, normally distributed noise) (Al-Jibory and El-Zaart 2013). A convolution mask based on the Gaussian distribution (Equation 1.6 and 1.7) is used for this processing step. Typically, convolution masks with a size between 3 × 3 and 5 × 5 pixels are used, as the sensitivity of the filter decreases with larger mask sizes (Maini and Aggarwal 2009).

$$f(x) = \frac{1}{\sigma\sqrt{2\pi}} e^{-\frac{1}{2}\left(\frac{x-\mu}{\sigma}\right)^2}. \tag{1.6}$$

$$\textit{Exemplary } 3 \times 3 \textit{ Gaussian convolution mask: } C = \frac{1}{16}[1\ 2\ 1\ 2\ 4\ 2\ 1\ 2\ 1]. \tag{1.7}$$

In the next step, the edge strength of each pixel is compared to a pair of set threshold values (t_{high} and t_{low}) (Al-Jibory and El-Zaart 2013). In this pixel-based segmentation process, pixels with a value above the high threshold are considered edge pixels, while pixels below the threshold are changed to background (black).

$$\textit{Strong edge pixels: } e > t_{high} \tag{1.8}$$

$$\textit{Weak edge pixel: } t_{high} \geq e \geq t_{low} \tag{1.9}$$

$$\textit{Background pixels: } e < t_{low} \tag{1.10}$$

MODERN METHODS FOR IMAGE PROCESSING

This section introduces further developments and extended versions of established applications for image processing. Following the general trend of processing techniques for different types of data, there are numerous neural network-based developments for high-quality medical images. Automated detection of known structures, anatomical features, and physiological processes, or even medical findings for support of radiologists and physicians are particularly frequent topics in current publications. The following subsections give an overview of techniques for graphically analysing images and present exemplary use cases for the automated detection of medically relevant image elements and findings.

Segmentation

Segmentation in medical image processing refers to the process of partitioning a medical image into multiple regions or segments that correspond to different structures or regions of interest (Bankman 2008). The goal of segmentation is to identify and isolate specific structures within the image, such as tumours, organs, bones, or tissues, and to extract useful information from them. The segmented regions can then be used for further analysis, such as quantifying their size, shape, or intensity, or for visualisation purposes, such as displaying a 3D reconstruction of a specific organ or structure.

There are various techniques for performing medical image segmentation, including manual methods, semi-automated methods, and fully automated methods (Pham, Xu, and Prince 2000). Manual methods involve a human expert manually tracing or outlining the structures of interest, while semi-automated methods involve a combination of manual and automated approaches. Fully automated methods, on the other hand, rely on computer algorithms to segment the image, typically by using image analysis techniques such as edge detection, region growing, or clustering.

Recent developments in the field of medical image segmentation include the use of artificial neural networks to achieve more accurate and efficient segmentation results. Artificial neural networks have a complex structure of neurons with the simplest form consisting of an input layer, one hidden layer, and an output layer. Additionally, the integration of machine learning algorithms with traditional image processing methods has improved the ability of automated segmentation methods to handle complex and challenging images, such as those that contain noise, low contrast, or large anatomical variations (Pham, Xu, and Prince 2000).

The algorithms and required processing steps are typically implemented using *Convolutional Neural Networks* (CNN), which are specifically well-suited to process image data (Narin, Kaya, and Pamuk 2021). Similar to classic segmentation techniques, a convolution filter is applied to the image data at one point of the processing workflow with the aim of preprocessing the image and optimising the result (Bhandari, Koppen, and Agzarian 2020). In order to create a suitable input for the artificial network, the image has to be converted into a numerical representation. A vector of a predefined number of features (*feature vector*) is computed by assigning a numerical value for each feature, whereby the features represent different image properties. A pixelwise computation is possible, as well as the creation of feature vectors for larger image regions of interest (Prokop et al. 1997). Based on the given input vectors, the CNN computes the respective output for each pixel or region. For the specific case of a segmentation task, the output is the assignment of each input (pixel or image region) to one of a number of predefined classes.

Which classes are available for selection depends on the medical question, e.g., differentiation of brain tissue in grey and white matter, tracking of vessels, or detection of a tumour in surrounding tissue. Computational power is a limiting factor for the use of CNNs for image segmentation (Wismüller et al. 2001). To reduce processing times, a wider image region presumably containing the structures of interest can be selected in advance.

Segmentation with Time Series Analysis

As described before, artificial neural networks have found their way into the discipline of medical image processing. As these systems operate completely independent from human input, they are especially well suited for data streams including large amounts of data. For instance, in functional MRI imaging, physiological processes are visualised, such as the accumulation of contrast agents in a tumour, neuronal activity in the brain after motor stimulation (fMRI), or perfusion imaging. With these techniques, image data is recorded with an additional temporal component – several images of the same slice at different time points. Thus, the information that can be gained from these streams is enormous, however, handling these amounts of data by humans also becomes more difficult (Bankman 2008).

Time series analysis is performed to realise the segmentation of structures and to be able to assign pixels or image regions to tissue categories (clusters). An exemplary method for clustering based on neural network time series analysis is described here. This algorithm is frequently applied to fMRI data. In functional MRI imaging, the brain's response to a motor or visual stimulus is recorded – more precisely the blood-oxygen-level-dependent (BOLD) signal is measured. When the neural activity increases due to a stimulus, the blood is enriched with oxygen and the blood flow in the active areas increases. Due to the increased oxygen level the relaxation times of the blood changes, which leads to a different signal intensity of the respective brain areas and a different image contrast (BOLD contrast) (Logothetis et al. 1999).

The goal of the neural network-based algorithms is to find pixels with similar behaviour and sort them into different clusters. For the special case of fMRI scans, the goal is to find pixels with increased activity and assort them to clusters representing different anatomical structures or image areas. For good clusters, the difference between the included data points should be as small as possible. An increase in neural activity can be mathematically described as a change in signal intensity over time for a considered data point. For magnetic resonance imaging, this is equivalent to a change of the PTC (pixel intensity over time, i.e., the sequential scans) (Fischer and Hennig 1999). To provide processible input for the NN, a data vector is created for each pixel in the scan sequence. This so-called feature vector p contains the intensity value for each scan in the sequence (n pixel intensity values I_n for n scans: $\vec{p} = \{I_1, I_2, \ldots, I_n\}$). The totality of all feature vectors forms the input data matrix. The feature vectors created for the individual pixels are mapped in the feature space. Pixels with a similar intensity change and therefore similar PTC will lay close together in the feature space (Fischer and Hennig 1999). For the actual task of forming clusters, a self-organising, i.e., unsupervised approach is frequently used. The number of desired clusters k is defined in advance. Based on the location of their feature vector in the feature space, the pixels are assigned to the clusters. Feature vectors located close to each other are assigned to the same cluster, whereby a variety of different distance measures can be used (Fischer and Hennig 1999). Each cluster is represented by a value for the cluster centre that is determined by an incremental calculation performed by the neural network (Wismüller et al. 2001). After a sufficient number of increments is passed, clusters split into smaller clusters, allowing for a more precise categorisation of the pixels (Wismüller et al. 2001). The number of increments can be chosen according to the medical question and the required cluster size. The identified clusters can finally be displayed in the initial MR image and indicate pixels with similar behaviour, which are likely to belong to the same type of tissue or connected areas of neural activity.

IMAGING MODALITIES

Computed Tomography

Computed tomography is a medical imaging technique that uses X-rays and computer processing to produce detailed images of internal organs, bones, and other tissues. CT scans are widely used for diagnostic purposes and provide valuable information for medical professionals in various fields, including radiology, oncology, and trauma surgery. Unlike traditional X-ray images that provide only a two-dimensional view of the body, CT scans produce cross-sectional images, providing a three-dimensional view of the inside of the body. These images are generated by taking multiple X-ray images of the body from different angles and combining them into a single, detailed image (Bankman 2008). CT scans are quick, non-invasive, and painless, making them an important tool in modern medicine. In particular, CT is well suited for imaging of dense body structures and tissues like bone. In addition to that, CT is the imaging modality of choice for time-critical medical emergencies due to its short examination times. CT imaging is the gold standard for initial imaging during the treatment of trauma patients. However, there are significant limitations of this modality, one being the high dose of ionising radiation and another being the insufficient representation of tissue other than bone.

CT scanning is a medical imaging method that produces detailed cross-sectional images of the body. A CT scanner has a modern X-ray machine mounted inside it and a digital detector on the opposite side. By rotating around the patient, single images, also known as "slices," are captured (Kalender 2011). By moving the patient table through the scanner, the entire body can be scanned in a spiral form (Mazzoni et al. 2021). CT imaging works by measuring how much X-rays are absorbed by the body. The more dense the tissue, the more the X-rays are absorbed, and this information is used to create an image of the inside of the body. The amount of X-rays absorbed by the tissue is called the "attenuation coefficient" μ_{tissue}. This information, along with the initial intensity of the X-rays and the residual intensity measured by the detector, is used to create a one-dimensional image data for each section of the image, known as a "voxel".

A *forward projection* of the attenuation profile of each image slice of the scanned object results in the first set of two-dimensional image data, the so-called *sinogram*. By recombining the sinogram with the spatial information (*back projection*), the image is reconstructed – in different grey values representing the respective CT-values. These CT-values are indicated in Hounsfield Units (HU) and are defined as shown in Equation 1.11 (Kalender 2011).

$$\text{CT} - \text{value:} = \frac{\mu_{tissue} - \mu_{water}}{\mu_{water} - \mu_{air}} \cdot 1000\, HU \tag{1.11}$$

Each CT-value can be directly mapped to a different tissue type, for an overview see (Toga, Mazziotta, and Mazziotta 2002). However, the resulting image is blurred. In order to create a richly detailed image, *filtered back projection* (FBP) is carried out, sharpening edges and increasing image contrast by applying different convolution kernels.

Newer developments led to faster and high-resolution imaging. Dual-Energy CTs are equipped with two X-ray tubes, allowing for acquisition from different angles and with different X-ray energies and therefore a better differentiation of different body tissues (Goo and Goo 2017). In addition, modern devices allow for multi-slice imaging. With one rotation they are able to acquire up to 128 slices at once due to multiple parallel rows of detectors (Goldman 2008).

Magnetic Resonance Imaging

Magnetic resonance imaging is a radiation-free imaging modality that allows for good soft tissue contrast. Because of these two characteristics, it is used for a variety of applications and medical questions. Drawbacks of this imaging technique are the long examination times, loud noise created by vibrations inside the device, electronic and metal implants as contraindicators, and possible uncomfortable nerve stimulation.

Magnetic resonance imaging uses a strong magnetic field and radio waves to produce images of the inside of the body. It works by detecting the presence of hydrogen nuclei, or protons, in tissues. These protons have a natural spinning motion, and when they are exposed to a strong magnetic field, they line up in a certain direction. The spinning motion of the protons creates a radio signal that can be detected and used to create an image. This is done by placing the patient inside a large, powerful magnet and using radio waves to stimulate the protons and create a signal. The magnetic field should be as uniform as possible to improve the quality of the images produced.

Two important properties relevant to image contrast are T1 time and T2 time. The T1 time is the so-called longitudinal relaxation time. Here, the T1 time constant describes the time period required for recovering 63% of the initial magnetisation. With the T2 time describing the transverse relaxation, the T2 constant is the duration until the transverse magnetisation is reduced by 63%.

Various parameters have an influence on the appearance of acquired images. Different combinations of parameter values are implemented in the various imaging sequences. Standard imaging options are T1-weighting and T2-weighting. Different tissues have different T1 and T2 relaxation times. Utilising the T1 relaxation times of the different tissues to create the image contrast creates T1-weighted images, while using the T2 constants of the respective tissues allows for T2-weighted images. Depending on the weighting of the image, the same tissue is displayed with different brightness.

New scientific and technical research concentrates on the creation of new imaging sequences and further developments of MR devices with the goal of making new applications available. Ultra-high and low tesla scanners, larger built bores, new technologies for functional imaging, faster imaging protocols for specific body regions, and advanced imaging for high-resolution images for different applications are just a few examples (Mazzoni et al. 2021; Y. Liu et al. 2021).

Positron Emission Tomography

CT and MRI are two highly efficient techniques for anatomical and structural imaging. Positron emission tomography on the other hand allows for the visualisation and imaging of metabolic processes (Bailey et al. 2005). This imaging modality is part of nuclear medicine with oncology being its largest field of application. Here PET is used for the detection of tumours and monitoring of tumour growth. To make imaging with PET possible, a slightly radioactive tracer is administered to the patient. As different metabolic processes and different tissue types use different kinds of molecules, the tracer is chosen based on the medical question. Compared to normal tissue, tumour cells have increased metabolic activity. The administered radioactive tracer therefore accumulates in a tumour, more than in cells of neighbouring tissue.

Similar to CT imaging, the acquired image data is stored in a sinogram (Bailey et al. 2005). Compared to CT and MRI, PET systems have a poorer image resolution. The resolution in PET is determined by the size of the scintillator detector elements; only the approximate location of any activity can be determined. More structural details would help to obtain information with improved significance from the acquired PET data. Hybrid imaging of PET/CT or PET/MR is the solution to this issue by providing anatomical and functional information about the imaged body region. Data acquisitions of both modalities are done consecutively. A superimposition of the structural scan and PET data is created as the final examination result. PET/CT is particularly well suited for the differentiation of tumour cells and healthy tissue, whereas PET/MR is mostly used for applications such as brain functionality or cardiovascular issues, as it works well for soft tissue (Cho et al. 2010). Back-to-back image acquisition saves time and due to the limited movement of the patient, image registration is easier.

Sonography

Sonography is an imaging modality based on ultrasound waves – sound waves between 1 and 30 MHz that cannot be detected by the human ear (Sanders and Winter 2006). The key element of a sonography system is the transducer. It functions as a transmitter and receiver of ultrasound waves. A piezo crystal inside the transducer generates ultrasonic waves that are then sent into the examined part of the body. On their way through the body, the largest portion of the sound waves is absorbed by the tissue, yet a portion of the waves is reflected at interfaces between different organs and tissues and in heterogeneous tissues.

The reflected ultrasound waves are received by the transducer where they collide with the piezo crystal, causing it to deform and generate an electrical signal. This signal is then transformed into a 2D sonographic image. Interfaces between structures with a great difference in density produce stronger echoes and therefore stronger signals. In a greyscale sonographic image, tissues with different densities can be better distinguished than neighbouring tissues with similar densities and structural properties (Sanders and Winter 2006).

DISCUSSION

Medical image processing is a rapidly growing field that plays a crucial role in modern medicine. It includes various techniques and algorithms that help improve the quality of medical images and make them more informative for doctors and clinicians (Gull, Akbar, and Khan 2021). Medical imaging is an indispensable tool in modern medicine, providing detailed information about the internal structure and function of the body. The images produced by techniques such as computed tomography, magnetic resonance imaging, positron emission tomography, and sonography are used to diagnose, monitor, and treat a wide range of medical conditions (Bankman 2008).

Over the past few years, a large number of research articles have been published on the search for new methods for automated detection of findings specialised for selected medical questions. Different experimental and advanced use cases and different body regions are covered, such as the brain, knee, liver, lung, and prostate. Recent CNN algorithms can detect brain tumours in MR images (Gull, Akbar, and Khan 2021). The CNN extracts the image features and performs a pixel-wise classification into the tumour and non-tumour tissue. A recent application is the classification of lung CT and X-ray images or even ultrasound images of COVID-19 patients. Similar to tumour detection in MR, a CNN is used for feature extraction and image classification (Kassania et al. 2021; McDermott et al. 2021). Binary classification into healthy and damaged lungs to filter out patients with lung infiltrates (Kassania et al. 2021) or multi-class classification with additional differentiation between types of pneumonia (Narin, Kaya, and Pamuk 2021) are possible. Such systems to assist radiologists could be of great use as the pandemic progresses.

Regardless of the use case, current algorithms achieve high accuracy, with NNs and radiologists performing equally well on a given task (Gull, Akbar, and Khan 2021; F. Liu et al. 2019). However, no AI will ever make the final decision on the medical findings but will serve as a tool to assist the physician in the diagnosis and save time.

Medical image processing has also opened up new possibilities for personalised medicine, allowing for individualised diagnoses and treatments based on the unique characteristics of each patient (Lambin et al. 2017). Hereby, the goal is to provide a comprehensive and quantitative characterisation of the imaging phenotype of a patient, which can be used to predict patient outcomes, diagnosis, treatment response, and disease progression. This offers a unique opportunity to bridge the gap between medical imaging and personalised medicine by providing an extensive and robust set of imaging biomarkers that can be used to guide personalised treatment strategies.

Medical image processing has great potential as the number of radiological examinations and the amount of data is increasing rapidly (Lambin et al. 2017; Narin, Kaya, and Pamuk 2021). Taking it a step further, novel AI systems based on neural networks can assist physicians by highlighting regions containing abnormalities and suggesting possible findings. Segmentation and object detection algorithms are able to process large image sets without missing details due to a different focus or a large amount of data.

CONCLUSION

The use of advanced AI algorithms in medical imaging is a great benefit to patients and physicians. Advanced processing techniques for all imaging modalities enable faster and more accurate diagnoses. Physicians are supported in handling the increasing amount of image data. Image processing is becoming more effective and less prone to error.

There is a growing number of new techniques based on the latest developments in AI and neural networks. Convolutional neural networks are used to analyse scans acquired with different imaging modalities. Automated detection of findings is possible for a variety of medical problems, with tumour detection and segmentation being particularly well developed. Segmentation of anatomical structures and clustering of image regions provide insight into the imaged body region without requiring a great deal of time and medical knowledge. Post-acquisition image quality enhancement using a variety of techniques supports all further tasks and makes modern medical imaging even more powerful. The use of artificial intelligence, especially neural networks, enables advanced processing of medical images and has the potential to replace conventional image processing techniques.

REFERENCES

Al-Jibory, W. K., and A. El-Zaart. 2013. "Edge Detection in X-Ray Computed Tomography Images Using Weibull Distribution." In *Proceedings of the International Conference on Image Processing, Computer Vision, and Pattern Recognition (IPCV)*, 1. The Steering Committee of The World Congress in Computer Science, Computer ....

Arenson, R. L., S. B. Seshadri, H. L. Kundel, D. DeSimone, F. Van der Voorde, W. B. Gefter, D. M. Epstein, W. T. Miller, J. M. Aronchick, and M. B. Simson. 1988. "Clinical Evaluation of a Medical Image Management System for Chest Images." *AJR. American Journal of Roentgenology* 150 (1): 55–59.

Bailey, D. L., M. N. Maisey, D. W. Townsend, and P. E. Valk. 2005. *Positron Emission Tomography*. London: Springer.

Bankman, I. 2008. *Handbook of Medical Image Processing and Analysis*. Elsevier.

Bhandari, A., J. Koppen, and M. Agzarian. 2020. "Convolutional Neural Networks for Brain Tumour Segmentation." *Insights into Imaging* 11 (1): 77.

Canny, J. 1986. "A Computational Approach to Edge Detection." *IEEE Transactions on Pattern Analysis and Machine Intelligence* 8 (6): 679–698.

Chen, Y., and H. An. 2017. "Attenuation Correction of PET/MR Imaging." *Magnetic Resonance Imaging Clinics of North America* 25 (2): 245–255.

Cho, Z. H., Y. D. Son, Y. B. Kim, and S. S. Yoo. 2010. "Fusion of PET and MRI for Hybrid Imaging." *Biomedical Image Processing*. https://link.springer.com/chapter/10.1007/978-3-642-15816-2_2.

Fischer, H., and J. Hennig. 1999. "Neural Network-Based Analysis of MR Time Series." *Magnetic Resonance in Medicine: Official Journal of the Society of Magnetic Resonance in Medicine/Society of Magnetic Resonance in Medicine* 41 (1): 124–131.

Goldman, L. W. 2008. "Principles of CT: Multislice CT." *Journal of Nuclear Medicine Technology*. https://tech.snmjournals.org/content/36/2/57.short.

Goo, H. W., and J. M. Goo. 2017. "Dual-Energy CT: New Horizon in Medical Imaging." *Korean Journal of Radiology: Official Journal of the Korean Radiological Society* 18 (4): 555–569.

Gull, S., S. Akbar, and H. U. Khan. 2021. "Automated Detection of Brain Tumor through Magnetic Resonance Images Using Convolutional Neural Network." *BioMed Research International* 2021 (November): 3365043.

Jünger, S. T., U. C. I. Hoyer, and D. Schaufler. 2021. "Fully Automated MR Detection and Segmentation of Brain Metastases in Non-small Cell Lung Cancer Using Deep Learning." *Journal of Magnetic Resonance.* https://onlinelibrary.wiley.com/doi/abs/10.1002/jmri.27741.

Kalender, W. A. 2011. "Computed Tomography: Fundamentals, System Technology, Image Quality, Applications." https://books.google.de/books?hl=en&lr=&id=gfLWmRjoyPMC&oi=fnd&pg=PP2&dq=Computed+Tomography:+Fundamentals,+System+Technology,+Image+Quality,+Applications&ots=Eu4e73xcsF&sig=JuQs8p3wQ3PJ5tBlohg69HOpMGc.

Kamalian, S., M. H. Lev, and R. Gupta. 2016. "Computed Tomography Imaging and Angiography - Principles." Edited by Joseph C. Masdeu and R. Gilberto González. *Handbook of Clinical Neurology* 135 (January): 3–20.

Kassania, S. H., P. H. Kassanib, M. J. Wesolowskic, K. A. Schneidera, and R. Detersa. 2021. "Automatic Detection of Coronavirus Disease (COVID-19) in X-Ray and CT Images: A Machine Learning Based Approach." *Biocybernetics and Biomedical Engineering* 41 (3): 867–879.

Kostelec, P. J., and S. Periaswamy. 2003. "Image Registration for MRI." *Modern Signal Processing.* http://library.msri.org/books/Book46/files/07kostelec.pdf.

Lambin, P., R. T. H. Leijenaar, T. M. Deist, J. Peerlings, E. E. C. de Jong, J. van Timmeren, S. Sanduleanu, et al. 2017. "Radiomics: The Bridge between Medical Imaging and Personalized Medicine." *Nature Reviews. Clinical Oncology* 14 (12): 749–762.

Liu, F., B. Guan, Z. Zhou, A. Samsonov, H. Rosas, K. Lian, R. Sharma, et al. 2019. "Fully Automated Diagnosis of Anterior Cruciate Ligament Tears on Knee MR Images by Using Deep Learning." *Radiology. Artificial Intelligence* 1 (3): 180091.

Liu, Y., A. T. L. Leong, Y. Zhao, L. Xiao, H. K. F. Mak, A. C. O. Tsang, G. K. K. Lau, G. K. K. Leung, and E. X. Wu. 2021. "A Low-Cost and Shielding-Free Ultra-Low-Field Brain MRI Scanner." *Nature Communications* 12 (1): 7238.

Logothetis, N. K., H. Guggenberger, S. Peled, and J. Pauls. 1999. "Functional Imaging of the Monkey Brain." *Nature Neuroscience* 2 (6): 555–562.

Maini, R., and H. Aggarwal. 2009. "Study and Comparison of Various Image Edge Detection Techniques." *International Journal of Image Processing (IJIP)* 3 (1): 1–11.

Mazzoni, L. N., M. Bock, I. R. Levesque, D. J. Lurie, and G. Palma. 2021. "New Developments in MRI: System Characterization, Technical Advances and Radiotherapy Applications." *Physica Medica: PM: An International Journal Devoted to the Applications of Physics to Medicine and Biology: Official Journal of the Italian Association of Biomedical Physics* 90 (October): 50–52.

McDermott, C., M. Łącki, B. Sainsbury, J. Henry, M. Filippov, and C. Rossa. 2021. "Sonographic Diagnosis of COVID-19: A Review of Image Processing for Lung Ultrasound." *Frontiers in Big Data* 4 (March): 612561.

Narin, A., C. Kaya, and Z. Pamuk. 2021. "Automatic Detection of Coronavirus Disease (COVID-19) Using X-Ray Images and Deep Convolutional Neural Networks." *Pattern Analysis and Applications: PAA* 24 (3): 1207–1220.

Perumal, S., and T. Velmurugan. 2018. "Preprocessing by Contrast Enhancement Techniques for Medical Images." *International Journal of Pure and Applied Mathematics: IJPAM*. https://www.researchgate.net/profile/Velmurugan-Thambusamy/publication/325361080_Preprocessing_by_contrast_enhancement_techniques_for_medical_images/links/5fc1ee66a6fdcc6cc6774288/Preprocessing-by-contrast-enhancement-techniques-for-medical-images.pdf.

Pham, D. L., C. Xu, and J. L. Prince. 2000. "Current Methods in Medical Image Segmentation." *Annual Review of Biomedical Engineering* 2: 315–337.

Prokop, M., H. O. Shin, A. Schanz, and C. M. Schaefer-Prokop. 1997. "Use of Maximum Intensity Projections in CT Angiography: A Basic Review." *Radiographics: A Review Publication of the Radiological Society of North America, Inc* 17 (2): 433–451.

Sanders, R. C., and T. C. Winter. 2006. *Clinical Sonography: A Practical Guide*. 4th ed. Philadelphia, PA: Lippincott Williams and Wilkins.

Sarkar, S., and A. Mandal. 2015. "Comparison of Some Classical Edge Detection Techniques with Their Suitability Analysis for Medical Images Processing." *International Journal of Computer Sciences*. https://www.researchgate.net/profile/Subhro-Sarkar-4/publication/307174169_Comparison_of_Some_Classical_Edge_Detection_Techniques_with_their_Suitability_Analysis_for_Medical_Images_Processing/links/57c4010a08ae32a03dac3fd1/Comparison-of-Some-Classical-Edge-Detection-Techniques-with-their-Suitability-Analysis-for-Medical-Images-Processing.pdf.

Shedbalkar, J., and K. Prabhushetty. 2021. "A Comparative Analysis of Filters for Noise Reduction and Smoothening of Brain MRI Images." *2021 6th International*. https://ieeexplore.ieee.org/abstract/document/9417979/.

Srinivasan, U., and B. Arunasalam. 2013. "Leveraging Big Data Analytics to Reduce Healthcare Costs." *IT Professional*. https://ieeexplore.ieee.org/abstract/document/6560016/?casa_token=BZ_0MCM9LqcAAAAA:QocNl-w9hh-3QMIQSB4nqWdYt-m40FDlLdcdhvXMQs4hH6tFXP3u8cf39srIrXgF27EYOX927Axz.

Toga, A. W., J. C. Mazziotta, and J. C. Mazziotta. 2002. "Brain Mapping: The Methods." https://books.google.de/books?hl=en&lr=&id=mBBYKlIGwZYC&oi=fnd&pg=PR4&dq=CT+Angiography+and+CT+Perfusion+Imaging.+In:+Toga,+A.W.,+Mazziotta,+J.C.+(Eds.)+Brain+Mapping:+The+Methods&ots=o8Qo4-0WlV&sig=-MDH5EswTj48h7G78ggH7X2-dcI.

Wahlang, I., G. Saha, and A. K. Maji. 2020. "A Comparative Analysis on Denoising Techniques in Brain Mri and Cardiac Echo." *Systems: I3CS 2020, NEHU, Shillong, India.* https://link.springer.com/chapter/10.1007/978-981-33-4084-8_36.

Wiens, J., S. Saria, M. Sendak, M. Ghassemi, V. X. Liu, F. Doshi-Velez, K. Jung, et al. 2019. "Do No Harm: A Roadmap for Responsible Machine Learning for Health Care." *Nature Medicine* 25 (9): 1337–1340.

Wismüller, A., O. Lange, D. R. Dersch, K. Hahn, and G. L. Leinsinger. 2001. "Neural Network Analysis of Dynamic Contrast-Enhanced MRI Mammography." In *Artificial Neural Networks — ICANN 2001*, 1000–1005. Springer Berlin Heidelberg.

Xue, Z., S. Antani, L. Rodney Long, D. Demner-Fushman, and G. R. Thoma. 2012. "Window Classification of Brain CT Images in Biomedical Articles." *AMIA ... Annual Symposium Proceedings/AMIA Symposium. AMIA Symposium* 2012 (November): 1023–1029.

CHAPTER 2

Smart Wearables in Healthcare

Eva van Weenen

INTRODUCTION

Technology has become increasingly ubiquitous in the recent era of digital transformation. Consequently, it is associated with the collection of large amounts of data, "big data". Particularly, wearable technology is a leading category in the Internet of Things (IoT), which allows for the non-intrusive collection of large amounts of longitudinal data of individuals.

Wearable technology is defined as small mobile electronic devices incorporated into gadgets, accessories, or clothes that can be worn in-, directly on-, or in close proximity to the human body. Wearable devices can be categorised into four categories: (i) *head-mounted* devices, such as headsets and neural interfaces; (ii) *body-worn* devices, subdivided into near-body (smart bands, activity trackers), on-body (EEG, ECG, EMG monitors) and in-body devices (implantables, smart tattoos); (iii) *lower-body* devices, such as smart shoes and belts; and (iv) *wrist-worn* devices, such as smartwatches and smart rings.

Through its design, wearable technology enables continuous or intermittent data collection, particularly in the field of physiological data monitoring (Ometov et al., 2021). Its monitoring is generally unobtrusive, thus allowing for data collection under free-living conditions of individuals. Besides data collection, wearable devices commonly have various data analytic tools integrated, thus providing aggregated insights to its user.

Within the medical domain, wearable technology has received wide interest due to its ability to provide long-term non-obtrusive patient

DOI: 10.1201/9781032699745-3

monitoring (Bonato, 2003). This interest was further promoted by the increasing ageing population, the prevalence of chronic illnesses, and continuously rising healthcare costs (Teng et al., 2008). The potential of wearable technology exists primarily in patient monitoring outside of constant clinical care through capturing (i) rare events of medical importance; (ii) physiological responses under free-living conditions that are more realistic indicators of a patient's health or response to an intervention; and (iii) circadian variation in physiological signals that may reflect the progression of a health condition (Binkley et al., 2003). Hence, representative, continuous, and high-resolution patient monitoring can be used to fill the information gap that exists in the recovery and deterioration phase of a patient outside of constant clinical care.

Adoptions of wearable technology in health care exist for various use cases, such as aiding patient assessment, treatment, and management. Specifically, non-invasive monitoring of vital signs has been of interest within the health care domain, such as the continuous monitoring of heart rate and heart rate variability, blood pressure, body temperature, respiratory rate, oxygen saturation, and motion detection. Combined with data on the wearer's context and other health indicators, this data may provide the physiological state of a patient (Tröster, 2005) and aid in personalised decision-making. Successful applications of wearable technology exist in the achievement of early diagnosis (e.g., for congestive heart failure), prevention and management of chronic diseases (e.g., diabetes, cardiovascular disease), improved clinical management of neurodegenerative conditions (e.g., Parkinson's disease), and the ability to promptly respond to emergency situations (e.g., seizures in patients with epilepsy and cardiac arrest in subjects undergoing cardiovascular monitoring) (Bonato, 2010). Hence, wearable medical systems may improve health decisions, health outcomes, and quality of life (Teng et al., 2008; Tröster, 2005; Lymberis, 2003).

Not only has wearable technology in health care been of interest to the practitioner, but also the patient plays a central role in wearable technology. This interest is supported by the paradigm shift from a hospital-centred healthcare system towards an individual-centred one emphasising personal risk prevention (Teng et al., 2008). Wearable technology allows for self-monitoring: empowering the patient through continuous information on their health status, giving insights into the effects of lifestyle choices, aiding in the management of chronic diseases, contributing to self-care, potentially decreasing clinical visits, and reducing waiting room burden. Consequently, the increasing demand for wearable technology has led to growth in this sector, particularly in the availability of consumer-grade wearable technology on the mass market. As opposed to clinical-grade wearable technology, which requires formal regulatory approval, consumer-grade wearable technology is more affordable, but far less accurate and does not qualify as a medical device. Particularly, machine learning (ML) has aided in the development of consumer-grade wearable technology, allowing for the extraction of meaningful information from the large amounts of data collected. In that way, wearable technology can be considered "smart": i.e., through complex ML algorithms, it can provide intelligent insights from the wearable sensor data collected, beneficial for clinical practice and public health. Accordingly, rather than relying on averages from the collective, as is traditional in medical practice, smart wearable technology can supply personalised data that can aid in diagnosis and treatment (Godfrey et al., 2018).

This Chapter provides a comprehensive overview of smart wearable technology in health care. The Chapter is structured as follows. First, we provide an overview of the types of wearable technologies used to monitor physiological signals. Following, we address the data storage, processing, and analysis, before listing successful applications of smart wearable technology in health care. Afterwards, we discuss the design, adoption, quality, reliability, security, privacy, and future of smart wearable technology in health care. Please note that we do not consider in-body or implantable devices in this Chapter's scope due to their relatively invasive nature. Furthermore, we will focus on wearable technology worn by the patient and thereby disregard wearable devices worn by the clinician.

HARDWARE

The primary functionality of wearable technology is sensing. In health care, wearable devices capture physiological signals, which can be translated into medical parameters informative of physiological state. The sensor is an essential type of hardware for measuring physiological signals with wearables. It is a technology that detects or measures a physical property and records, indicates, or responds to it electrically. In other words, a sensor turns a phenomenon into an electric quantity that can be resolved, discretised, and processed. Various types of sensors exist, such as magnetic, mechanical, chemical, electromagnetic, thermal, and acoustic sensors, and we will further discriminate between them in this Section. In terms of the remaining hardware, today's wearable devices are generally a commodity: consisting of a lithium-ion battery, one or more sensors, actuators (visual, auditory, or haptic feedback), external flash data storage, a microprocessor and a wireless interface (Williamson et al., 2015).

In this Section, we give a high-level overview of the different types of wearable technology in health care and the respective physiological signals that they measure. Please note that this overview entails merely a selection of the most common non-invasive wearable sensing technologies used for health care purposes. Hence, technologies that are not widely adopted are excluded from this overview. As a reference, Table 2.1

TABLE 2.1 Overview of the Different Types of Wearable Sensing Technologies in Health Care and the Respective Physiological Signals That They Measure

Technology	*Sensor Type*	*Physiological Signals*
Electrophysiology	*Electrical*	*Biopotentials*
Electrocardiography (ECG)	Electrical	Cardiac activity
Electroencephalography (EEG)	Electrical	Brain activity
Electromyography (EMG)	Electrical	Neuromuscular activity
Electrodermal activity (EDA)	Electrical	Sympathetic nervous system activity
Plethysmography		*Fluctuations in blood or air volume*
Photoplethysmography (PPG)	Optical	Cardiac activity, oxygen saturation, blood pressure
Respiratory inductive plethysmography (RIP)	Mechanical	Respiratory activity
Inertial and magnetic measurement unit (IMMU)	*Mechanical*	*Motion*
Accelerometer	Mechanical	Proper acceleration
Gyroscope	Mechanical	Angular velocity
Magnetometer	Mechanical	Magnetic field and orientation
Biochemical sensors	*Chemical*	*Metabolism*
Environmental sensors		
Barometer	Mechanical	Air pressure and altitude
Global Positioning System (GPS)	Electromagnetic	Location
Microphone	Mechanical	Acoustics
Temperature	Optical	Temperature
Humidity	Chemical	Humidity
Radiation	Electromagnetic	Radiation

provides an overview of the different wearable sensing technologies in health care, and their associated sensor types, measurement frequencies, and the respective physiological signals that they measure.

Electrophysiology

Electrophysiology involves recording biopotentials, i.e., electrical signals from physiological processes in the body generated by biological cells and tissue. These biopotentials essentially result from different ion concentrations inside and outside of cell membranes and are typically produced by the electrochemical activity of excitable cells. Excitable cells can be found in the nervous system, muscles, and endocrine system and can be categorised into sensor neurons (transduction of signals from sensory organs to central nervous system), motor neurons (transduction of signals from central nervous system to effector cells), as well as interneurons (existing within the central nervous system connecting motor- and sensor neurons), and neurons in the brain (Thakor, 2014).

Electrophysiological recording of biopotentials can be achieved *intracellular*, i.e., invasively with needles, or *extracellular*, i.e., non-invasively on the skin. In this Chapter, we focus on the latter: non-invasive recording of biopotentials. Extracellular recording of biopotentials generally involves measuring the electric potential of multiple electrodes (commonly silver-chloride electrodes) placed on the skin or living tissue and is sometimes referred to as *electrography* (Tröster, 2005). Electrograms may inform about the localisation, timing, and waveform generation of signals produced by the excitable cells of interest (Oreggioni et al., 2017). Electrography exists in various modalities, such as electrocardiography (ECG; measuring the electric activity of the heart), electroencephalography (EEG; measuring the electric activity of the brain with extracranial electrodes), and electromyography (EMG; measuring the electric activity of the muscles). Other electrography techniques exist, such as electrooculography (EOG) and electrogastrography (EGG), but they are less common. Further details on the most common electrography techniques, ECGs, EEGs, and EMGs, are described below.

Electrocardiography (ECG)

Electrocardiography (ECG) is the graphic recording of *cardiac activity*. It records the electrical activity produced by the conduction system and myocardium of the heart during its depolarisation and repolarisation

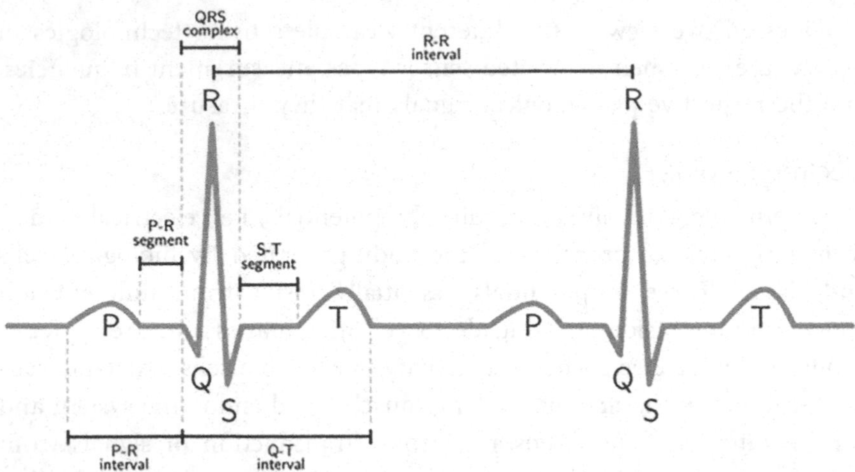

FIGURE 2.1 Illustration of an electrocardiography (ECG) signal.

cycle. Its signal can be used to infer metrics for cardiovascular activity, such as *heart rate (HR)* and *heart rate variability (HRV)*. Continuous ECG monitoring provides a realistic report of a patient's heart rhythm during daily activity, allows the capture of rare events in the cardiac cycle (arrhythmia), and may help identify related cardiovascular conditions.

ECGs are typically recorded by attaching two electrodes to the skin, where the signal is obtained from the potential difference between the two electrodes. The ECG records the depolarisation and repolarisation of the cardiac muscle during a cardiac cycle and its signal can be decomposed into five phases: P, Q, R, S, and T, as shown in Figure 2.1. The P wave corresponds to atrial contraction and depolarisation, the QRS complex corresponds to contraction and depolarisation of the ventricles, and the T wave corresponds to ventricular repolarisation and relaxation. The R-R interval is indicative of heart rate and heart rate variability.

Electroencephalography (EEG)

Electroencephalography (EEG) is the graphic recording of *brain activity*. It records the electrical activity of the brain generated by neurons in the cerebral cortex. This technique can be used to aid in the diagnosis of epilepsy, as well as for long-term monitoring of sleep, and the diagnosis of brain-related disorders.

EEGs are typically recorded by attaching multiple electrodes to fixed locations of the scalp. The EEG signal reflects the summation of synchronous activity of a large number of neurons in similar orientations, representing itself in neural oscillations. The various frequency ranges of these oscillations correspond to different states of brain functioning, e.g., *deep sleep* (delta rhythm, < 4Hz), *unconsciousness* and *arousal* (theta rhythm, 4–8Hz), *relaxed* (alpha, 8–13Hz), *active* (beta, 18–30Hz), *highly active* (gamma, > 30Hz) (Tatum IV, 2021; Groppe et al., 2013).

Electromyography (EMG)

Electromyography (EMG) is the graphic recording of *muscle activity.* It records the electrical activity of the neuromuscular system, generated when muscle cells are neurologically activated. The technology can be applied to identify neuromuscular disease and abnormalities and to support physical therapy. Additionally, the EMG technology can be used in prosthetic devices and as assistive technology for individuals with paralysis or loss of speech.

The measurement principle of EMGs is similar to that of ECGs and EEGs. In a wearable, non-invasive setting, EMGs are recorded by attaching multiple electrodes to the surface of the skin surrounding a muscle. The EMG signal reflects the time and intensity of neuromuscular activity (Chowdhury et al., 2013).

Electrodermal Activity (EDA)

Electrodermal activity (EDA), also known as galvanic skin response (GSR), is measured through *skin impedance* or *skin conductance.* Changes in the activity of the sympathetic nervous system will lead to changes in EDA due to eccrine sweat gland activity, which can be an indicator of *arousal, stress, activity,* and *pain.* Potential applications for EDA in health care are measuring anxiety in patients with autism spectrum disorder, epileptic seizure detection, the detection of hypoglycemia in patients with diabetes, and monitoring sleep disorders (Fletcher et al., 2010).

Contrary to the electrography techniques mentioned previously, in which electrical activity is directly generated by biological tissue, it is worth noting that EDA is an *indirect* biopotential. That is, the EDA signal is only obtained after applying a current to the skin.

EDA is measured by applying a constant voltage between two electrodes onto the skin. The changes in skin resistance are indicative of EDA. The EDA signal can be decomposed into tonic and phasic activity. Tonic activity is a slowly fluctuating component related to arousal, whereas phasic activity is a faster-varying component related to stimulus reactions.

Plethysmography

Plethysmography is a technique for measuring fluctuations in blood or air volume within an organ or whole body. Its detection of blood volume changes in the microvascular tissue can be used to infer cardiac activity, for which PPG is commonly used. Additionally, RIP can be used to infer respiratory activity. Alternative plethysmography techniques exist, such as impedance plethysmography (IPG). Here we will not discuss IPG due to its controversy regarding reliability for cardiac activity (Malmivuo, 1995).

Photoplethysmography (PPG)

Photoplethysmography (PPG) is an optical sensing technology often used to measure *changes in blood volume.* A PPG signal is obtained through the illumination of the skin's surface using a green or red light-emitting diode (LED) and the subsequent recording of its optical absorption or reflection. The variation in optical reflection and absorption can finally be transformed into a physical quantity. Due to its small size, low cost, and portability, a PPG sensor can be easily incorporated into a wearable device and can be commonly found in smartwatches. Vital signs that can be measured with PPG are *cardiac activity*, such as *heart rate* and *heart rate variability*, as well as *pulse oximetry*, such as *partial pressure of oxygen* (PO_2) and *oxyhemoglobin saturation* (SpO_2).

Comparisons of ECG and PPG recordings in healthy subjects show a high degree of correlation between obtained heart rate and heart rate variability (Lu et al., 2009; Weiler et al., 2017). Nevertheless, most PPG sensors require direct contact with the skin and are affected by skin colour and moisture (Bayoumy et al., 2021). Furthermore, low perfusion and motion artifacts may reduce the accuracy of the sensor. When ECG and PPG signals are combined, they can be used to infer *blood pressure.* The pulse transit time (PTT), defined as the time between the R-peak of the ECG and the characteristic point of the PPG, serves as an estimation for blood pressure.

Respiratory inductive plethysmography (RIP)

Respiratory inductive plethysmography (RIP) is a technique for detecting changes in air volume, particularly *respiration activity.* Respiration is associated with the kinematics of the chest due to changes in pulmonary volume. RIP leverages this principle by measuring the movement of the chest and abdominal wall. It includes the placement of two wires worn circumferentially around the ribcage and abdomen, which can be embedded into clothes. Respiratory motions will alter the self-inductance of the wires, which can be measured with any type of magnetometer or displacement sensor, to obtain an estimate of *changes in pulmonary volume*, as well as *respiration rate* (Teng et al., 2008; Tröster, 2005). Please note that there are various alternative methods for determining respiration rate as well, for instance, through ECG (known as ECG-derived respiration (EDR)) (Orphanidou et al., 2013), from modulations of the PPG signal (Karlen et al., 2013; Zhu et al., 2015), or from accelerometer sensors (Haescher et al., 2016).

Inertial and Magnetic Measurement Unit (IMMU)

Inertial and magnetic sensors, such as accelerometers, gyroscopes, and magnetometers, measure the *motion* (*proper acceleration*, *angular velocity*, and *orientation*, respectively) of their respective wearable device. Together, the 3-axis sensors make up the inertial and magnetic measurement unit (IMMU). In a healthcare setting, obtaining complex motion patterns can provide insights into activity (e.g., exercise and sleep patterns) and physiological status and can help detect motor fluctuations in patients with Alzheimer's disease (Tröster, 2005; Haghi et al., 2017). Moreover, it can be used to denoise other signals, such as ECG (Tröster, 2005). The placement of the IMMU sensors with respect to the human body affects their accuracy, where a central placement on the torso is the preferred site for accurate motion detection (Bayoumy et al., 2021).

The IMMU in wearable technology is typically fabricated as microelectromechanical systems (MEMS). MEMS are microscopic (1–100µm) devices consisting of electric and mechanical elements that convert mechanical energy into electrical energy and thereby provide an electrical signal from a physical property. Many MEMS have been developed and widely adopted over the past decades. The main advantages of this technology are miniaturisation, mass production, and low costs. Two of the most common types of MEMS sensors are capacitive and piezoresistive sensors. Piezoresistive sensors make use of the piezoresistive effect (i.e., a change in resistivity of the material due to applied strain) and thus measure a change in resistance when there is a change in gauge dimension. Capacitive sensors consist of fixed and moving conducting plates, and measure a change in capacitance due to changing distances between the plates (PRIME Faraday Partnership, 2002).

Accelerometers

Accelerometers measure three-dimensional *proper acceleration*, i.e., acceleration with respect to the rest frame of the device and not to an established coordinate system. MEMS accelerometers commonly consist of a seismic mass and supporting silicon spring. The displacement of the mass due to acceleration induces a change in capacitance between the mass and fixed electrodes and thus a measurable signal (capacitive accelerometer; Maenaka, 2008; Yazdi et al., 1998).

Gyroscopes

Gyroscopes measure three-dimensional changes in rotational motion (*angular velocity*). Gyroscopes have a similar structure as accelerometers but instead, measure the Coriolis force generated by angular velocity affecting a vibrating mass supported by springs. By design, the change in capacitance due to angular velocity generates a measurable electrical signal (Maenaka, 2008; Söderkvist, 1994).

Magnetometers

Magnetometers measure *magnetic fields* and can thus provide *orientation* with respect to the Earth's magnetic field. Whereas inertial sensors (accelerometer and gyroscopes) can only measure with respect to the rest frame of the device, magnetometers can provide *absolute* orientation. MEMS magnetometers generally make use of the Hall effect. That is, in the presence of a magnetic field, charge flowing through a conductive plate will undergo a Lorentz force, which will result in a change in voltage of the measurable signal.

Biochemical Sensors

Various biochemical sensors exist for monitoring chemicals related to *metabolism*. These chemicals can be measured either in human body fluids, such as tears, saliva, sweat, and interstitial fluids, or in human body odour from exhaled breath or skin secretion. Chemicals measured from body fluids include glucose, lactate, alcohol, nitrite, pH, Na^+, K^+, uric acid, and creatinine. Chemicals in exhaled breath are commonly volatile organic compounds (VOCs) indicative of biochemical processes and may present diseases. Chemical sensors can be applied to diagnose kidney dysfunction (Voss et al., 2005), diabetes (Ping et al., 1997), respiratory disease (Dragonieri et al., 2017), liver dysfunction (Voss et al., 2022), and cancer (Baldini et al., 2020). Chemical sensors can be designed as skin patches, tattoos, contact lenses, and textiles. Body fluids can be extracted through microneedles or reverse iontophoresis, where a low-voltage current is applied on the skin to extract charged molecules. Single chemical sensors are typically made for a specific chemical compound and cannot measure multiple chemicals simultaneously. A widely implemented chemical sensor is the continuous glucose monitoring (CGM) sensor for diabetes patients, consisting of a needle in the interstitial fluid. In this Chapter, we do not widely discuss biochemical sensors due to their invasiveness in measuring interstitial fluids and general limitations, such as high sensitivity, potential oxidation reactions, and the need for regular recalibration.

Environment Sensors

Environmental sensors are commonly integrated into wearable technology, with applications ranging from measurement of the environment and interaction with the user to calibration and enhancement of other sensors. Various environmental sensors are also based on MEMS, making them suitable for integration into wearable technology.

Barometers

Barometers are piezoresistive pressure sensors (strain gauges) used to measure *atmospheric pressure*. Piezoresistive pressure sensors consist in essence of a semiconducting material that changes its resistance when stretched or compressed. Generally, this material is a silicon-based Wheatstone-Bridge.

Barometers give insight into environmental factors and can complement *indoor navigation* for fitness and calorie tracking. Besides providing accurate indications of *local weather changes*, barometers are also commonly used for *position monitoring*. A typical implementation of a MEMS barometer is a *barometric altimeter* to detect vertical position. When properly calibrated, a barometric altimeter determines *altitude* by matching the measured air pressure levels to corresponding known levels of atmospheric pressure at certain altitudes (Bolanakis, 2016). The altitude obtained can be used for indoor navigation and enhancing GPS (Global Positioning System) signals. In a medical context, barometric information may be helpful for fall detection and fitness and calorie tracking through enhanced step and stair counting. The accuracy of barometers is prone to environmental changes, where a natural change in temperature or pressure may be mistaken for a change in altitude (Bayoumy et al., 2021).

Global Positioning System (GPS)

Global Positioning System (GPS) sensors are used to determine outdoor positions and are commonly used in combination with barometers to assess horizontal and vertical distances travelled with physical activity. GPS makes use of 4 out of at least 24 orbital satellites that broadcast GHz-frequency signals to determine location at a 5-metre accuracy.

Acoustics

Acoustic sensors (microphones) are used to record audio signals and can be used in health care for cough detection in pulmonary disease (Barata et al., 2019) or in the form of a wearable stethoscope for acoustic heart rate monitoring. Various implementations of MEMS acoustic sensors exist, both mechanical and optical. Optical MEMS acoustic sensors can be implemented as a Fabry-Pérot cavity that changes length under acoustic waves (Zhu et al., 2015).

Other Techniques

Sensors commonly integrated into wearable devices but not discussed so far are **temperature and radiation** sensors. For instance, temperature sensors are able to measure the temperature of the skin. Within health care, this may be useful for monitoring fever or the menstrual cycle. Moreover, radiation sensors can measure the UV exposure of the skin.

DATA

Wearable technology is associated with the collection of large amounts of data. This Section describes the various processes that are involved in the collection, transfer, storage and processing of this data. In particular, we look at data collection, data preprocessing, data transfer and storage, data processing, and data analysis.

Data Collection

Data from wearable technology is collected by sensors. The previous Section describes the different types of sensors used in wearable technology for health care. Sensors transform a physical phenomenon into an electrical signal. The analogue-to-digital (A/D) converter transforms the *analogue* signal, continuous in time and amplitude, to a *digital* signal, discrete in time and amplitude. Digitisation involves two aspects: (i) *sampling*, the A/D conversion of time, where the signal is recorded in discrete intervals defined by the sampling rate [samples/second]; and (ii) *quantisation*, the A/D conversion of amplitude, involving the discretisation of the continuous voltage defined by the quantisation level [bits/sample]. Together, the sampling rate and quantisation level determine the amount of data collected per second. Note that there exists a minimum sampling rate, the *Nyquist sampling rate* equal to two times the highest frequency of a signal, to prevent distortion known as *aliasing*.

Therefore, in wearable technology, data can be collected at both high (many times per minute) and low (once every few minutes) *sampling frequencies*, depending on measurement requirements (Godfrey et al., 2018). In practice, battery and memory capabilities prevent wearable technology from collecting data at high frequencies at all times. Due to their design and operating requirements, it is often not feasible for wearable devices to operate continuously at high sampling frequencies. Therefore, a common approach of wearable devices is to sample continuously at lower frequencies and dynamically adjust towards higher sampling frequencies after detecting a certain event of interest (Williamson et al., 2015). Through collaborative sensing, it is even possible for the receiving device to assist in detecting such events, sending a signal to the wearable device to increase sampling frequencies when an event is detected (Williamson et al., 2015). Moreover, some studies adopt a strategy of monitoring individuals at low frequencies over prolonged time periods, such that conclusions can still be drawn through repeated measurements (Godfrey et al., 2018).

Data Preprocessing

The initial form of the data collected by a wearable is its *raw* form. Raw data are essentially the quantised voltages measured at their original sampling frequency. Raw data contain errors, statistical outliers, inconsistencies, and noise and require initial cleaning, thereby discarding unnecessary data to maximise computational resources in the following stages. The initial cleaning and preprocessing are commonly done on the wearable device by a lower-power embedded microprocessor. Moreover, the raw data is often compressed before transmission to limit transmission energy (Williamson et al., 2015; Ometov et al., 2021).

MEMS sensors require cleaning and continuous calibration. In particular, MEMS gyroscopes are sensitive to sensor drift (where error accumulates over time), MEMS magnetometers require continuous hard and soft iron corrections, MEMS barometers are sensitive to temperature, and all MEMS sensors are sensitive to environmental effects such as temperature, humidity, altitude, and magnetic field distortion (Williamson et al., 2015). Other sensors require calibration and cleaning as well. In particular, motion artifacts are problematic for sensors such as PPG and barometers.

Data Transfer and Storage

Wearable devices often rely on a receiving device with a connection to the internet in order to safely store and further process their collected data. Transfer of data to external storage allows for more powerful processing of data that is not possible on the wearable device itself. Commonly, the receiving device is the wearer's own smartphone and the storage location of the data is either *local* (on the receiver itself) or *remote* (on a remote server in the cloud).

Due to the emergence and widespread adoption of Bluetooth Low Energy (BLE) technology, data is commonly transferred from wearable device to receiver using this technology, operating within a relatively short range of 10m (Mukhopadhyay et al., 2022). However, Most wearable devices are equipped with at least two wireless interfaces for short- and medium-range connectivity (Ometov et al., 2021), where Wireless Fidelity (Wi-Fi), for instance, can be used for data transfer within a 250m range. Alternative transmission technologies include Near Field Communication (NFC), ZigBee, and Low-Power Wide Area Network (LPWAN). A summary of short-range wireless communication technologies used for wearable communication can be found in Table 2.2.

Data Processing

After the raw or preprocessed data has been transferred, the following data processing steps consist of filtering and transforming the data to reduce noise, remove outliers, and increase data quality. For instance, ECG and PPG sensors suffer from noise due to baseline drifts, external

TABLE 2.2 Overview of Short-Range Communication Technologies for Wearable Communication (i.e., Cao et al., 2022; Ometov et al., 2021)

Technology	*Range*	*Frequency*	*Data Rate*	*Power Consumption*
Near Field Communication (NFC)	*20cm*	*13.56MHz*	*424 kbps*	*10mA*
Bluetooth Low Energy (BLE)	*10m*	*2.4GHz*	*24 Mbps*	*20mA*
ZigBee	*100m*	*2.4GHz*	*250 kbps*	*5mA*
Wi-Fi	*250m*	*2.5, 5GHz*	*1200 Mbps*	*10–50mA*

interference, muscle noise, etc. (Khan et al., 2020). Limiting the signal to specific frequency bands (filtering) is a common way to remove periodic noise from the signal and is an attempt to recover its original shape. Retrieving a noise-less signal is helpful for feature extraction, such as QRS detection in the ECG signal or counting heel strikes for step-count detection from accelerometer data. Data processing can be done in batches, in real-time, or online.

Advanced processing and heavy computations are not computationally feasible on the wearable itself. In the recent era of wearable technology, the smartphone acts as the gateway between the wearable device and the internet and provides access to further computational resources. Hence, most of the computations described in this subsection are performed on devices other than the wearable itself. Computing paradigms followed by wearable devices today are *Cloud, Edge, and Fog computing*, and they define the location in the network of devices where the computations should be carried out and where data should be managed and stored.

Filtering and Fourier Transforms

Filtering is a widely used technique for removing periodic noise from signal data. When the noise is periodic, the frequency of that noise can be filtered out. In signal processing, filtering requires three steps: (1) transforming the signal into its frequency domain; (2) multiplication of a filter function with the frequency domain of the signal; and (3) transforming the signal back into its time domain.

The aforementioned steps can be mathematically described as follows.

1. **Transformation to frequency domain:** A continuous signal can be described as a continuous one-dimensional function of time $f(t)$. To obtain a function of the frequency domain $F(x)$, i.e., a function of the different frequencies x of the signal, we use the *Fourier transform*

   $$F(x) = \int_{-\infty}^{\infty} f(t)e^{-2\pi ixt}dt.$$

   $F(x)$ can also be interpreted as the *spectrum* of the signal.

2. **Multiplication with filter function:** The filter is implemented relying on the Convolution Theorem, using the equation below

$$G(x) = H(x)F(x).$$

It is a multiplication of the Fourier transform $F(x)$ and a filter function $H(x)$. This filter function determines which frequencies can be let through (*passed*) or should be reduced, and which can remain.

3. **Inverse transformation to time domain:** The filtered signal in the frequency domain $G(x)$ should be transformed back to the time domain $g(t)$, using the *Inverse Fourier transform*

$$g(t) = \int_{-\infty}^{\infty} G(x)e^{2\pi ixt}dx.$$

Please note that for signals in wearable data, we do not directly use the continuous Fourier transform as described above, but rather its discrete form, also referred to as the discrete Fourier transform (DFT). The *filter function* $H(x)$ determines which frequencies to filter and is characterised by a specific *cut-off frequency*. For instance, *low-pass* filters let lower frequencies pass, and *high-pass* filters let higher frequencies pass. Applying these filters to data collected by wearable technology, high-pass filters can be used to filter out the gravity component in accelerometer data, whereas low-pass filters can be used to filter out high-frequency noise. Low-pass filters can be implemented as *finite impulse response* (FIR; moving averages) or *infinite impulse response* (IIR; running averages, considering the entire signal history). A *Butterworth* filter is a specific type of low-pass filter commonly used in physiological signal recording. It is an IIR filter with a maximally flat frequency response in the passband, which simultaneously causes an inherent delay to the signal.

With the increasing number of sensor modalities in wearables today, a wide range of wearable devices produced, and a plethora of different filter functions that could be used to process this data, standardisation of data processing in wearable data is highly recommended and useful to distinguish the quality of algorithms on the same data. Föll et al. (2021) took an initial step in this direction by proposing standardisation for ECG, PPG, and accelerometer data.

Data Fusion

Wearable devices commonly contain a range of different sensors (*sensor modalities*). These sensor modalities can be combined to improve the quality of the signal. For instance, artifacts and errors in the data can be removed by leveraging data from other sensors that capture these errors. For example, various sensors suffer from *motion artifacts*, i.e., increased sensor error due to increased motion of the sensor. Typically, these artifacts can be removed by using frequency domain heuristic methods or transformations. Alternatively, the accelerometer signal can be leveraged to remove motion artifacts from sensors, assuming the artifact is a linear addition (Teng et al., 2008).

Data Aggregation

The data gathered by wearable devices are time series, sometimes recorded at high frequencies. However, presenting the processed time series in its sparse form may be less relevant to the user or subsequent algorithm, presenting difficulties in extracting the relevant information from these enormous amounts of data collected by wearable devices. Data aggregation can be a solution here, where sparse data is aggregated on lower dense levels to summarise the time series data.

Data aggregation for time series is commonly done on a *(rolling-) window* basis and is defined by the following parameters: the aggregation window, aggregation frequency, and aggregation functions. In this rolling-window approach, a rolling window of a particular size slides over the time series data with a specific frequency (step size) and applies an aggregation function over the data window.

Aggregation functions for time series data exist in the time-, frequency-, and time-frequency domains, whereby aggregation in the frequency domain first requires transformation using the DFT. Examples of aggregation functions are the mean, standard deviation, minimum, maximum, sum, percentiles, energy function, entropy, power density, number of peaks, peak width, and peak-to-peak range. Moreover, custom aggregation functions also exist, combining data from multiple signals to obtain variables such as step count and sleep quality.

Data Analysis

The large amounts of non-intrusively collected data from wearable devices are well-suited for subsequent analysis. In particular, machine learning (ML) has been widely integrated into physical sensing systems. The considerable potential of ML has given wearable technology the opportunity to be "smart": its complex algorithms allow for intelligent insights that can be used for clinical practice and public health.

ML encompasses many models, ranging from *white-box* (interpretable) to *black-box* (non-interpretable). The objective of ML is to find a relation f between the observed data x and a variable of interest or chosen outcome y, where $y = f(x)$. The chosen outcome y can be continuous or discrete, where the task at hand is referred to as a *regression* or *classification* task, respectively. Moreover, as the variable of interest y_t and the observed data x_t are functions of time, finding a relation between x_t and y_t with the same time labels may be referred to as *detection* ($y_t = f(x_t)$), whereas a positive difference ($n > 0$) in time labels of x_t and y_{t+n} may be referred to as *prediction* or *forecasting* ($y_{t+n} = f(x_t)$).

State-of-the-art parametric- and non-parametric ML methods include support vector machines (SVMs), decision trees, random forests, gradient boosting, and neural networks, including multilayer perceptrons (MLPs), long short-term memory (LSTM) networks and convolutional neural networks (CNNs). Moreover, various ML methods exist for clustering and dimensionality reduction, such as k-means and principal component analysis (PCA). Similar to regression approaches, the objective of *supervised* parametric ML models is to approximate the function f, a function between the observed data x and a variable of interest y. However, the difference to classical regression is that these models contain a much larger number of parameters in different structures, allowing for more complex and non-linear relationships. For a complete discussion on the comparison of white-box with black-box artificial intelligence (AI), we kindly refer you to the chapter on interpretable AI in health care in this book.

The contribution of ML to wearable technology lies mainly in its potential for scalability and interpretability of data. As wearable technology allows for massive data collection from many individuals in their natural environment, ML facilitates the processing and analysis of this data, thereby providing meaningful insights that otherwise would not have been possible.

A particular application of ML is finding *biomarkers* from data gathered by wearable technology. When data from data streams other than those of the wearable device are collected simultaneously, ML can be leveraged to find a relation between wearable data characteristics and external data. Once this relation is established with sufficient accuracy/sensitivity/specificity, the wearable data can serve as a biomarker for the external data, thus not requiring this external data collection in the future. This approach is beneficial for data that is difficult to collect due to its recording being invasive (e.g., continuous glucose monitoring) or requiring effort from the user (e.g., daily sleep quality assessments through questionnaires or food diaries). Further applications of ML include anomaly detection and time series forecasting. For an overview of successful applications of these ML models, we refer you to the next Section of this Chapter.

The application of ML for wearable data presents various challenges. For instance, an imbalance in the data poses limitations on the generalisability and validation of ML models. This imbalance may occur in the variable of interest (e.g., an infrequent occurrence of a symptom) or as a result of the observational nature of this data, where the patient population may not be representative (e.g., a rare health condition). Data augmentation has been proposed as a solution, but this may raise other issues, such as an unrealistic representation of the data. Finally, a big challenge of wearable technology is its limited computational resources, thus limiting the computational complexity of the ML models.

APPLICATIONS

Wearable technology in health care can be applied to monitor diseases, provide interventions and improve understanding of health conditions. In the following Section, we describe applications of smart wearable technology in health care. These applications range from various disorders, such as Parkinson's disease and diabetes mellitus, to mental-, public- and personal health.

Wearable technology for health care purposes can be categorised according to three issues they address: (i) criticality of the information gathered; (ii) wearing duration and timing; and (iii) rapidity of transferring the collected data to a remote site and the associated intervention (Bonato, 2010). Hence, some applications are designed to perform long-term patient monitoring of uncritical data without direct interventions or responses, whereas others are designed to provide acute interventions or responses in emergency situations.

In applications of wearable technology in health care, AI and ML are commonly used to build models that associate data collected by the sensors of wearable devices to a specific health outcome, such as motor fluctuations in Parkinson's disease and sleep quality for patients with obstructive sleep apnea. Moreover, ML may be used to obtain proxies for vital signs that are otherwise difficult or costly to capture (e.g., through using PPG instead of RIP for respiration rate). In that way, AI and ML allow for real-time, remote, and continuous patient monitoring of specific health outcomes. Ultimately, this may enable patients to self-monitor their health conditions and improve their prognosis. Data processing in the cloud allows for direct involvement of healthcare providers and appropriate interventions, improving treatment timelines (Xie et al., 2021).

Vital Signs Monitoring

Vital signs monitoring is a crucial part of hospital care, facilitating early detection of physiological deterioration. Clinical-grade wearable technology allows for monitoring vital signs outside of clinical care, where vital signs include heart rate and heart rate variability, respiratory rate, oxygen saturation, blood pressure, and temperature. Various applications have been designed for the monitoring of vital signs, in the form of patches (Intelsens Zensor), clothing (Hexoskin, VivoMetrics LifeShirt), chest straps (Polar H7, Zephyr BioHarness, EQ02 LifeMonitor), or wristbands (ViSi Mobile). Finally, consumer-grade vital sign monitoring is a rising market, mainly in the design of wearable fitness wristbands (FitBit, Apple Watch, empatica e4) (Iqbal et al., 2016; Soon et al., 2020).

Cardiovascular Disease

Within vital signs monitoring, particular emphasis has been on cardiac activity. The consumer-grade wearable technology mentioned above primarily measures heart rate through PPG sensors, optionally augmented with a single-lead ECG. In cardiovascular medicine, wearable technology can be applied for risk assessment and lifestyle interventions, screening and diagnosis, and patient monitoring.

A high resting heart rate, impaired heart rate during recovery after exercise, and HRV have been associated with an increased risk of coronary artery disease and all-cause death, as well as increased adverse cardiovascular events (Bayoumy et al., 2021; Singh et al., 2018; Sydó et al., 2018; Fox et al., 2008; Zhang et al., 2016). Moreover, physical activity measured by wearable devices has been inversely associated with all-cause mortality (Bayoumy et al., 2021). Wearable technology measuring physical activity, HR, HRV, and blood pressure allows for continuous longitudinal cardiovascular risk assessment.

Hypertension is associated with the risk of cardiovascular disease. Continuous blood pressure measurements through wearable devices allow for early detection of hypertension, particularly during phases in which traditional devices are not practical, such as exercise and sleep (e.g., using Omron HeartGuide).

Moreover, longitudinal monitoring through wearable devices may be of use for other cardiovascular conditions, such as *atrial fibrillation (AF)* and *arrhythmias*. AF has been associated with stroke and heart failure. Smart wearable technology may enable early detection of AF through continuous PPG monitoring. Various studies have been conducted in this area, such as the Apple Heart study (Perez et al., 2019), with 419,297 participants enroled to predict AF through irregular pulse detection from the Apple Watch PPG sensors with a positive predictive value of 84%. Other studies using deep neural networks (DNNs) for AF detection from smartwatch data report a C-statistic of 0.97 (Tison et al., 2018) and a sensitivity and specificity of 95.4% and 99.7%, respectively (Fan, 2019). Furthermore, DNNs have been demonstrated to perform cardiologist-level detection and classification of arrhythmias for ambulatory ECG sensors (Hannun et al., 2019).

Finally, DNNs have demonstrated benefits for other cardiovascular conditions as well. For instance, in the DeepHeart study (Ballinger et al., 2018), an LSTM demonstrates C-statistics of 0.74 and 0.81 for detecting *high cholesterol* and *high blood pressure*, respectively, from data collected from popular consumer-grade smartwatches. Furthermore, *asymptomatic left ventricular dysfunction* could be identified in patients with a convolutional neural network (CNN) from ECG data with a C-statistic of 0.93. Finally, low-energy algorithms for the real-time detection of *myocardial infarction* report an accuracy of 90% (Sopic et al., 2018).

Effective control and monitoring of risk factors of cardiovascular disease influence its outcome. An additional application of wearable technology for cardiovascular disease is long-term *patient monitoring* to detect a worsening patient status and to intervene in case the patient deteriorates. Various remote monitoring interventions have been assessed in randomised control trials for *heart failure* (Abraham et al., 2011; Ong et al., 2016), *established AF* (Zado et al., 2019; Stavrakis et al., 2017), and *coronary artery disease* (Marvel et al., 2019).

Neurological Conditions

Parkinson's disease requires extensive monitoring outside of clinical care, including the timing, duration, and severity of different types of motor fluctuations, which cannot be reliably self-monitored by patients themselves. Smart wearable technology may capture the severity and potential deterioration of symptoms over time and thus facilitate clinical management of symptoms and consequent medication titration. Common applications of wearable technology for Parkinson's disease consist of wrist-based accelerometers to capture and classify the severity of motor fluctuations (tremor, bradykinesia, and dyskinesia) using neural networks (Keijsers et al., 2000; Keijsers et al., 2003; Hoff et al., 2001) or other ML techniques (Patel et al., 2009; Bonato et al., 2004).

Alternative neurological disorders that may benefit from wearable technology include *epilepsy*, for instance, through seizure detection by wearable EEG sensors (Shoeb et al., 2007) or by accelerometers (Nijsen et al., 2005), and *Alzheimer's disease* through location monitoring with GPS (e.g., with Everon Vega).

Pulmonary Disease

In various pulmonary diseases, long-term continuous monitoring of symptoms is a relevant aspect. Wearable technology allows for the monitoring of multiple vital signs, such as oxygen saturation (from PPG sensors), respiratory activity (through RIP or from ECG, PPG, or accelerometer sensors), heart rate and heart rate variability (from ECG or PPG), and temperature. Applications exist for patients with chronic obstructive pulmonary disease (COPD), obstructive sleep apnea (OSA), and asthma.

In patients with *chronic obstructive pulmonary disease (COPD)*, wearable technology may aid in the remote monitoring of symptoms and, thereby, early detection of physiological deterioration. Most applications focus on monitoring vital signs through smart vests with multiple sensors attached to the chest, such as Colantonio et al., 2015, or VivoMetrics LifeShirt. Moreover, for patients with COPD undergoing pulmonary rehabilitation, motor activity and activity levels may be detected and classified using accelerometer data (Sherrill et al., 2005; Steele et al., 2000). Full disease management platforms such as WELCOME (Chouvarda et al., 2014) and CHRONIOUS (Rosso et al., 2010) have been developed, allowing for COPD management at home.

Similarly, monitoring vital signs is also relevant for the early detection of *asthma* deterioration. For asthma patients in particular, breathing rate and airflow sound are relevant indicators and are either measured directly or indirectly from ECG and PPG sensors or chest movements. Other relevant vital signs for asthma include blood oxygen saturation, temperature, blood pressure, verbal sound, and pain response. Furthermore, environmental sensors measuring air quality may be useful (Talyor et al., 2022).

Another condition for which its patients may benefit from wearable technology is *obstructive sleep apnea (OSA)*. Various applications using AI have been used for diagnosing OSA from ambulatory signals. For instance, Nikkonen et al. (2019) use artificial neural networks to estimate the apnea-hypopnea index and the oxygen desaturation index from SpO_2 signals, obtaining an accuracy of >90% for correct classification into OSA severity categories. Moreover, Korkalainen et al. (2020) obtained an accuracy of 83.7% (76.5% and 84.5% for individuals with and without diagnosed OSA, respectively) for the classification of sleep stages using convolutional and LSTM neural networks from EEG data, facilitating diagnosis of sleep disorders such as OSA. Other studies are more targeted towards long-term sleep quality and OSA monitoring, such as Surrel et al., 2017, providing online detection of the sleep apnea score from single-channel ECG from a wearable device with an accuracy of up to 88.2%, as well as the Sleepcare Kit (Jeon et al., 2019), providing real-time monitoring of sleep quality and potential emergency situations. Furthermore, as a low-cost alternative to the current state-of-the-art, Cinel et al. (2020) propose a system for monitoring OSA by tracking the respiration rate from an accelerometer on the stomach or temperature sensor in the nose.

Finally, acoustics can be leveraged for various pulmonary diseases involving the detection of breathing patterns and sounds from audio data. For instance, *cough detection* through audio recordings is commonly implemented on smartphones, but (Barata et al., 2019) demonstrated that it could also be applied to other mobile devices.

Public Health

Besides applications for clinical and personal health, wearable technology has also been used to support public health. One of the most famous recent examples of leveraging wearables for public health may be the *COVID-19* pandemic, where smart wearable technology can assist in large-scale early detection, diagnosis, and monitoring at a distance through monitoring of vital signs such as HR, respiratory rate, SpO_2 and temperature (Tavakoli et al., 2020; Cheong et al., 2022). Other applications for public health are preventing *mosquito-born diseases* through KitePatch, dispersing VOCs as mosquito repellant, or monitoring Malaria symptoms through the TermoTell bracelet. Furthermore, various environmental sensors can monitor air quality (e.g., through TZOA, AirBeam, and Lapka PEM) and ultraviolet (UV) radiation to prevent *skin cancer* by providing alerts.

Personal Health and Wellness

A large stream of wearable technology for consumers focuses on personal health and wellness. Consumer-grade wearables provide insights into activity, stress, and sleep and provide personalised recommendations for health and behaviour, such as reminders to move, stand, or walk.

Physical activity in consumer-grade wearables is tracked by the IMMU in combination with potential barometers and GPS sensors, allowing for the detection of complex motion patterns and trajectories. A common way to present activity in consumer-grade wearables is through step counting (*pedometry*). Enhanced by heart rate through PPG, these devices can aid in monitoring exercise and sports and undertaking specific training.

Various consumer-grade wearables report *stress levels*, for instance, based on accelerometer, EDA, and PPG data (e.g., Sano et al., 2013), giving users feedback on their behaviour. Moreover, similar sensors are used for the measurement of the *sleep cycle*. In reference to the gold standard for sleep cycle monitoring (polysomnography) that leverages EEG, EMG, and EOG sensors, sleep cycle monitoring in consumer-grade wearables commonly makes use of accelerometer data and is therefore referred to as *actigraphy* (Ancoli-Israel et al., 2003). As these devices are not designed for clinical or research purposes, their accuracy is often limited.

DISCUSSION

In this Chapter, we provide an overview of the technologies used in wearable devices for healthcare purposes. We discuss the different technologies for monitoring physiological signals and the algorithms and techniques for data collection, processing, transfer, and analysis. Moreover, we discuss successful applications of wearable technology in health care, both in clinical practice and for public health. Finally, we discuss the design, adoption, quality, reliability, privacy, security, and future of wearable technology in health care.

Design

Wearable technology design is highly relevant for its adoption and further usage. The device's design should meet the requirements of its purpose while simultaneously being technologically feasible. General system requirements of wearable technology include remote (physiological) data collection and storage, a (graphical) user interface for interaction with- and feedback to the user, and wireless communication technology. A general limitation is battery capacity. Moreover, secondary system criteria include wearability, compactness, durability, reliability, robustness, and invasiveness.

To promote the adoption of consumer-grade wearable technology, on-body wearable devices are commonly embedded in items of clothing or gadgets that one would have customarily worn. Examples include smart watches (e.g., Garmin, Apple Watch), -rings (e.g., Oura Ring), -glasses (e.g., Google Glass), and -bracelets (e.g., Fitbit), but also smart textiles, -belts, and -shoes. The purpose of these designs is to reduce obtrusiveness and thereby promote accessibility, acceptance, and adoption of wearable technology.

Moreover, the miniaturisation of accelerometers, gyroscopes, and magnetometers with low power consumption through MEMS has transformed the field of activity and motion monitoring, allowing for the seamless integration of these sensors into wearable technology (Bonato, 2010). Hence, most wearables today contain a combination of various sensor modalities.

In this Chapter, we mainly focused on non-invasive wearable devices. A category of wearable devices that we have not reviewed is in-body or implantable devices. Implantable devices are (partially) inside the human body and are therefore more invasive. They allow for more local monitoring of the physiological signal. A famous and widely used example of an implantable device is a CGM device, where a needle is implanted in the skin and transmits glucose measurements to a receiving device. Other implantables include insertable cardiac monitors and insertable drug delivery systems (IDDS). As these invasive devices allow for targeted physiology and metabolism monitoring, these devices offer exciting opportunities for wearable technology-based chronic disease management (Milani et al., 2016). Nevertheless, the current issues of data reliability, privacy, and security should still be addressed (Xie et al., 2021).

An important aspect of the design of wearable technology is the delivery of information and feedback to the user. User information and feedback include information on data aggregates, such as step count, time spent in heart rate zones, and hours slept. However, wearable technology can also be used as a decision support system, providing insights into the choices of ML models and giving relevant recommendations for lifestyle adjustments. Perceived user benefit can be influenced by the usefulness of the information presented. Future generations of wearable technology may also incorporate medical history and user preferences to provide personalised feedback (Loncar-Turukalo et al., 2019).

A major challenge of wearable technology is energy consumption. Due to its compact size, battery capacity remains limited in wearable devices and hence also provides restrictions on the computations that can be carried out on the device. Battery life is one of the top selection criteria for individuals selecting a wearable device. Power consumption can be minimised using low-power sensors, advanced battery techniques such as lithium-ion batteries, and energy harvesting (Ometov et al., 2021). Energy harvesting involves extracting energy from the environment through energy sources such as motion, temperature, light, and electromagnetic radiation, generated by the human body, the sun, or other energy sources. Nevertheless, energy harvesting has limited capabilities in wearable devices due to their constraints on size and weight (Ghomian et al., 2019).

Adoption

Following the Technology Acceptance Model (Davis et al., 1989), the adoption of wearable technology is based on perceived usefulness and perceived ease of use (Page, 2015). Commonly mentioned factors that limit the adoption of wearable technology mentioned in literature are intrusiveness, i.e., a general feeling of discomfort or stress caused by the wearable technology, as well as concerns about data privacy and ownership.

Perceived usefulness and perceived ease of use of wearable technology have been influenced by marketing. Consumer-grade wearable technology for healthcare purposes has been marketed as "technology-assisted self-care" (Schüll, 2016) and a valuable aid to informing healthy living (Godfrey et al., 2018) and thanks its success to consumerism stimulated by marketing (Godfrey et al., 2018). Purchases of consumer-grade wearable technology often lead to short-term engagement, as users may grow disinterested over time. Moreover, social acceptance may limit adoption, highlighting the purpose of integration into clothing or implantable devices (Godfrey et al., 2018; Loncar-Turukalo et al., 2019).

A key factor in the adoption of wearable technology is a cohort-specific design, specifically regarding generational differences. It has been shown that the adoption of wearable technology is lower for older generations for various reasons. Concerns about data privacy, potential dangers, and robustness are mentioned as potential issues. Moreover, the technical skills of older generations may be limited (relating to perceived ease of use) and they may find it harder to rationalise their usage (relating to perceived usefulness), as opposed to the younger generations that benefited from early exposure to technology. Resistance to change in technology in the older generations is a consequence thereof (e.g., Page, 2015; Shin et al., 2019; Godfrey et al., 2018). However, the usefulness of wearable technology for older generations remains, as they suffer more often from health conditions. Hence, to stimulate adoption among all groups of users, wearable technology should be designed to align with their personal preferences instead of a one-fits-all design concept (Shin et al., 2019).

Quality and Reliability

In the discussion of the quality and reliability of wearable technology, it is essential to distinguish between consumer-grade and clinical-grade wearable devices. Clinical-grade wearable devices have high enough quality and reliability to be used in medical applications and have often been approved by authorities such as the US Food and Drug Administration (FDA). Consequently, this technology often comes at a higher price. On the other hand, consumer-grade wearable devices aim to sell wearable technology to the mass market at a lower cost, thereby making a trade-off between price and quality. As consumer-grade wearable technology has become more mainstream over the last decade, there is increasing adoption of consumer-grade wearable technology in clinical studies. Therefore, its quality and reliability should be considered accordingly.

In consumer-grade wearable technology, lack of standardisation is a major issue. Sensors vary from manufacturer to manufacturer and a wide range of data processing algorithms is deployed on them. Pre-processing protocols exist, but inherent errors and discrepancies between devices still remain. As a result, the physiological values obtained from consumer-grade wearable technology may vary or change over time after the implementation of a software update. Best practice guidelines or standards for data processing are recommended for researchers working with data from wearables. To address this issue from the research side, e.g., Föll et al. (2021) propose a processing pipeline for EDA, HR, and accelerometer sensor modalities from commonly used wearable devices. Nevertheless, further research on this topic is still required.

Clinical-grade wearable devices must at all times warrant the safety of their usage. Users of clinical-grade wearable technology may depend on these systems for their medical safety and health, for which there is no room for errors. Failure of medical technology can cost lives. Thus the existence of false negatives is not accepted. Even though devices often have to make a trade-off between sensitivity and specificity, the number of false positives should be small, as it negatively influences user trust and may hamper user adherence (Loncar-Turukalo et al., 2019). Therefore, clinical-grade wearable technology must comply with strict standards and regulations, such as the IEC 62366-1:2015 standard in the EU.

Machine learning (ML) and artificial intelligence (AI) have transformed the field of wearable technology. These techniques enable real-time advanced data processing to retrieve meaningful and actionable information. Nevertheless, the generalisability of such algorithms is often limited, as they are commonly tested by simulation, under fixed conditions, or on a homogeneous population (Baig et al., 2017). Hence, their accuracy generally does not suffice for clinical-grade wearable devices, and scalability and broader integration prove to be a challenge for the reliability and accuracy of wearable technology. Considering that there exists no regulation for the validation of ML in wearable technology for health care and that the algorithms deployed on consumer-grade wearable technology and their validation procedures are not transparent, the adoption of consumer-grade wearable technology in health care should be treated with caution.

A direct and previously under-reported issue in wearable technology is the reduced reliability of various optical sensors, such as photoplethysmography (PPG), for individuals with darker skin tones (Fallow et al., 2013; Shcherbina et al., 2017). The resulting racial bias in wearable health technology is highly concerning and directly results from the validation of wearable technology on homogeneous populations, such as individuals with lighter skin tones. Due to the ongoing transition in the usage of consumer-grade wearable technology for healthcare applications and consequent FDA approval of the associated algorithms, this issue requires particular attention from the industry and the scientific community (Colvonen et al., 2020).

Privacy and Security

Data privacy, security, and associated patient confidentiality are rising concerns for wearable technology. Wearable devices collect, store, and transfer large amounts of sensitive data and are therefore vulnerable to security attacks. Therefore sufficient encryption and authentication are vital for ensuring data safety to prevent the misuse of personal health data. Moreover, privacy also involves control over one's data and should always be guaranteed due to the sensitive nature of the collected data.

Various security issues and data breaches related to medical or wearable devices have been reported over the last few years (e.g., Chen et al., 2016; Davis, 2019; McKeon, 2021). There are multiple ways in which malicious parties can access sensitive data, such as *eavesdropping* (intercepting unencrypted data when it is transferred), data modification, replay attacks, *denial of service* attacks (flooding system traffic), *man-in-the-middle* attacks, and masquerading attacks. Prevention of such attacks can be implemented through data encryption, two-factor authentication, security of the receiving device (acting as a gateway to the internet), and authentication with multiple credentials, such as passwords, certificates, and biometrics (Alkeem et al., 2015), potentially moderated by block-chain technology (Xie et al., 2021).

Privacy concerns of wearable technology users arise mainly from ambiguity over authorisation of the collected data stored in the cloud. In particular, it may be unclear to users by which parties and in which way certain personal data is used. Concerns range from collecting unnecessary personal data to data sharing with third parties or misuse of the data shared for personal benefit (Kapoor et al., 2020). The General Data Protection Regulation (GDPR) was enacted in the EU in 2016 to assure data privacy and protection for all its citizens. In particular, the following proposals should be considered by organisations working with wearable technology to ensure user privacy: (i) *respect for context* – "consumers have a right to expect that companies will collect, use, and disclose personal data in ways that are consistent with the context in which consumers provide the data"; (ii) *risk-benefit analysis* – assessment of the benefits of using certain data against the risk of consumer privacy; (iii) *transparency* about how personal data is used; (iv) *de-identification* – decoupling personal identity from data; (v) *reasonable individual access* for user engagement with their data; (vi) *appropriate security* as mentioned above; and (vii) development of *codes of conduct* to ensure privacy compliance (Wolf et al., 2016).

CONCLUSION

The market for wearable technology in health care is surging. Current developments in wearable technology show a focus on multi-functional wearables with a large number of integrated sensors. Nevertheless, in this era of rapid growth of technological developments, it is uncertain how wearable technology will develop in the future. Future technological developments may present more invasive wearable technology, such as smart tattoos, contact lenses, swallowable gadgets, implantables and other wearable devices that invade personal space, indicating a need for increased security regulations. Moreover, the limitation of battery capacity in wearable devices may be addressed by techniques such as energy harvesting. Furthermore, the future of wearable technology may offer a multitude of specialised wearable devices dedicated to a specific health benefit, possibly collectively *interoperable* (i.e., seamlessly cooperating and interacting with each other, following the IoT paradigm, to achieve their full potential). Consumer interest in this direction is already expressed through the simultaneous use of various wearable technologies, observed in consumers wearing a smartwatch for activity monitoring and as a personal assistant, a smart ring (e.g., Oura ring) for sleep tracking, and a continuous glucose monitoring device (e.g., Supersapiens) for energy management associated with physical exercise, while concurrently using a smartphone with various health apps, such as a food diary and a meditation aid.

The potential of wearable technology lies in its ability to collect enormous amounts of data ("big data"). Large amounts of highly personalised data can be non-intrusively collected using wearable technology and potentially used for personal interventions, as well as for health benefits of the overall population (Wu, 2019). AI and ML can be leveraged to process and analyse these complex amounts of data to find valuable insights for clinical diagnosis and treatment, creating "smart" wearable technology for health care. Yet, it is questionable whether industry and the scientific community can keep up with the exponential growth of varying data gathered by wearable technology that still needs to be interoperable within the Wearable Internet of Things.

REFERENCES

Abraham, W. T., P. B. Adamson, R. C. Bourge, M. F. Aaron, M. R. Costanzo, L. W. Stevenson, W. Strickland, et al. 2011. "Wireless Pulmonary Artery Haemodynamic Monitoring in Chronic Heart Failure: A Randomised Controlled Trial." *The Lancet* 377 (9766): 658–666.

Alkeem, E. A. L., C. Y. Yeun, and M. J. Zemerly. 2015. "Security and Privacy Framework for Ubiquitous Healthcare IoT Devices." 2015 10th International Conference for Internet Technology and Secured Transactions (ICITST).

Ancoli-Israel, S., R. Cole, C. Alessi, M. Chambers, W. Moorcroft, and C. P. Pollak. 2003. "The Role of Actigraphy in the Study of Sleep and Circadian Rhythms." *Sleep* 26 (3): 342–392. 10.1093/sleep/26.3.342.

Baig, M. M., H. GholamHosseini, A. A. Moqeem, F. Mirza, and M. Lindén. 2017. "A Systematic Review of Wearable Patient Monitoring Systems - Current Challenges and Opportunities for Clinical Adoption." *Journal of Medical Systems* 41 (7): 115.

Baldini, C., L. Billeci, F. Sansone, R. Conte, C. Domenici, and A. Tonacci. 2020. "Electronic Nose as a Novel Method for Diagnosing Cancer: A Systematic Review." *Biosensors* 10 (8): 84.

Ballinger, B., J. Hsieh, A. Singh, N. Sohoni, J. Wang, G. Tison, G. Marcus, et al. 2018. "DeepHeart: Semi-Supervised Sequence Learning for Cardiovascular Risk Prediction." Proceedings of the AAAI Conference on Artificial Intelligence 32 (1).

Barata, F., K. Kipfer, M. Weber, P. Tinschert, E. Fleisch, and T. Kowatsch. 2019. "Towards Device-Agnostic Mobile Cough Detection with Convolutional Neural Networks." 2019 IEEE International Conference on Healthcare Informatics (ICHI), 1–11.

Bayoumy, K., M. Gaber, A. Elshafeey, O. Mhaimeed, E. H. Dineen, F. A. Marvel, S. S. Martin, et al. 2021. "Smart Wearable Devices in Cardiovascular Care: Where We Are and How to Move Forward." *Nature Reviews Cardiology* 18 (8): 581–599.

Binkley, P. F., W. Frontera, D. G. Standaert, and J. Stein. 2003. "Predicting the Potential of Wearable Technology." *IEEE Engineering in Medicine and Biology Magazine* 22 (3): 23–27.

Bolanakis, D. E. 2016. "MEMS Barometers in a Wireless Sensor Network for Position Location Applications." 2016 IEEE Virtual Conference on Applications of Commercial Sensors (VCACS), 1–8.

Bonato, P. 2010. "Advances in Wearable Technology and Its Medical Applications." 2010 Annual International Conference of the IEEE Engineering in Medicine and Biology 2010, 2021–2024.

Bonato, P. 2003. "Wearable Sensors/Systems and their Impact on Biomedical Engineering." *IEEE Engineering in Medicine and Biology Magazine* 22 (3): 18–20.

Bonato, P., D. M. Sherrill, D. G. Standaer, S. S. Salles, and M. Akay. 2004. "Data Mining Techniques to Detect Motor Fluctuations in Parkinson's Disease." The 26th Annual International Conference of the IEEE Engineering in Medicine and Biology Society 2, 4766–4769.

Cao, S., X. Chen, and B. C. Yuan. 2022. "Overview of Short-range Wireless Communication Protocol." 2022 7th International Conference on Computer and Communication Systems (ICCCS) 00, 519–523.

Chen, X., X. F. Wang, X. Huang, C. Wang, X. Guo, Y. Wang, Y. Chen, and B. Liu. 2016. "Friend or Foe?" Proceedings of the 11th ACM on Asia Conference on Computer and Communications Security, 189–200.

Cheong, S. H. R., Y. J. X. Ng, Y. Lau, and S. T. Lau. 2022. "Wearable Technology for Early Detection of COVID-19: A Systematic Scoping Review." *Preventive Medicine* 162: 107170.

Chouvarda, I., N. Y. Philip, P. Natsiavas, V. Kilintzis, D. Sobnath, R. Kayyali, J. Henriques, et al. 2014. "WELCOME - Innovative Integrated Care platform using Wearable Sensing and Smart Cloud Computing for COPD patients with Comorbidities." 2014 36th Annual International Conference of the IEEE Engineering in Medicine and Biology Society 2014, 3180–3183.

Chowdhury, R. H., M. B. I. Reaz, M. A. B. M. Ali, A. A. A. Bakar, K. Chellappan, and T. G. Chang. 2013. "Surface Electromyography Signal Processing and Classification Techniques." *Sensors* 13 (9): 12431–12466.

Cinel, G., E. A. Tarim, and H. C. Tekin. 2020. "Wearable respiratory rate sensor technology for diagnosis of sleep apnea." *2020 Medical Technologies Congress (TIPTEKNO)* 00: 1–4.

Colantonio, S., L. Govoni, R. L. Dellacà, M. Martinelli, O. Salvetti, and M. Vitacca. 2015. "Decision Making Concepts for the Remote, Personalized Evaluation of COPD Patients? Health Status." *Methods of Information in Medicine* 54 (03): 240–247.

Colvonen, P. J., P. N. DeYoung, N.-O.A Bosompra, and R. L. Owens. 2020. "Limiting Racial Disparities and Bias for Wearable Devices in Health Science Research." *Sleep* 43 (10): zsaa159.

Davis, F. D., R. P. Bagozzi, and P. R. Warshaw. 1989. "User Acceptance of Computer Technology: A Comparison of Two Theoretical Models." *Management Science* 35 (8): 982–1003.

Davis, J. 2019. *277,000 Patients Impacted in Medical Device Vendor Breach.* Accessed November 24, 2022. https://healthitsecurity.com/news/277000-patients-impacted-in-medical-device-vendor-breach.

Dragonieri, S., G. Pennazza, P. Carratu, and O. Resta. 2017. "Electronic Nose Technology in Respiratory Diseases." *Lung* 195 (2): 157–165.

Fallow, B. A., T. Tarumi, and H. Tanaka. 2013. "Influence of Skin Type and Wavelength on Light Wave Reflectance." *Journal of Clinical Monitoring and Computing* 27 (3): 313–317.

Fan, Y.-Y. L. 2019. "Diagnostic Performance of a Smart Device With Photoplethysmography Technology for Atrial Fibrillation Detection: Pilot Study (Pre-mAFA II Registry)." *JMIR Mhealth Uhealth* 7 (3): e11437

Fletcher, R. R., M.-Z. Poh, and H. Eydgahi. 2010. "Wearable Sensors: Opportunities and Challenges for Low-cost Health Care." 2010 Annual International Conference of the IEEE Engineering in Medicine and Biology 2010, 1763–1766.

Föll, S., M. Maritsch, F. Spinola, V. Mishra, F. Barata, T. Kowatsch, E. Fleisch, and F. Wortmann. 2021. "FLIRT: A Feature Generation Toolkit for Wearable Data." *Computer Methods and Programs in Biomedicine* 212: 106461.

Fox, K., I. Ford, P. G. Steg, M. Tendera, M. Robertson, and R. Ferrari. 2008. "Heart Rate as a Prognostic Risk Factor in Patients with Coronary Artery Disease and Left-ventricular Systolic Dysfunction (BEAUTIFUL): A

Subgroup Analysis of a Randomised Controlled Trial." *The Lancet* 372(9641): 817–821.

Ghomian, T., and S. Mehraeen. 2019. "Survey of Energy Scavenging for Wearable and Implantable Devices." *Energy* 178:33–49.

Godfrey, A., V. Hetherington, H. Shum, P. Bonato, N. H. Lovell, and S. Stuart. 2018. "From A to Z: Wearable Technology Explained." *Maturitas* 113:40–47.

Groppe, D. M., S. Bickel, C. J. Keller, S. K. Jain, S. T. Hwang, C. Harden, and A. D. Mehta. 2013. "Dominant Frequencies of Resting Human Brain Activity as Measured by the Electrocorticogram." *NeuroImage* 79:223–233.

Haescher, M., J. Trimpop, D. J. C. Matthies, and B. Urban. 2016. "SeismoTracker." Proceedings of the 2016 CHI Conference Extended Abstracts on Human Factors in Computing Systems, 2209–2216.

Haghi, M., K. Thurow, and R. Stoll. 2017. "Wearable Devices in Medical Internet of Things: Scientific Research and Commercially Available Devices." *Healthcare Informatics Research* 23 (1): 4–15.

Hannun, A. Y., P. Rajpurkar, M. Haghpanahi, G. H. Tison, C. Bourn, M. P. Turakhia, and A. Y. Ng. 2019. "Cardiologist-level arrhythmia detection and classification in ambulatory electrocardiograms using a deep neural network." *Nature Medicine* 25 (1): 65–69.

Hoff, J. I., A.A. v/d Plas, E. A. H. Wagemans, and J. J. van Hilten. 2001. "Accelerometric assessment of levodopa-induced dyskinesias in Parkinson's disease." *Movement Disorders* 16 (1): 58–61.

Iqbal, M. H., A. Aydin, O. Brunckhorst, P. Dasgupta, and K. Ahmed. 2016. "A review of wearable technology in medicine." *Journal of the Royal Society of Medicine* 109 (10): 372–380.

Jeon, Y. J., and S. J. Kang. 2019. "Wearable Sleepcare Kit: Analysis and Prevention of Sleep Apnea Symptoms in Real-Time." *IEEE Access* 7:60634–60649.

Kapoor, V., R. Singh, R. Reddy, and P. Churi. 2020. "Privacy Issues in Wearable Technology: An Intrinsic Review." *SSRN Electronic Journal.*

Karlen, W., S. Raman, J. M. Ansermino, and G. A. Dumont. 2013. "Multiparameter Respiratory Rate Estimation From the Photoplethysmogram." *IEEE Transactions on Biomedical Engineering* 60 (7): 1946–1953.

Keijsers, N. L. W., M. W. I. M. Horstink, J. J. van Hilten, J. I. Hoff, and C. C. A. M. Gielen. 2000. "Detection and Assessment of the Severity of Levodopa-induced Dyskinesia in Patients with Parkinson's Disease by Neural Networks." *Movement Disorders* 15 (6): 1104–1111.

Keijsers, N. L. W., M. W. I. M. Horstink, and S. C. A. M. Gielen. 2003. "Automatic Assessment of Levodopa-induced Dyskinesias in Daily Life by Neural Networks." *Movement Disorders* 18 (1): 70–80.

Khan, S., S. Parkinson, L. Grant, N. Liu, and S. Mcguire. 2020. "Biometric Systems Utilising Health Data from Wearable Devices." *ACM Computing Surveys (CSUR)* 53 (4): 1–29.

Korkalainen, H., J. Aakko, S. Nikkonen, S. Kainulainen, A. Leino, B. Duce, I. O. Afara, S. Myllymaa, J. Tyrs, and T. Leppnen. 2020. "Accurate Deep Learning-Based Sleep Staging in a Clinical Population With Suspected

Obstructive Sleep Apnea." *IEEE Journal of Biomedical and Health Informatics* 24 (7): 2073–2081.

Loncar-Turukalo, T., E. Zdravevski, J. M. da Silva, I. Chouvarda, and V. Trajkovik. 2019. "Literature on Wearable Technology for Connected Health: Scoping Review of Research Trends, Advances, and Barriers." *J Med Internet Res* 21 (9): e14017.

Lu, G., F. Yang, J. A. Taylor, and J. F. Stein. 2009. "A Comparison of Photoplethysmography and ECG Recording to Analyse Heart Rate Variability in Healthy Subjects." *Journal of Medical Engineering & Technology* 33 (8): 634–641.

Lymberis, A. 2003. "Smart Wearable Systems for Personalised Health Management: Current R&D and Future Challenges." Proceedings of the 25th Annual International Conference of the IEEE Engineering in Medicine and Biology Society (IEEE Cat. No.03CH37439) 4, 3716–3719.

Maenaka, K. 2008. "MEMS Inertial Sensors and Their Applications." 2008 5th International Conference on Networked Sensing Systems, 71–73.

Malmivuo, J. 1995. "Impedance Plethysmography." In *Bioelectromagnetism: Principles and Applications of Bioelectric and Biomagnetic Fields*, 405–419. Oxford University Press.

Marvel, F. A., E. M. Spaulding, M. Lee, W. Yang, and S. S. Martin. 2019. "Abstract 26: The Corrie Myocardial infarction, COmbined-device, Recovery Enhancement (MiCORE) Study: 30-Day Readmission Rates and Cost-Effectiveness of a Novel Digital Health Intervention for Acute Myocardial Infarction Patients." *Circulation: Cardiovascular Quality and Outcomes* 12 (Suppl_1).

McKeon, J. 2021. 61M Fitbit, Apple Users Had Data Exposed in Wearable Device Data Breach. Accessed November 24, 2022. https://healthitsecurity.com/news/61m-fitbit-apple-users-had-data-exposed-in-wearable-device-data-breach.

Milani, R. V., R. M. Bober, and C. J. Lavie. 2016. "The Role of Technology in Chronic Disease Care." *Progress in Cardiovascular Diseases* 58 (6): 579–583.

Mukhopadhyay, S. C., N. K. Suryadevara, and A. Nag. 2022. "Wearable Sensors for Healthcare: Fabrication to Application." *Sensors (Basel, Switzerland)* 22 (14): 5137.

Nijsen, T. M. E., J. B. A. M. Arends, P. A. M. Griep, and P. J. M. Cluitmans. 2005. "The Potential Value of Three-dimensional Accelerometry for Detection of Motor Seizures in Severe Epilepsy." *Epilepsy & Behavior* 7 (1): 74–84.

Nikkonen, S., I. O. Afara, T. Leppänen, and J. Töyräs. 2019. "Artificial Neural Network Analysis of the Oxygen Saturation Signal Enables Accurate Diagnostics of Sleep Apnea." *Scientific Reports* 9 (1): 13200.

Ometov, A., V. Shubina, L. Klus, J. Skibinska, S. Saafi, P. Pascacio, L. Flueratoru, et al. 2021. "A Survey on Wearable Technology: History, State-of-the-art and Current Challenges." *Computer Networks* 193:108074.

Ong, M. K., P. S. Romano, S. Edgington, H. U. Aronow, A. D. Auerbach, J. T. Black, T. D. Marco, et al. 2016. *"Effectiveness of Remote Patient Monitoring After Discharge of Hospitalized Patients With Heart Failure: The Better Effectiveness After Transition-Heart Failure (BEAT-HF) Randomized Clinical Trial."* *JAMA Internal Medicine* 176 (3): 310.

Oreggioni, J., A. A. Caputi, and F. Silveira. 2017. "Biopotential Monitoring." In *Encyclopedia of Biomedical Engineering*, 296–304. Elsevier.

Orphanidou, C., S. Fleming, S. A. Shah, and L. Tarassenko. 2013. "Data Fusion for Estimating Respiratory Rate from a Single-lead ECG." *Biomedical Signal Processing and Control* 8 (1): 98–105.

Page, T. 2015. "A Forecast of the Adoption of Wearable Technology." *International Journal of Technology Diffusion (IJTD)* 6 (2): 12–29.

Patel, S., K. Lorincz, R. Hughes, N. Huggins, J. Growdon, D. Standaert, M. Akay, J. Dy, M. Welsh, and P. Bonato. 2009. "Monitoring Motor Fluctuations in Patients with Parkinson's Disease Using Wearable Sensors." *IEEE Transactions on Information Technology in Biomedicine* 13 (6): 864–873.

Perez, M. V., K. W. Mahaffey, H. Hedlin, J. S. Rumsfeld, A. Garcia, T. Ferris, Vi. Balasubramanian, et al. 2019. "Large-Scale Assessment of a Smartwatch to Identify Atrial Fibrillation." *New England Journal of Medicine* 381 (20): 1909–1917.

Ping, W., T. Yi, X. Haibao, and S. Farong. 1997. "A Novel Method for Diabetes Diagnosis Based on Electronic Nose." *Biosensors and Bioelectronics* 12 (9-10): 1031–1036.

PRIME Faraday Partnership. 2002. *Technology Watch: An Introduction to MEMS (Micro-electromechanical Systems)*. Loughborough University.

Rosso, R., G. Munaro, O. Salvetti, S. Colantonio, and F. Ciancitto. 2010. "CHRONIOUS: An Open, Ubiquitous and Adaptive Chronic Disease Management Platform for Chronic Obstructive Pulmonary Disease (COPD), Chronic Kidney Disease (CKD) and Renal Insufficiency." 2010 Annual International Conference of the IEEE Engineering in Medicine and Biology 2010, 6850–6853.

Sano, A., and R. W. Picard. 2013. "Stress Recognition using Wearable Sensors and Mobile Phones." 2013 Humaine Association Conference on Affective Computing and Intelligent Interaction, 671–676.

Schüll, N. D. 2016. "Data for life: Wearable Technology and the Design of Self-care." *BioSocieties* 11 (3): 317–333.

Shcherbina, A., C. M. Mattsson, D. Waggott, H. Salisbury, J. W. Christle, T. Hastie, M. T. Wheeler, and E. A. Ashley. 2017. "Accuracy in Wrist-Worn, Sensor-Based Measurements of Heart Rate and Energy Expenditure in a Diverse Cohort." *Journal of Personalized Medicine* 7 (2): 3.

Sherrill, D. M., M. L. Moy, J. J. Reilly, and P. Bonato. 2005. "Using Hierarchical Clustering Methods to Classify Motor Activities of COPD Patients from Wearable Sensor Data." *Journal of NeuroEngineering and Rehabilitation* 2 (1): 16.

Shin, G., M. H. Jarrahi, Y. Fei, A. Karami, N. Gafinowitz, A. Byun, and X.-a. Lu. 2019. "Wearable Activity Trackers, Accuracy, Adoption, Acceptance and Health Impact: A Systematic Literature Review." *Journal of Biomedical Informatics* 93:103153.

Shoeb, A., B. Bourgeois, S. T. Treves, S. C. Schachter, and J. Guttag. 2007. "Impact of Patient-Specificity on Seizure Onset Detection Performance." *2007 29th Annual International Conference of the IEEE Engineering in Medicine and Biology Society* 2007: 4110–4114.

Singh, N., K. J. Moneghetti, J. W. Christle, D. Hadley, V. Froelicher, and D. Plews. 2018. "Heart Rate Variability: An Old Metric with New Meaning in the Era of Using mHealth Technologies for Health and Exercise Training Guidance. Part Two: Prognosis and Training." *Arrhythmia & Electrophysiology Review* 7 (4): 1.

Söderkvist, J. 1994. "Micromachined Gyroscopes." *Sensors and Actuators A: Physical* 43 (1-3): 65–71.

Soon, S., H. Svavarsdottir, C. Downey, and D. G. Jayne. 2020. "Wearable Devices for Remote Vital Signs Monitoring in the Outpatient Setting: An Overview of the Field." *BMJ Innovations* 6 (2): 55.

Sopic, D., A. Aminifar, A. Aminifar, and D. Atienza. 2018. "Real-Time Event-Driven Classification Technique for Early Detection and Prevention of Myocardial Infarction on Wearable Systems." *IEEE Transactions on Biomedical Circuits and Systems* 12 (5): 982–992.

Stavrakis, S., J. A. Stoner, J. Kardokus, P. J. Garabelli, S. S. Po, and R. Lazzara. 2017. "Intermittent vs. Continuous Anticoagulation Therapy in Patients with Atrial Fibrillation (iCARE-AF): A Randomized Pilot Study." *Journal of Interventional Cardiac Electrophysiology* 48 (1): 51–60.

Steele, B. G., L. Holt, B. Belza, S. Ferris, S. Lakshminaryan, and D. M. Buchner. 2000. "Quantitating Physical Activity in COPD Using a Triaxial Accelerometer." *Chest* 117 (5): 1359–1367.

Surrel, G., A. Aminifar, F. Rincn, S. Murali, and D. Atienza. 2017. "Online Obstructive Sleep Apnea Detection on Medical Wearable Sensors." *IEEE Transactions on Biomedical Circuits and Systems* 12 (4): 762–773.

Sydó, N., T. Sydó, K. A. Gonzalez Carta, N. Hussain, S. Farooq, J. G. Murphy, B. Merkely, F. Lopez-Jimenez, and T. G. Allison. 2018. "Prognostic Performance of Heart Rate Recovery on an Exercise Test in a Primary Prevention Population." *Journal of the American Heart Association* 7 (7): e008143.

Talyor, L., X. Ding, D. Clifton, and H. Y. Lu. 2022. "Wearable Vital Signs Monitoring for Patients with Asthma: A Review." *IEEE Sensors Journal.*

Tatum IV, W. O. 2021. *Handbook of EEG interpretation*. Springer Publishing Company.

Tavakoli, M., J. Carriere, and A. Torabi. 2020. "Robotics, Smart Wearable Technologies, and Autonomous Intelligent Systems for Healthcare During the COVID-19 Pandemic: An Analysis of the State of the Art and Future Vision." *Advanced Intelligent Systems* 2 (7): 2000071.

Teng, X.-F., Y.-T. Zhang, C. C. Y. Poon, and P. Bonato. 2008. "Wearable Medical Systems for p-Health." *IEEE Reviews in Biomedical Engineering* 1: 62–74.

Thakor, N. V. 2014. "Biopotentials and Electrophysiology Measurement." In *Measurement, Instrumentation, and Sensors Handbook*, edited by CRC Press. Taylor & Francis Group.

Tison, G. H., J. M. Sanchez, B. Ballinger, A. Singh, J. E. Olgin, M. J. Pletcher, E. Vittinghoff, et al. 2018. "Passive Detection of Atrial Fibrillation Using a Commercially Available Smartwatch." *JAMA Cardiology* 3 (5): 409.

Tröster, G. 2005. "The Agenda of Wearable Healthcare." *Yearbook of Medical Informatics* 14 (01): 125–138.

Voss, A., V. Baier, R. Reisch, K. von Roda, P. Elsner, H. Ahlers, and G. Stein. 2005. "Smelling Renal Dysfunction via Electronic Nose." *Annals of Biomedical Engineering* 33 (5): 656–660.

Voss, A., R. Schroeder, S. Schulz, J. Haueisen, S. Vogler, P. Horn, A. Stallmach, and P. Reuken. 2022. "Detection of Liver Dysfunction Using a Wearable Electronic Nose System Based on Semiconductor Metal Oxide Sensors." *Biosensors* 12 (2): 70.

Weiler, D. T., S. O. Villajuan, L. Edkins, S. Cleary, and J. J. Saleem. 2017. "Wearable Heart Rate Monitor Technology Accuracy in Research: A Comparative Study Between PPG and ECG Technology." *Proceedings of the Human Factors and Ergonomics Society Annual Meeting* 61 (1): 1292–1296.

Williamson, J., Q. Liu, F. Lu, W. Mohrman, K. Li, R. Dick, and L. Shang. 2015. "Data Sensing and Analysis: Challenges for Wearables." The 20th Asia and South Pacific Design Automation Conference, 136–141.

Wolf, C., J. Polonetsky, and K. Finch. 2016. "A Practical Privacy Paradigm for Wearables." *Future of Privacy Forum*.

Wu, M. 2019. "Wearable Technology Applications in Healthcare: A Literature Review | HIMSS." *Online Journal of Nursing Informatics* 23 (3): 1–16.

Xie, Y., L. Lu, F. Gao, S.-j. He, H.-j. Zhao, Y. Fang, J.-m. Yang, Y. An, Z.-w. Ye, and Z. Dong. 2021. "Integration of Artificial Intelligence, Blockchain, and Wearable Technology for Chronic Disease Management: A New Paradigm in Smart Healthcare." *Current Medical Science* 41 (6): 1123–1133.

Yazdi, N., F. Ayazi, and K. Najafi. 1998. "Micromachined Inertial Sensors." *Proceedings of the IEEE* 86 (8): 1640–1659.

Zado, E. S., M. Pammer, T. Parham, D. Lin, D. S. Frankel, S. Dixit, and F. E. Marchlinski. 2019. "'As Needed' Nonvitamin K Antagonist Oral Anticoagulants for Infrequent Atrial Fibrillation Episodes Following Atrial Fibrillation Ablation Guided by Diligent Pulse Monitoring: A Feasibility Study." *Journal of Cardiovascular Electrophysiology* 30 (5): 631–638.

Zhang, D., W. Wang, and F. Li. 2016. "Association Between Resting Heart Rate and Coronary Artery Disease, Stroke, Sudden Death and Noncardiovascular Diseases: A Meta-Analysis." *Canadian Medical Association Journal* 188 (15): E384–E392.

Zhu, T., M. A. F. Pimentel, G. D. Clifford, and D. A. Clifton. 2015. "Bayesian Fusion of Algorithms for the Robust Estimation of Respiratory Rate from the Photoplethysmogram." 2015 37th Annual International Conference of the IEEE Engineering in Medicine and Biology Society (EMBC) 2015, 6138–6141.

ACRONYMS

A/D	analog-to-digital
AF	atrial fibrillation
AI	artificial intelligence
BLE	Bluetooth Low Energy
CGM	continuous glucose monitoring
CNN	convolutional neural network
COPD	chronic obstructive pulmonary disease
DFT	discrete Fourier transform
DNN	deep neural network
ECG	electrocardiography
EDA	electrodermal activity
EDR	ECG-derived respiration
EEG	electroencephalography
EGG	electrogastrography
EMG	electromyography
EOG	electrooculography
FDA	Food and Drug Administration
FIR	finite impulse response
GDPR	General Data Protection Regulation
GPS	global positioning system
GSR	galvanic skin response
HR	heart rate
HRV	heart rate variability
IDDS	insertable drug delivery system
IIR	infinite impulse response
IMMU	inertial and magnetic measurement unit
IoT	Internet of Things
IPG	impedance plethysmography
LED	light-emitting diode
LPWAN	Low-Power Wide Area Network
LSTM	long short-term memory

MEMS	microelectromechanical systems
ML	machine learning
MLP	multilayer perceptron
NFC	Near Field Communication
OSA	obstructive sleep apnea
PCA	principal component analysis
PO_2	partial pressure of oxygen
PPG	photoplethysmography
PTT	pulse transit time
RIP	respiratory inductive plethysmography
SpO_2	oxyhemoglobin saturation
SVM	support vector machine
UV	ultraviolet
VOC	volatile organic compound
Wi-Fi	Wireless Fidelity

CHAPTER 3

Causal AI in Personalised Healthcare

Tobias Hatt

MOTIVATION

The goal of personalised healthcare is to tailor treatment decisions to each individual patient. This means considering how a treatment will affect a specific patient, rather than treating all patients the same. For instance, when deciding whether to prescribe a treatment to a patient, it is important to consider whether that specific patient will benefit from the treatment. It is known that different patients can have different responses to the same treatment, based on their characteristics and circumstances. Therefore, it is important for both patients and doctors to understand how a treatment will affect an individual patient. Personalised healthcare can improve health outcomes by focusing on treating only those patients who will benefit from a treatment (e.g., Tschernutter et al. 2022), taking into account factors such as the patient's medical history, lifestyle, and environment.

Personalisation in healthcare has gained significant attention in recent years. However, the concept of tailoring treatment decisions to the individual patient dates back centuries, with examples such as blood typing being used to guide transfusions as early as the 1900s (National Research Council et al. 2011; Collins and Varmus 2015). The renewed interest in personalisation is largely due to the desire for improved healthcare decision-making. It has been observed that a significant number of patients receive treatments that do not improve their health, and some treatments may even be harmful (Currie et al. 2006). In fact, the top ten

DOI: 10.1201/9781032699745-4

highest-grossing medical drugs in the United States only benefit between 4% and 25% of patients (Schork 2015). Personalised healthcare aims to address this issue by considering the unique characteristics of each individual patient, thereby optimising treatment decisions and reducing the risk of suboptimal or harmful prescriptions (Sanders et al. 2016; Neumann and Ollendorf 2021).

Recent technological advancements, such as the availability of large-scale biologic databases (e.g., the human genome sequence) and patient characterisation tools (e.g., electronic health records), have provided the necessary foundation for personalised healthcare. These advances, coupled with the use of AI, allow for the creation of a comprehensive view of each individual patient and the integration of this information into data-driven decision-making processes (Collins and Varmus 2015; Topol 2019).

The potential value of personalised healthcare, recent advancements in data collection, and analysis have contributed to the increased attention and investment in this field. This has resulted in an acceleration of research (Mullard 2015; Oezyurt et al. 2021), investment (Fleisch et al. 2021), and regulatory changes (FDA 2016; FDA 2017; FDA 2020) with the goal of advancing personalised healthcare.

CHALLENGES

Despite recent advancements in personalised healthcare, the full potential of this field has yet to be realised. There are numerous challenges that must be addressed in order to achieve personalised healthcare (e.g., Alyass et al. 2015; Schork 2015). One such challenge is the ability to estimate the effect of a treatment on an individual patient. In conventional medicine, clinical trials are used to assess the efficacy and safety of a treatment. However, these trials are not designed to provide individualised treatment effects, which are necessary for personalised healthcare. To understand the limitations of clinical trials in this regard, it is important to first understand how these trials are conducted.

Clinical trials are a widely accepted method for evaluating the effectiveness and safety of a treatment in patients (e.g., Schulz and Grimes 2018). The results of these trials are used to support marketing approval by regulatory bodies such as the U.S. Food and Drug Administration (FDA) and to inform healthcare decision-making by medical practitioners. Clinical trials can take various forms but typically consist of three phases, with a potential fourth phase called a post-approval trial, which is conducted after marketing approval and aims to further understand the long-term effects of the treatment.

One key feature of clinical trials is that they are conducted in a highly controlled setting, where the trial investigator can control which subjects receive the treatment and which do not. Subjects are often divided into two groups: a treatment group that receives the experimental treatment and a control group that receives a placebo (or "sham") treatment with no therapeutic effect. The difference in outcomes between the two groups is then measured.

To ensure that the difference in outcomes is solely due to the experimental treatment, the treatment and control groups must be identical except for the prescribed treatment. Randomisation is often used to achieve this, with subjects being randomly assigned to the treatment or control group (e.g., Barton 2000). These types of clinical trials, known as randomised controlled trials (RCTs), are considered the gold standard for assessing treatment safety and efficacy due to the controlled nature of the study and the use of randomisation to eliminate the effects of confounding variables.

While RCTs are an effective method for estimating treatment effects in a general population, they are not suitable for estimating individualised treatment effects, which is required for personalised healthcare. This is because RCTs are highly controlled studies and, therefore, very costly to conduct. As a direct result, the size of RCTs is usually small and, as such, RCTs may not capture all possible individual variations in patient outcomes. However, since the goal of personalised healthcare is to tailor the treatment decision to the individual patient, these individual variations are central to estimating the individual treatment effect.

To overcome this limitation, alternative study designs and methods are needed to estimate individualised treatment effects in personalised medicine. These methods may include using data from electronic health records or real-world observations to estimate treatment effects at the individual level, or using machine learning techniques to identify patient subgroups that are most likely to benefit from a particular treatment.

In summary, while RCTs are a well-established method for evaluating treatment effects in a general population, they are not suitable for estimating individualised treatment effects, which are required for personalised healthcare. Alternative study designs and methods, such as estimating treatment effects at the individual level or identifying patient subgroups likely to benefit from a treatment, must be employed to estimate individualised treatment effects in personalised healthcare.

THE POTENTIAL OF REAL-WORLD DATA

Real-world data (RWD), which are generated outside of traditional clinical trials and may come from sources such as electronic health records, insurance data, product and disease registries, and wearable devices, have the potential to facilitate the estimation of individualised treatment effects and address the limitations of traditional randomised controlled trials (RCTs) (Makady et al. 2017; Yang and Yu 2021, Frauen et al. 2022). RWD have traditionally been used by regulatory institutions to monitor the long-term safety and rare adverse effects of marketed drugs (Jernberg et al. 2015), but have more recently been embraced by healthcare decision-makers as a key source of evidence in the drug development process due to advances in digital technologies, new incentives for pharmaceutical companies to adopt RWD strategies, and the shift towards personalised healthcare (Szlezak et al. 2014; Corrigan et al. 2018).

RWD have the potential to create a holistic view of individual patients and facilitate personalised healthcare (Topol 2019). In particular, RWD is often available in large quantities due to advances in digital technologies and can be collected at a lower cost than RCT data. This large quantity of data, when analysed with advanced AI techniques, can reveal individual variations across a wide range of patients. Additionally, RWD represent patients in real-world settings, as they are collected outside of clinical settings, and may have greater external validity than RCTs.

To fully utilise the potential of real-world data (RWD) and effectively generate useful evidence from them, it is important to not only have high-quality RWD, but also the ability to analyse these data effectively. Since RWD is collected outside of controlled clinical trials, it is not guaranteed that the various health outcomes observed in patients are solely due to the prescribed treatment. As a result, standard statistical tools may not accurately estimate treatment effects when applied to RWD. This is because treatment effects are inherently causal effects, and it is necessary to use analytics tools that can distinguish causation from correlation when analysing RWD (e.g., Rosenbaum 2002; Rosenbaum 2010, Schulz and Grimes 2018). Developing valid advanced AI techniques that can accurately retrieve causal effects from RWD is therefore critical to fully leveraging the potential of this data.

A CAUSAL AI APPROACH

In this chapter, we aim to introduce novel methods from the field of causal AI that can leverage real-world data (RWD) to approach personalised healthcare. Causal AI is a branch of AI that focuses on estimating causal effects, rather than just correlations (e.g., Johansson et al. 2016; Chernozhukov et al. 2018; Peters et al. 2017; Shalit et al. 2017; Wager and Athey 2018, Hatt and Feuerriegel 2021). This is a relevant approach for personalised healthcare, as it allows for the estimation of treatment effects on an individual patient, rather than just estimating correlations. Estimating such treatment effects from RWD is a challenging task, as it requires the use of advanced methods that can distinguish causation from correlation. Therefore, our use of causal AI methods aims at accurately estimating treatment effects from RWD.

CAUSAL AI FOR REAL-WORLD DATA

In this section, we give a broad overview of common methods for causal inference from RWD. To do so, we follow the famous Neyman-Rubin framework (Rubin 2011). For this, we consider a binary treatment (i.e., taking the drug vs. not taking the drug), indicated by the variable T (T = 1 for taking the drug and T = 0 for not taking the drug). Each individual has two potential outcomes, one under each possible treatment scenario. We denote the pair of potential outcomes as Y(1) and Y(0), where 1 indicates taking the drug and 0 indicates not taking the drug. Then, we can define causal effects at different levels clearly. For instance:

- Average treatment effect (ATE): $E[Y(1) - Y(0)]$, for the entire population.
- Conditional average treatment effect (CATE): $E[Y(1) - Y(0)|X]$, for a specific individual defined by covariates X.

The ATE is the causal effect a treatment has on average in the population. The CATE is the causal effect of a treatment on a specific individual (specified by covariates X).

Unfortunately, the potential outcomes are not observed in reality (hence, the name 'potential'). In particular, we can only see one outcome as the subject receives the treatment or does not receive the treatment. Therefore, estimating causal effects requires more assumptions than what is usually required for estimating correlations in common statistical analysis. The most important assumption is the so-called '*strong ignorability assumption*', which assumes that whether or not a subject receives the treatment does not depend on the potential outcomes when all relevant covariates are controlled for. This assumption holds true in randomised experiments since the treatment assignment is randomised and, hence, does not depend on any covariates. However, in RWD, this assumption may break down, which makes controlling for confounding a challenging undertaking. It consists of two components: (i) control of observed (i.e., measured) confounding, as important observed covariates may be distributed differently between treatment and control group, and (ii) control of unobserved confounding (hidden bias), as not all relevant covariates are observed in RWD. For (i), controlling observed confounding, well-established statistical methods exist. However, for (ii), controlling for unobserved confounding, there are much fewer methods and they have been much less used since it remains difficult to control for unobserved confounding.

Controlling for Observed Confounding

In RWD subjects are not randomly assigned to treatment and control groups. In fact, the subject itself (or their medical doctor) makes the decision to take a treatment or not. Without a random assignment mechanism, some subjects are more likely than others to receive the treatment due to differences in individual characteristics (e.g., age, gender, genetics). Since the assignment mechanism is broken in RWD (due to the lack of randomisation), it is natural to develop tools to fix this. Therefore, careful statistical adjustments are needed to estimate the causal effect based on RWD.

Propensity Score Methods for Average Treatment Effects

The propensity score is a technical tool that addresses the treatment assignment issue. In particular, it can balance the observed covariate distributions between treatment and control groups and, as such, simulate a randomisation-like scenario in terms of treatment assignment. As a result, propensity score methods are used to reduce the bias in treatment effect estimation induced by observed confounding. Mathematically, for a binary treatment T and covariates X, the propensity score is defined by

$$e(X) = P(X)$$

In randomised experiments, the propensity score is usually known and, often, constant if the subjects are assigned randomly. When using RWD, the propensity score is usually not known and, hence, needs to be estimated via a logistic regression or a more advanced machine learning method. In the remainder of this section, we provide more details about several popular methods for estimating the ATE using the propensity score.

Inverse Propensity Score Weighting

Inverse Propensity score weighting (IPSW) is a popular method for estimating the ATE. The idea is to create a pseudo-population in which all covariates are balanced at the population level. Due to this, subjects in the treatment group are weighted by the inverse of the propensity score. Subjects in the control group are weighted with the inverse of 'one minus the propensity score'.

Mathematically, the ATE can be written as

$$ATE = E\left[Y(1) - Y(0)\right] = E\left[\frac{T}{e(X)}Y - \frac{1 - T}{1 - e(X)}Y\right]$$

where Y is the outcome that was observed. Hence, in order to estimate the ATE using the inverse propensity score weighting method, we first estimate the propensity score from the RWD, which yields $\hat{e}(X)$. Then, we plug it into the above equation, which yields the following estimator for the ATE:

$$\widehat{ATE} = \frac{1}{n}\sum_{i=1}^{n}\left(\frac{T_i}{\hat{e}(X_i)}Y_i - \frac{1 - T_i}{1 - \hat{e}(X_i)}Y_i\right)$$

While the IPSW method yields unbiased estimates for the ATE, it may lead to high variance. Moreover, since we need to estimate the propensity score, there is always a chance that the propensity score is not estimated correctly. Both shortcomings can be addressed by the augmented inverse propensity score weighting (AIPSW) method. This method reduces the variance and is 'doubly robust' since it combines the propensity score and a regression model to improve performance (Bang and Robins 2005).

Propensity Score Matching

Propensity score matching is an alternative popular method for estimation of the ATE. The idea is to match two subjects with the same covariates X, one of which is from the treatment group and the other one is from the control group. Ideally, we want to match exactly on every covariate to remove the observed confounding. However, matching on many covariates can be computationally infeasible. As a remedy, it was found that it is sufficient to match subjects with the same propensity score. This creates a study sample with balanced covariate distributions in the treatment and control groups. The simplest way to match subjects based on their propensity score is via a nearest-neighbour algorithm. Once we matched the subjects, we needed to check the covariate balance. From a practical perspective, this can be done by checking the covariate mean differences (via standardised differences) and the variance difference (via logarithm of standard deviation ratio) for each covariate, before and after matching. If the balance is sufficient, we can proceed to estimate the ATE by taking the difference between the average outcome in the treatment group and the average outcome in the control group.

Propensity Score Stratification

Another well-known method for estimating the ATE is Propensity score stratification. The idea behind this method is similar to propensity score matching. We create mutually exclusive strata and assign each subject to a stratum based on its (estimated) propensity score. Then, in each stratum, we take the difference of average outcomes. A weighted average across all strata yields the final estimate of the ATE. Propensity score stratification is easy to implement and use. However, there may be some residual confounding left in each stratum, which can lead to biased estimates. To circumvent this, further propensity score adjustment can be used in each stratum. In practice, 5–10 strata often remove most (~90%) of the bias due to observed confounding.

The above methods were all developed for estimating the average treatment effect and, hence, do not give insights into how different individuals respond to a treatment. In the next section, we discuss methods from the causal AI literature that address this gap.

Causal AI Methods Conditional Average Treatment Effect

The goal of personalised healthcare is to prescribe patients a treatment if the patient responds positively to the treatment. For this, we need to know the causal effect of a treatment on a specific individual (as opposed to the average effect). This requires estimating the conditional average treatment effect (CATE). As a reminder, the CATE is defined as follows:

$$E[Y(1) - Y(0)|X]$$

Which describes the effect of a treatment on an individual specified by covariates X. Estimating the CATE requires a different set of methods. In the following, we introduce two popular methods from the causal AI literature; one method based on trees and one method based on deep learning.

CAUSAL FOREST

Causal forests were introduced by Wager and Athey 2018 and, as the name suggests, extend random forests to the causal inference setting. In random forests, the data is repeatedly split in order to minimise the prediction error of an outcome variable. Causal forests are built similarly, although with one difference: at every split, we consider the reduction in treatment effect error, not the prediction error of an outcome variable. For this, we build on the intuitive idea that similar subjects have similar treatment effects and, hence, in a small enough subset of subjects the treatment effect is approximately constant. Then, for a new potential split, we can estimate the (constant) treatment effect in each leaf using residual-residual regression (Robinson 1988) and, from there, proceed as in random forests. Causal forests have shown great potential for estimating conditional average treatment effect and are, therefore, often used in practice.

COUNTERFACTUAL REGRESSION

Another popular method is the counterfactual regression, which was developed by Shalit et al. 2017. They incorporate two ideas about CATE estimation into their algorithm. First, although the treated outcome, Y(1), and the untreated outcome, Y(0), are different, it is reasonable to assume that they are related. As such, in order to learn both outcomes, they use a deep learning architecture inspired by multi-task learning. Their architecture learns both outcomes in an end-to-end procedure by allowing some layers to be shared among the two outcomes (which learn the similarities) and some layers to be separate (which learn the differences). This type of deep learning architecture is called the Treatment-Agnostic Representation Network (TARNet). Second, their algorithm accounts for the covariate imbalance between the treatment and control groups. For this, in every learning step, the imbalance between the treatment and control group in one of the shared layers is computed (via some probabilistic metric, e.g., maximum mean discrepancy). Then, the loss function is penalised with this imbalance. This forces the algorithm to learn a deep learning model that accounts for the covariate imbalance while still being predictive of the outcomes. Counterfactual regression is one of the main deep-learning methods for estimating the CATE. It is one of the building blocks of causal AI research and motivated many further methods (e.g., Berrevoets 2020; Curth and van der Schaar 2021; Kuzmanovic et al. 2021; Hatt et al. 2022).

Controlling for Unobserved Confounding

Controlling for unobserved confounding is much more difficult than controlling for observed confounding. The reason for this is that when confounding variables are not observed it is difficult to control for them (as opposed to the observed confounders, where propensity score methods can be used). As such, there exist fewer methods that can control for unobserved confounding. In this section, we introduce two common methods that can account for unobserved confounding. Finally, we point out some novel ideas that are ongoing research, but which are promising and should be considered when controlling for unobserved confounding.

SENSITIVITY ANALYSIS

Sensitivity analysis, as the name suggests, analyses how sensitive our conclusion about the treatment effect is to unobserved confounding. In particular, we assume a model for the influence of a potentially unobserved confounder and, then, investigate how strong this influence would need to be to alter our conclusion about the treatment effect (i.e., flipping a positive treatment effect to a negative one and vice-versa). Formally, we introduce a binary variable U as a proxy for the unmeasured confounder. With U, we restore the strong ignorability assumption. That is, the treatment assignment is independent of the potential outcomes given the observed covariates X and the binary indicator U. In order to analyse the impact of U on the treatment assignment, we pose the following logistic regression model:

$$logit\,(P\,(T = 1|X,\,U)) = \kappa\,(X) + \gamma U$$

$\kappa(X)$ is a nuisance part and represents the impact of observed covariates. This part could be balanced, for instance by propensity score matching. The parameter γ is the sensitivity parameter and describes the influence of the unobserved confounder (here, it is assumed to be linear). With this model, we can investigate how much the propensity score changes given a value for the sensitivity parameter γ. As we have seen in the previous section, changes in the propensity score directly translate into changes in the treatment effect estimate. For instance,

when $\gamma = 0$, this is the conventional propensity score model and there is no unobserved confounding. When $\gamma > 0$, there is unobserved confounding. Technically, γ captures the association between treatment assignment and U in the odds ratio scale. For instance, if $e^{\gamma} = 2$, two units in the matched pair that appear similar with regards to the observed covariates, X, could differ in their odds of receiving the treatment by as much as a factor of 2. Then, one of them might be twice (on the odds ratio scale) as likely as the other to receive the treatment, due to the unobserved confounder. If this factor is also related to the outcome via, for instance, propensity score weighting, the estimated treatment effect with adjustment only for observed covariates might be mitigated if U is accounted for. A study is highly sensitive to unobserved confounding if the conclusion changes for e^{γ} just barely greater than 1, and it is robust or insensitive if the conclusion changes only for quite large values of e^{γ}.

INSTRUMENTAL VARIABLE ANALYSIS

Another popular method for estimating treatment effects in the presence of unobserved confounding is instrumental variable analysis (Imbens and Angrist 1994). In this case, we can estimate the treatment effect if we can find a so-called instrumental variable. An instrumental variable is a variable that affects the treatment assignment but is independent of the unobserved confounders. Moreover, the instrumental variable only influences the outcome indirectly via the treatment assignment. In this case, we can disentangle the effect of the treatment from the effect of the unobserved confounder. This works since we can decompose the effect from the instrument on the outcome into the effect from the treatment on the outcome and from the instrument on the treatment. We can then estimate the effect from the instrument on the outcome and the effect from the instrument on the treatment from the RWD. The remainder, the effect from the treatment on the outcome, can then be implied directly from those two quantities. Instrumental variable analysis is a highly effective and well-established method. However, we need to find an instrumental variable and, then, justify why this variable is independent from the unobserved confounder and only affects the outcome indirectly via the treatment.

ON-GOING RESEARCH

The field of causal AI has grown tremendously over the past few years. As such, more methods were developed that, among others, address the issue of observed and unobserved confounding. While the majority of research focuses on the less challenging problem of observed confounding, there is a growing literature that accounts for unobserved confounding. Broadly speaking, there are three promising approaches for accounting for unobserved confounding. First, latent variable approaches try to use the observed data to recover latent variables that can be used as unobserved confounders. They either consider the observed covariates to be noise measurements of the unobserved confounders and, then, use those to recover a latent variable (e.g., Louizos et al. 2018; Kallus et al. 2018; Kuzmanovic et al. 2021). Or they use the treatment assignment to recover latent variables that can be used as substitutes for the unobserved confounders (e.g., Wang and Blei 2018; Bica et al. 2020; Hatt and Feuerriegel 2021). The latent variable approach shows promising results and can sometimes provably recover valid substitutes for the unobserved confounders. However, these approaches may not be robust to violations of the underlying assumptions. Second, inspired by sensitivity analysis of treatment effects, another approach to accounting for unobserved confounding is to derive bounds for the estimated treatment effect (e.g., Kallus et al. 2019; Hatt et al. 2022). That is, we can derive bounds for the ATE and CATE, which allows considering the impact of unobserved confounding. This can be used in the final decision-making as a measure of uncertainty and to study whether potential unobserved confounding could alter the conclusion. Third, most relevant for the medical domain, is the combination of experimental data and RWD (e.g., Kallus et al. 2018; Hatt et al. 2022). While there is no unobserved confounding in experimental data, this type of data is usually of small size. Hence, it is difficult to use for estimating complex models such as deep learning approaches. RWD is usually of large size, but there may be unobserved confounding. Hence, a recent approach develops an algorithm that can learn from both types of data.

As such, using small amounts of experimental data can account for the unobserved confounding in RWD. This approach yields very good results but requires experimental data, which may not be feasible to collect in some domains. While these approaches seem to be promising, further research has to be conducted to make them applicable to practice.

CONCLUSION

In this chapter, we have seen how causal AI can help on the journey to personalised healthcare. In particular, we discussed that in order to make personalised healthcare happen, we must move away from estimating average treatment effects, which only give insights about the average patient to estimating individualised treatment effects, which give insights about how a specific patient may respond to a treatment. To do so, we must leverage new sources of data in the form of RWD, which are available in large quantities and allow us to capture great variations in patients. Since RWD is not collected in a controlled clinical environment, estimating treatment effects from RWD is challenging and requires more advanced AI techniques. Since treatment effects are inherently causal effects, these AI techniques originate from the field of causal AI. Causal AI is the intersection of causality and AI and aims at estimating causal effects rather than correlations. We introduced several popular methods for estimating the average treatment effect (ATE) and the conditional average treatment effect (CATE), where the latter describes the effect of a treatment on the individual. Among others, these methods account for observed or unobserved confounding. While there exist several well-established methods that account for observed confounding, there are not many methods that can account for unobserved confounding. For this, there are several promising methods currently studied in the causal AI community that can potentially push towards more robustness with respect to unobserved confounding.

REFERENCES

Alyass A., Turcotte M., Meyre D. 2015. From big data analysis to personalized medicine for all: challenges and opportunities. *BMC medical genomics*, 8(1):1–12

Barton S. 2000. Which clinical studies provide the best evidence?: The best RCT still trumps the best observational study. *Bmj*, 321(7256):255–256

Bang H., Robins J. M. 2005. Doubly robust estimation in missing data and causal inference models. *Biometrics*

Berrevoets J., Jordon J., Bica I., Gimson A., van der Schaar M. 2020. OrganITE: Optimal transplant donor organ offering using an individual treatment effect, *Neural Information Processing System*

Bica I., Alaa A. M., van der Schaar M. 2020. Time series deconfounder: Estimating treatment effects over time in the presence of hidden confounders. International Conference on Machine Learning

Chernozhukov V., Chetverikov D., Demirer M., Duflo E., Hansen C., Newey W., Robins J. 2018. Double/debiased machine learning for treatment and structural parameters. *The Econometrics Journal*, 21(1):C1–C68

Collins F. S., Varmus H. 2015. A new initiative on precision medicine. *New England Journal of Medicine*, 372(9):793–795

Corrigan-Curay J., Sacks L., Woodcock J. 2018. Real-world evidence and real-world data for evaluating drug safety and effectiveness. *JAMA*, 320 (9):867–868

Currie G. P., Lee D. K. C., Lipworth B. J. 2006. Long-acting β2-agonists in asthma. *Drug Safety*, 29(8):647–656

Curth A., van der Schaar M. 2021. On inductive biases for heterogeneous treatment effect estimation. Conference on Neural Information Processing Systems

FDA. 2016. 21st century cures act. Retrieved from https://www.fda.gov/regulatory-information/selected-amendments-fdc-act/21st-century-cures-act

FDA. 2017. Use of real-world evidence to support regulatory decision-making for medical devices. Retrieved from https://www.fda.gov/regulatory-information/search-fda-guidance-documents/use-real-world-evidence-support-regulatory-decision-making-medical-devices

FDA. 2020. Submitting documents using real-world data and real-world evidence to FDA for drugs and biologics guidance for industry. Retrieved from https://www.fda.gov/media/124795/download

Fleisch E., Franz C., Herrmann A. 2021. *The digital Pill: what everyone should know about the future of our healthcare system*. Emerald Group Publishing

Frauen D., Hatt T., Melnychuk V., Feuerriegel S. 2022. Estimating average causal effects from patient trajectories. AAAI Conference on Artificial Intelligence

Hatt T., Feuerriegel S. 2021. Estimating average treatment effects via orthogonal regularization. International Conference on Information and Knowledge Management

Hatt T., Tschernutter D., Feuerriegel S. 2022. Generalizing off-policy learning under sample selection bias. Conference on Uncertainty in Artificial Intelligence

Imbens G., Angrist J. 1994. Identification and estimation of local average treatment effects. *Econometrica: Journal of the Econometric Society*

Jernberg T., Hasvold P., Henriksson M., Hjelm H., Thuresson M., Janzon M. 2015. Cardiovascular risk in post-myocardial infarction patients: nationwide real-world data demonstrate the importance of a long-term perspective. *European Heart Journal*, 36(19):1163–1170

Johansson F. D., Shalit U., Sontag D. 2016. Learning representations for counterfactual inference. International Conference on Machine Learning

Kallus N., Puli A. M., Shalit U. 2018. Removing hidden confounding by experimental grounding. *Advances in Neural Information Processing Systems*

Kallus N., Mao X., Zhou A. 2019. Interval estimation of individual-level causal effects under unobserved confounding. International Conference on Artificial Intelligence and Statistics

Kuzmanovic M., Hatt T., Feuerriegel S. 2021. Deconfounding temporal autoencoder: estimating treatment effects over time using noisy proxies. *Machine Learning for Health*

Louizos C., Shalit U., Mooij J. M., Sontag D., Zemel R., Welling M. 2018. Causal effect inference with deep latent-variable models. *Advances in Neural Information Processing Systems*

Makady A., de Boer A., Hillege H., Klungel O., Goettsch W., et al. 2017. What is real-world data? a review of definitions based on literature and stakeholder interviews. *Value in Health*, 20(7):858–865

Mullard A. 2015. $215 million precision-medicine initiative takes shape. *Nature Reviews Drug Discovery*, 14(3):155–156

National Research Council et al. 2011. *Toward precision medicine: building a knowledge network for biomedical research and a new taxonomy of disease.* National Academies Press

Neumann P. J., Cohen J. T., Ollendorf D. A. 2021. *The right price: a value-based prescription for drug costs.* Oxford University Press

Oezyurt Y., Kraus M., Hatt T., Feuerriegel S. 2021. AttDMM: An attentive deep Markov Model for risk scoring in intensive care units. International Conference on Knowledge Discovery and Data Mining

Peters J., Janzing D., Schölkopf B. 2017. *Elements of causal inference: foundations and learning algorithms.* The MIT Press

Rosenbaum P. R. 2002. Overt bias in observational studies. *In Observational Studies.* Springer

Rosenbaum P. R. et al. 2010. *Design of observational studies*, volume 10. Springer

Rubin D. 2011. Causal inference using potential outcomes. *Journal of the American Statistical Association*

Robinson P. 1988. Root-N-consistent semiparametric regression. *Econometrica: Journal of the Econometric Society*

Sanders G. D., Neumann P. J., Basu A., Brock D. W., Feeny D., Krahn M., Kuntz K. M., Meltzer D. O., Owens D. K., Prosser L. A., et al. 2016. Recommendations for conduct, methodological practices, and reporting of cost-effectiveness analyses: second panel on cost-effectiveness in health and medicine. *JAMA*, 316(10):1093–1103

Schork N. J. 2015. Personalized medicine: time for one-person trials. *Nature*, 520(7549):609–611

Schulz K., Grimes D. A. 2018. Essential concepts in clinical research: randomised controlled trials and observational epidemiology. *Elsevier Health Sciences*

Shalit U., Johansson F. D., Sontag D. 2017. Estimating individual treatment effect: Generalization bounds and algorithms. In International Conference on Machine Learning

Szlezak N., Evers M., Wang J., Pérez L. 2014. The role of big data and advanced analytics in drug discovery, development, and commercialization. *Clinical Pharmacology & Therapeutics*, 95(5):492–495

Topol E. J. 2019. High-performance medicine: the convergence of human and artificial intelligence. *Nature Medicine*, 25(1):44–56

Tschernutter D., Hatt T., Feuerriegel S. 2022. Interpretable off-policy learning via hyperbox search. International Conference on Machine Learning

Wang Y., Blei D. M. 2018. The blessings of multiple causes. *Journal of the American Statistical Association*

Wager S., Athey S. 2018. Estimation and inference of heterogeneous treatment effects using random forests. *Journal of the American Statistical Association*, 113(523):1228–1242

Yang H., Yu B. 2021. *Real-world evidence in drug development and evaluation*. CRC Press

CHAPTER 4

Interpretable AI in Healthcare

Kevin Kohler and Mathias Kraus

INTRODUCTION

Healthcare is a high-stakes domain where poor assessment of patient conditions can entail catastrophic consequences. However, the majority of decision-making processes performed by caregivers are still based on standard procedures or practical experience. Systematic consideration of a patient's medical specifics could prove beneficial, with potential use cases such as accurate diagnosis classification, mortality likelihood assessment, or length of stay prediction.

This chapter provides a review of fundamental concepts for interpretable AI in healthcare, highlighting the currently relevant literature on healthcare analytics, intelligible models, the interpretability-accuracy trade-off, and hybrid approaches, such as explainable or interpretable machine learning models.

The core concept of healthcare analytics is presented first, by illustrating the efficiency challenge in the health domain, a potential solution in the form of analytics methods performed on extensive medical data as well as the recent emergence of machine learning in the field. Second, it is attempted to define and quantify the still vague concept of model interpretability, before its necessity is evaluated from both a legislative and a practical viewpoint. The third subsection briefly recaps the interpretability-accuracy trade-off and categorises machine learning algorithms based on the transparency of their inner mechanics: presented are non-linear black-box models, simpler interpretable models, as well as

DOI: 10.1201/9781032699745-5

hybrid model approaches, which in turn consist of the subtypes; explainable and additive hybrid models.

Machine Learning in the Healthcare Realm

Healthcare analytics systems are increasingly utilised for various applications across the medical sector. Taking into account the individual features of a patient (such as blood markers indicating disease progression over time) and comparing them to statistically evaluated patterns, such systems aim to provide caregivers with well-founded information for better decision-making. Once started as simple rule-based expert systems like MYCIN in 1972 (Shortliffe & Buchanan, 1975), medical decision support systems have since then evolved to apply techniques from the machine learning realm to healthcare tasks. For example, neural networks can be used to recognise malign tissue from X-ray scans or assess risk factor significance in cardiovascular diseases (Al-antari et al., 2018; Hsu, 2018).

The recent adoption of machine learning methods like neural networks within healthcare boasts a number of advantages, one of the most significant is that machines perform better than humans in various cases of clinical decision support (Ozaydin et al., 2021). This is because human judgement is impaired by perceptual biases and limited cognitive capacity - humans cannot process data fast enough or rapidly enough to compete with machines, and present-day algorithmic architectures can already surpass doctors in terms of predictive accuracy (Richens et al., 2020; Rudin, 2019).

Non-Intelligible Models in High-Stakes Domains

Advanced machine learning models like neural networks have a central shortcoming that hinders their widespread use in the medical sector so far: these models are non-intelligible, which means that the internal calculus processes from which they draw their conclusions are not understandable at an ordinary human level. This can be attributed to large numbers and complex combinations of parameters (Babic et al., 2021).

In a mission-critical environment such as healthcare, this is particularly obstructive, given that medical professionals are expected to build trust in a black-box system whose assessments they cannot critically evaluate. Moreover, it is likely that public authorities regulating healthcare might hesitate to accept this kind of decision-support system, showing reluctance to any diagnostic approach lacking a clinical link (Kundu, 2021). For example, the European Union's General Data

Protection Regulation obliges organisations using patient data for predictions to provide on-demand explanations, a request that can entail penalties but is often unfulfillable for said organisations (Ahmad et al., 2018; Buiten, 2019). As a result, the question of whether predictive models in the healthcare domain must be interpretable or not is met with increasing scientific attention.

Discussions on Interpretability versus Accuracy

Despite the fact that this subject is still disputed among researchers, two different viewpoints have emerged. The first one suggests that interpretability is fundamental to ensure trust towards results, transparent approaches, confidence in deploying results, and maintenance qualities of solutions, where needed (Kolyshkina & Simoff, 2021). They propose solutions sometimes referred to as interpretable artificial intelligence, where the connection between input and output variables of the predictive algorithm can be fully or at least partially comprehended. Interpretability is considered significant particularly for users to improve their faith in the system (Agarwal & Das, 2020).

Going even further, some researchers demand the discard of non-intelligible machine learning approaches under most conditions, at least in critical areas like medical analytics. They argue that models must be inherently interpretable and postulate that a black-box model should not be deployed if an interpretable model with the same level of performance exists (Rudin, 2019).

The opposite view disregards the importance of interpretability in at least some fields where machine learning is applied. It is argued that especially in time-critical use cases such as the prediction of cardiac arrhythmia, model understanding is secondary when a black box achieves higher accuracy than a white box model. Instead, healthcare professionals should strive for a deeper understanding of machine learning systems in general and educate themselves further on the topic (Babic et al., 2021). Moreover, some authors are sceptical of the concept of interpretability itself. They criticise both a current lack of definitional agreement among researchers and the absence of a technical operationalisation of the term (Krishnan, 2020; Lipton, 2018).

Approaches towards Interpretable and Accurate Models

Aiming to alleviate the trade-off between accuracy and interpretability, there are also hybrid approaches placed between aforesaid viewpoints.

These are designed to combine the predictive performance of non-linear, highly recursive models like neural networks with the interpretability of simpler approaches, for example, first-order logic rules (Hu et al., 2016).

The underlying mechanics of such hybrid architectures can be designed in various ways, but one central approach emerging is to let as much of the prediction as possible be performed by interpretable models. Black-box algorithms such as deep learning are only then applied when no sufficiently accurate prediction could be achieved by exclusive use of the simpler model (T. Wang & Lin, 2021). Yet most of the existing hybrid solutions have drawbacks as well: either only a subset of the feature space can be used for prediction or the simpler model's results are not utilised for further improvement, instead merely approximating the black-box function.

HEALTHCARE ANALYTICS: FUNDAMENTALS AND CURRENT DEVELOPMENTS

The Healthcare Efficiency Challenge

According to the World Health Organization, health systems can be defined as the entirety of all organisations, people, and actions whose primary intent is to promote, restore, or maintain health (Organization, 2007; Senn et al., 2021). Operating in a high-stakes environment, these systems face a variety of challenges affecting all aspects of healthcare provision: inconsistent quality and timeliness of medical care provision, a demographic shift demanding more resources per patient as well as administrative topics, ranging from staff insufficiency over rising treatment costs to medical infrastructure shortages. The former is among the most prominent healthcare issues which appear to occur simultaneously, thereby receiving considerable attention in research (Roncarolo et al., 2017).

What becomes evident is that a comprehensive improvement of all these issues is limited since their required solution approaches are partially contradictory: for example, swift access to medical services requires sufficient staffing, which in turn increases costs. Therefore, there is a necessity to balance access, cost and quality within the health system, referred to as the "iron triangle" by Khamis (Khamis, 2019).

Analytics as a Potential Remedy

One of the most promising approaches to alleviate the aforementioned trade-off and balance the iron triangle is the utilisation of data analytics in healthcare. Defined as the systematic use of data combined with quantitative as well as qualitative analysis to develop insights and make decisions (Islam et al., 2018; Simpao et al., 2014), data analytics have found their way into the medical realm as well: for instance, analytical approaches such as machine learning are utilised for imaging-based disease diagnostics or length of stay prediction at hospitals, in many cases obtaining performances on a par with certified professionals (Miotto et al., 2017). As a result, they enable caregivers to provide both patient-centred and resource-efficient treatment alike - doctors can identify those patients most likely in need of monitoring or surgery, avoid dangerous, expensive malpractice of healthy patients and estimate staff requirements based on expected occupancy of intensive care units (Falavigna, 2020).

The Increasing Availability of Medical Data

A vital precondition for these procedures to perform successfully is the utilisation of extensive volumes of biomedical and related data (Pramanik et al., 2020). The broad adoption of electronic health record systems (Choi et al., 2016; Gotz & Borland, 2016) within various healthcare domains makes an abundant source of (semi-)structured data available: initially, intensive care collects patients' biomarkers (such as blood pressure, glucose levels or heart rate) and monitors them over time, while logistics- and finance-related data ranging from length of stay to treatment costs are also recorded (Ghabra et al., 2019; Tomar, 10 2013). The aforementioned various types of medical-related data are increasingly bundled and stored in the form of electronic medical records, a storage format beneficial for data analytics approaches thanks to its emphasis on standardisation and accessibility (Kwon et al., 2019). Based on these aggregated training data covering thousands of patients' diagnoses, medications and procedures, algorithms learn to generalise from the information contained and make predictions or classifications, amongst others (Choi et al., 2016; Shah et al., 2019).

Machine Learning Developments in Healthcare

Applying statistics-based techniques like machine learning to extensive medical data is the foundation of healthcare analytics. In this field, one of the most significant developments that have emerged over the last years is the advent of neural networks, especially deep learning - a technique allowing us to find correlations too complex to render using previous machine learning algorithms (Bohr & Memarzadeh, 2020). Despite having been applied to medical problems for at least 20 years, neural networks have only recently experienced a surge in popularity thanks to advancements in computational capabilities and improvements in methodology (Choi et al., 2016; Miotto et al., 2017). A special case within neural networks, deep learning is able to optimise predictive loss functions exceptionally well due to a high number of hidden layers and can thus further enhance the prediction accuracy of traditional, less complex algorithms (Shamshirband et al., 2021).

Despite the predictive proficiency these algorithms demonstrate, as well as their versatility towards various medical prediction tasks, they are still only hesitantly adopted in high-stakes environments like practical healthcare. This is because neural networks, and particularly deep learning algorithms, have the pivotal impediment of pursuing a "black-box" approach (Ahmad et al., 2018). This refers to a lack of interpretability, implying missing transparency behind an algorithm's behaviour which leaves users with little to no understanding of how particular decisions are made by a model (Du et al., 2019). The absence of interpretability causes scepticism among legal authorities and practitioners alike (Agarwal & Das, 2020), posing a core obstacle to the adoption of various advanced machine learning techniques. The concept of interpretability will be explained in detail in the following subsection.

MODEL INTERPRETABILITY: DEFINITIONAL, LEGAL AND PRACTICAL VIEWPOINTS

Defining Model Interpretability

When it comes to defining model interpretability, it must be stated that there is no universally accepted definition or quantification available - interpretability is often used as an umbrella term enclosing a broad, rather poorly defined concept (Murdoch et al., 2019). This might be explainable by the fact that only in the last half-decade has interpretability started gaining some traction as a research field (Carvalho et al., 2019). As a result of this lack of common understanding (for instance in the form of an ontology), interpretability is often defined only model-specifically by researchers, without a claim for universal applicability in the first place (T. Wang & Lin, 2021).

However, one popular definition approach provided by Rudin et al. should be mentioned, which is due to its frequent adoption in citations and close alignment with multiple other authors' stances on the topic of interpretability: This definition refers to "interpretable predictive models, which are constrained so that their reasoning processes are more understandable to humans, are much easier to troubleshoot and to use in practice" (Rudin et al., 2022). Such constraints can, for example, take the form of "pruning" techniques where less important nodes or weights are removed from an initial, oversized tree-like decision model. In doing so, the creation of a more easily comprehensible model which is less prone to overfitting can be achieved, thereby improving its predictive accuracy (J. Wang et al., 2018).

In contrast, non-interpretable or so-called black-box models lack transparency and accountability according to Rudin, a shortcoming that can entail severe consequences especially in critical environments like healthcare (Rudin, 2019) - this is, for example, if algorithms are subject to undetected fallacies and misclassify endangered patients as healthy.

Quantifying Model Interpretability

Besides agreeing upon a widely accepted definition of interpretability such as Rudin's, quantifying the term is also still a research gap. This poses a challenge, since mathematical operationalisation could be necessary to compare the degree of interpretability between different model architectures, instead of merely classifying them as "interpretable" or "black-box". Some authors address the lack of standardised interpretability metrics by creating their own indicators, for example using the inverse of the sum of all utilised model parameters as a degree of complexity (Gosiewska et al., 2021). Others resort to less concrete measures, instead, they put a heavier emphasis on providing quantifiable subsets of conditions necessary for interpretability: these include sparsity of features, linearity, monotonicity or ability to explain feature interactions (ElShawi et al., 2020; Jovanovic et al., 2016; Ramchandani et al., 2020). Both the aforesaid and numerous other approaches to quantify interpretability have their justification, and more universal frameworks to address this question can be expected in the near future. Despite the still persisting shortcomings in defining and quantifying model interpretability, the concept has already found entrance in both legislation as well as practical application.

Interpretability as a Legal Requirement

When it comes to legal regulation of algorithmic interpretability, public authorities have mainly resorted to guidelines as well as initial regulatory frameworks in recent years (Carrillo, 2020; Fournier-Tombs, 2021). Although there is a necessity to regulate issues in machine learning interpretability, legally binding regulation is still in its infancy - and most statements issued by public authorities are mere recommendations or directives, which is not surprising given the complexity and novelty of the matter (Goodman & Flaxman, 2017): for example, public agencies like the White House Office of Science and Technology Policy as well as the French government have both issued guidelines in this regard, outlining the demand for artificial intelligence to be transparent and understandable by users (Carvalho et al., 2019; Chen et al., 2020). When it comes to official legislation though, it is mainly the European Union which has made an early attempt to enforce a "right to explanation" in the wake of the General Data Protection Regulation from 2018 onwards (Kolyshkina & Simoff, 2021). In addition to those measures issued, it will be necessary to both adjust existing and enact new legislation, in order to properly and timely regulate an evolving, high-stakes discipline like healthcare analytics (Pesapane et al., 2018).

Interpretability as a Practical Necessity

Aside from legislative topics, the requirement of model interpretability for practical application must also be taken into account. Lack of interpretability is a key factor that limits the wider adoption of machine learning in healthcare: this is mainly because practitioners find it challenging to trust complex models, as the former (often only designed and tested on certain diseases in limited environments) require additional knowledge in statistics and machine learning (Stiglic et al., 2020). Despite the recent advancements in medical artificial intelligence, caregivers will most probably still have the last say if treatment is performed or not, especially in a field as critical as healthcare. In this regard, interpretable machine learning systems can give users reasons to accept or reject predictions and recommendations by explaining their reasoning (Ahmad et al., 2018). Concluding, machine learning methodologies should be designed to seamlessly integrate with a user's abilities and knowledge in a certain domain, which entails the demand for interpretable solutions in order to reduce risks and make sound decisions (Coussement & Benoit, 2021).

Closely related to winning caregivers' acceptance of machine learning models is not only the necessity to make inner mechanics transparent, but also enabling users to detect potential fallacies they can critically evaluate before application. An example showcasing the importance of the former requirement is provided in a study that applies machine learning models to pneumonia datasets, aiming to predict pneumonia mortality risks (Cooper et al., 2005): using an interpretable rule-based learning system amongst others, it could be detected that a relationship was identified by the model between the presence of asthma and a lower risk of dying from pneumonia. Although the learning system identified causality prevalent in the data, the rule found is counterintuitive and even dangerous as the saying "correlation does not imply causation" applies: it was simply that those patients suffering from asthma received stricter care than others when admitted to the hospital, resulting in a lower mortality risk (Caruana et al., 2015; Cooper et al., 2005). Without the perks of an interpretable model (such as sparsity of features and low dimensionality), it cannot be expected from practitioners to detect such fallacies on time, before making potentially critical patient treatment decisions.

In conclusion, it can be stated that model interpretability is required for practical application in high-stakes domains like healthcare, entrusting caregivers and giving them the opportunity to cross-check predictions made by the model.

DESIGN APPROACHES FOR INTERPRETABLE AND ACCURATE MODELS

Unconstrained Black-Box Approaches

As previously stated, the relationship between model interpretability and predictive performance is often considered a trade-off in applied artificial intelligence (Du et al., 2019): in most use cases, non-interpretable models such as neural networks or ensemble methods outperform interpretable approaches like decision trees and logistic regression in terms of predictive accuracy (Linardatos et al., 2020; Stiglic et al., 2020). The reason for non-interpretable approaches like said deep learning to provide better predictive results is that they iteratively undergo several layers of non-linear transformations, thereby being able to capture actual data patterns beyond simpler or even linear structures (Chakraborty et al., 2021).

With a number of connected neurons jointly implementing this complex nonlinear mapping from input to output, such black-box models learn through thousandfold adaption of each neuron's weight via error propagation and related mechanisms (Montavon et al., 2018; Rumelhart et al., 1986). As these models are flexible enough to capture any form of functions (like arbitrary curves) upon proper network configuration, they can closely approximate underlying, often non-linear patterns present in data which eventually leads to superior predictive performance (Yang et al., 2021).

Worth mentioning is that non-linearity does not per se make a model opaque, but a series of non-linear operations often prevent users from understanding a model's inner workings. Furthermore, as these models are usually unaffected by explicit regularisation measures aimed at preventing overparameterisation, architectures like neural networks are largely unconstrained in complexity and their internal structure is not inherently decomposable. Hence, their internal reasoning (mainly the contribution of an input feature value to a specific outcome) is largely intransparent to humans and cannot be easily cross-checked by users (Caruana et al., 2015; Rudin et al., 2022). This limits the application range of non-interpretable models in critical environments such as healthcare (Kolyshkina & Simoff, 2021; Stiglic et al., 2020).

Linear Interpretable Approaches

In stark contrast, interpretable models such as linear regression provide users with a much simpler approximation of underlying data patterns, purposefully limited by constraints such as feature sparsity or monotonicity (Du et al., 2019; Stiglic et al., 2020). Due to their less complex architecture, as opposed to models like deep learning, many interpretable models can even be considered "frugal" (Linardatos et al., 2020). For instance, models like linear regression can be interpreted by using the covariate weights to evaluate the relative importance of the features on model predictions (Chakraborty et al., 2021). This procedure is highly transparent as the algorithm attempts to model a relationship between variables by fitting a simple linear equation, whose parameters could be described as representing the strength of association between each feature and an outcome or label (Lipton, 2018).

When it comes to predictive performance though, linear models are often oversimplified as they approximate non-linear relationships and complex surfaces with linear explanations, resulting in poor performance (Du et al., 2019). Moreover, the assumption of normally distributed errors inherent in these models is often violated in practice, which contributes to poor prediction accuracy (Thongpeth et al., 2021). This comparable loss in predictive performance is often accepted when utilising machine learning in high-stakes domains like healthcare, since the central question of these models is to be trusted by clinicians while still performing reasonably well (Boulesteix & Schmid, 2014; Kruppa et al., 2014; Linardatos et al., 2020). Apart from critical environments like medical care though, model interpretability is often not a top priority since black-box models are rather trained to optimise a single objective, namely predictive performance (T. Wang & Lin, 2021). Some authors even suggest that emphasising the indispensability of interpretability throughout all application areas could spark further mistrust towards algorithms, instead advocating for robust procedures, regulations and best practices when testing models (Krishnan, 2020).

Needless to say, there have been numerous attempts to combine the "best of both worlds", culminating in the effort to develop both accurate as well as interpretable models (De et al., 2020). Two main branches of research have emerged, which differ with respect to the underlying mechanics they apply to create accurate algorithms understandable by users.

Explainable Hybrid Approaches

The first branch is titled "Explainable Artificial Intelligence" (XAI) and has regained widespread popularity after years of scientific attention devoted rather to predictive accuracy than to interpretability (Barredo Arrieta et al., 2020; Gunning & Aha, 2019; Linardatos et al., 2020). Explainable models pursue the main objective of balancing the accuracy-interpretability trade-off: their underlying idea is to make complex models understandable to human users without the need to constrain these models, in order to keep their high predictive performance intact (Du et al., 2019; Yang et al., 2021).

A core feature of most explainable approaches is that they focus on post-hoc analysis, where an already fitted, opaque model (such as a deep neural network) is approximated using external tools: for instance, these can be partial dependence plots, local interpretable model-agnostic explanations, additive explanations or Heatmap visualisations, which attempt to approximate the opaque model's predictions as close as possible (T. Wang & Lin, 2021; Yang et al., 2021). The post-hoc approximation principle is where explainable models significantly differ from inherently interpretable models such as simple tree-based algorithms, since the latter have interpretability directly incorporated into their model structure due to aforesaid structural constraints (Margot & Luta, 2021). There are multiple approaches emerging with regard to explainable algorithms, usually classified as global or local, each of them entailing certain advantages.

Global explanatory models attempt to interpret the overall relationship between input variables and response variables over the entire model space, including techniques like Shapley additive explanations (Davazdahemami et al., 2022). Such global approaches aim to summarise the impact of a complete set or subset of input features on the model as a whole (Lundberg et al., 2020). In the global domain, particularly model-agnostic or model-independent approaches such as permutation feature importance are considered versatile when applied to non-interpretable algorithms, usually displaying robust and efficient implementation (Du et al., 2019). In comparison, local explanations focus on revealing the impact of input features on individual predictions or single samples, thereby aiming to provide local faithfulness to the original model (Lundberg et al., 2020). The reasoning behind this approach is that in locally confined areas, the predictions can only linearly or monotonously depend on a few features, rather than showing complex dependencies that require non-linear approaches (Carvalho et al., 2019). As such, explainable models can partially be broken down to instance level, where explanations about an individual observation in the data (like a single patient's outcome) should be able to generate actionable explanations for end users (De et al., 2020). Concepts typically used for local explanations are local interpretable model-agnostic explanations, which approximate classifiers locally with simpler models like sparse linear models or decision trees (Mishra et al., 2017).

Irrespective of their exact design, one of the main advantages of post-hoc explanation approaches is that they keep their underlying, non-interpretable model's accuracy mostly intact. This enables them to partly steer away from the constraints of interpretable models and their limited performance, hence they are principally enabled to reach their black-box model's predictive performance (Du et al., 2019). Also, according to some researchers, there are explainable models already which are intelligible enough to provide a window into the underlying data they utilise and the predictions they make. In this regard, they could spark further scientific and practical interest in the topic, thereby fostering the development of more advanced analyses such as causal reasoning for Generalized Additive Models (Caruana et al., 2015).

Therefore, it is to be expected that explainable models will enjoy increasing popularity in the near future, despite a number of shortcomings that could decisively compromise their safe application in high-stakes environments like healthcare. This could coincide with the observations of some researchers that users may form an inaccurate understanding when explanations are merely presented in the form of information transmission, implying the human bias towards simpler but more inaccurate explanations (Chromik, 2021). At first, explainable models only serve as a summarised surrogate with a more interpretable approximation, which is why they are necessarily an inaccurate representation of the original model in parts of the feature space (Rudin, 2019; Stiglic et al., 2020). This can result in impaired performance, where other models alone often still prove to be superior - in certain use cases, even those simple interpretable approaches that explainable artificial intelligence attempts to overcome are on par with the latter (Loyola-Gonzalez, 2019; Rudin & Radin, 2019).

Furthermore, even in cases where a black-box model makes a correct prediction and its explainer is correct in the approximation of the black box, it is possible that explanations leave out so much information that they have to be rendered meaningless for a human trying to understand a model's inner mechanics. This is particularly obstructive when explanations lull users into a false sense of confidence, as can happen when explainable models only indicate which data have been used for a correct prediction - all while lacking an explanation for both those data utilised in wrong predictions and the black-box model's inner mechanics: for instance, an explainer of a multiclass classification could provide similar or same explanations for each class even if all classifications of the model are wrong, but when only the explanation of the actually correct class is shown, users wrongly consider model and approximation to be useful (Rudin & Radin, 2019).

Eventually, explainable models show a tenuous connection between explainability and accountability, which becomes critical once an explainable algorithm makes a mistake and needs investigation: as they rely on imperfectly approximated post-hoc rationales, explainable models can obfuscate developers (and even worse, caregivers under pressure) onto wrong paths in case of an error - a problem that is aggravated by the fact that modern machine learning systems are often comprised of multiple connected black-boxes at once (Babic et al., 2021).

Additive Hybrid Approaches

Considering the shortcomings of explainable artificial intelligence, the emergence of a second branch of low-constrained architectures aimed to be understandable for humans can be observed: other than explainable approaches, these algorithms attempt to provide interpretability to users without the need to fall back on post-hoc explanations or overly constrained model architectures. One of the most prominent model classes of this category is generalised additive models, which are interpretable by humans as they can easily add together and visualise the impact of each feature on the prediction (Chang et al., 2021). Generalised additive models can be considered a further development of generalised linear models and replace a strictly linear function graph with a sum of smooth functions or splines for some predictors.

Therefore, they are no longer constrained to mere linear approximation and instead can use iterative "backfitting" to fit the model and smooth out partial residuals (Hastie & Tibshirani, 1986). Generalised additive models thus allow for arbitrary functions to model the influence of each covariate on an exponential family response in a multivariate regression setting. Hybrid approaches like the aforementioned generalised additive models have proven to be applicable in high-stakes use cases of healthcare like mortality risk prediction, primarily because they are sufficiently flexible and precise to model such complex nonlinear dynamics while offering a high degree of interpretability (Feng, 2021). Advanced developments in generalised additive models can especially be observed when it comes to pairwise interactions of explanatory variables or fitting with decision trees, aiming to increase the accuracy of predictions (Hegselmann et al., 07–08 Aug 2020; Karatekin et al., 2019). Reaching back as far as 1986, generalised additive models can be said to have laid the foundation of those machine learning models that iteratively optimise a linear function via nonlinear adjustments whenever this is beneficial to predictive performance (Hastie & Tibshirani, 1986).

CONCLUSION

Interpretable AI can foster practical adoption and make artificial intelligence a useful tool for medical decision support, provided user acceptance is sufficiently catered for. User acceptance depends on the ability of the model to be understood by users of all levels of knowledge. Therefore, it is necessary to separate involved persons' knowledge levels from their interpretability needs in this regard. This is because intelligible predictions are not only required by experienced domain experts with significant responsibilities.

However, experienced professionals and less proficient users may appreciate algorithm-based judgement differently: while the latter (such as apprentices and first responders) tend to rely more heavily on algorithmic decision support, the former (such as specialists and researchers) tend to take less advice from it (Logg et al., 2019).

Therefore, models must be deployed with these differing requirements in mind: on one hand, professionals should be motivated to think of decision support as a "crosscheck" to prevent serious misclassifications. Individuals with less expertise should receive intelligible information about the model's inner mechanics, its feature selection, and other aspects, to support their already strong algorithmic trust.

REFERENCES

Agarwal, N., & Das, S. 2020. Interpretable Machine Learning Tools: A Survey. *2020 IEEE Symposium Series on Computational Intelligence (SSCI)*, 1528–1534.

Ahmad, M. A., Eckert, C., & Teredesai, A. 2018. Interpretable Machine Learning in Healthcare. *Proceedings of the 2018 ACM International Conference on Bioinformatics, Computational Biology, and Health Informatics*. 10.1145/3233547.3233667

Al-antari, M. A., Al-masni, M. A., Choi, M.-T., Han, S.-M., & Kim, T.-S. 2018. A fully integrated computer-aided diagnosis system for digital X-ray mammograms via deep learning detection, segmentation, and classification. *International Journal of Medical Informatics, 117*, 44–54.

Babic, B., Gerke, S., Evgeniou, T., & Cohen, I. G. 2021. Beware explanations from AI in health care. *Science, 373*(6552), 284–286.

Barredo Arrieta, A., Díaz-Rodríguez, N., Del Ser, J., Bennetot, A., Tabik, S., Barbado, A., Garcia, S., Gil-Lopez, S., Molina, D., Benjamins, R., Chatila, R., & Herrera, F. 2020. Explainable Artificial Intelligence (XAI): Concepts, taxonomies, opportunities and challenges toward responsible AI. *An International Journal on Information Fusion, 58*, 82–115.

Bohr, A., & Memarzadeh, K. 2020. The rise of artificial intelligence in healthcare applications. In *Artificial Intelligence in Healthcare* (pp. 25–60). Elsevier.

Boulesteix, A.-L., & Schmid, M. 2014. Machine learning versus statistical modeling. *Biometrical Journal. Biometrische Zeitschrift, 56*(4), 588–593.

Buiten, M. C. 2019. Towards intelligent regulation of artificial intelligence. *European Journal of Risk Regulation, 10*(1), 41–59.

Carrillo, M. R. 2020. Artificial intelligence: From ethics to law. *Telecommunications Policy, 44*(6), 101937.

Caruana, R., Lou, Y., Gehrke, J., Koch, P., Sturm, M., & Elhadad, N. 2015. Intelligible Models for HealthCare. *Proceedings of the 21th ACM SIGKDD International Conference on Knowledge Discovery and Data Mining.* 10.1145/2783258.2788613

Carvalho, D. V., Pereira, E. M., & Cardoso, J. S. 2019. Machine learning interpretability: A survey on methods and metrics. *Electronics, 8*(8), 832.

Chakraborty, D., Başağaoğlu, H., & Winterle, J. 2021. Interpretable vs. non-interpretable machine learning models for data-driven hydro-climatological process modeling. *Expert Systems with Applications, 170*, 114498.

Chang, C.-H., Tan, S., Lengerich, B., Goldenberg, A., & Caruana, R. 2021. How interpretable and trustworthy are GAMs? In *Proceedings of the 27th ACM SIGKDD Conference on Knowledge Discovery & Data Mining* (pp. 95–105). Association for Computing Machinery.

Chen, P., Dong, W., Wang, J., Lu, X., Kaymak, U., & Huang, Z. 2020. Interpretable clinical prediction via attention-based neural network. *BMC Medical Informatics and Decision Making, 20*(S3). 10.1186/s12911-020-1110-7

Choi, E., Bahadori, M. T., Kulas, J. A., Schuetz, A., Stewart, W. F., & Sun, J. 2016. RETAIN: An Interpretable Predictive Model for Healthcare Using Reverse Time Attention Mechanism. *Proceedings of the 30th International Conference on Neural Information Processing Systems*, 3512–3520.

Chromik, M. 2021. *Human-centric explanation facilities* [Ludwig-Maximilians-Universität München]. 10.5282/EDOC.28238

Cooper, G. F., Abraham, V., Aliferis, C. F., Aronis, J. M., Buchanan, B. G., Caruana, R., Fine, M. J., Janosky, J. E., Livingston, G., Mitchell, T., Monti, S., & Spirtes, P. 2005. Predicting dire outcomes of patients with community-acquired pneumonia. *Journal of Biomedical Informatics, 38*(5), 347–366.

Coussement, K., & Benoit, D. F. 2021. Interpretable data science for decision-making. *Decision Support Systems, 150*, 113664.

Davazdahemami, B., Zolbanin, H. M., & Delen, D. 2022. An explanatory machine learning framework for studying pandemics: The case of COVID-19 emergency department readmissions. *Decision Support Systems*, 113730.

De, T., Giri, P., Mevawala, A., Nemani, R., & Deo, A. 2020. Explainable AI: A hybrid approach to generate human-interpretable explanation for deep learning prediction. *Procedia Computer Science, 168*, 40–48.

Du, M., Liu, N., & Hu, X. 2019. Techniques for interpretable machine learning. *Communications of the ACM, 63*(1), 68–77.

ElShawi, R., Sherif, Y., Al-Mallah, M., & Sakr, S. 2020. Interpretability in healthcare: A comparative study of local machine learning interpretability techniques. *Computational Intelligence. An International Journal, 37*(4), 1633–1650.

Falavigna, G. 2020. Prediction of general medical admission length of stay with natural language processing and deep learning: A pilot study. *Internal and Emergency Medicine, 15*(6), 917–918.

Feng, C. 2021. Spatial-temporal generalized additive model for modeling COVID-19 mortality risk in Toronto, Canada. *Spatial Statistics*, 100526.

Fournier-Tombs, E. 2021. Towards a United Nations internal regulation for artificial intelligence. *Big Data & Society, 8*(2), 205395172110394.

Ghabra, H., White, W., Townsend, M., Boysen, P., & Nossaman, B. 2019. Use of biomarkers in the prediction of culture-proven infection in the surgical intensive care unit. *Journal of Critical Care, 49*, 149–154.

Goodman, B., & Flaxman, S. 2017. European Union Regulations on algorithmic decision-making and a "right to explanation." *AI Magazine, 38*(3), 50–57.

Gosiewska, A., Kozak, A., & Biecek, P. 2021. Simpler is better: Lifting interpretability-performance trade-off via automated feature engineering. *Decision Support Systems, 150*, 113556.

Gotz, D., & Borland, D. 2016. Data-driven healthcare: Challenges and opportunities for interactive visualization. *IEEE Computer Graphics and Applications, 36*(3), 90–96.

Gunning, D., & Aha, D. 2019. DARPA's Explainable Artificial Intelligence (XAI) program. *AI Magazine, 40*(2), 44–58.

Hastie, T., & Tibshirani, R. 1986. Generalized additive models. *Statistical Science: A Review Journal of the Institute of Mathematical Statistics, 1*(3). 10.1214/ss/1177013604

Hegselmann, S., Volkert, T., Ohlenburg, H., Gottschalk, A., Dugas, M., & Ertmer, C. 2020. An evaluation of the doctor-interpretability of generalized additive models with interactions. In F. Doshi-Velez, J. Fackler, K. Jung, D. Kale, R. Ranganath, B. Wallace, & J. Wiens (Eds.), *Proceedings of the 5th Machine Learning for Healthcare Conference* (Vol. 126, pp. 46–79). PMLR.

Hsu, W.-Y. 2018. A decision-making mechanism for assessing risk factor significance in cardiovascular diseases. *Decision Support Systems, 115*, 64–77.

Hu, Z., Ma, X., Liu, Z., Hovy, E., & Xing, E. 2016. Harnessing Deep Neural Networks with Logic Rules. *Proceedings of the 54th Annual Meeting of the Association for Computational Linguistics (Volume 1: Long Papers)*, 2410–2420.

Islam, M., Hasan, M., Wang, X., Germack, H., & Noor-E-Alam, M. 2018. A Systematic Review on Healthcare Analytics: Application and Theoretical Perspective of Data Mining. *HealthcarePapers, 6*(2), 54.

Jovanovic, M., Radovanovic, S., Vukicevic, M., Van Poucke, S., & Delibasic, B. 2016. Building interpretable predictive models for pediatric hospital readmission using Tree-Lasso logistic regression. *Artificial Intelligence in Medicine, 72*, 12–21.

Karatekin, T., Sancak, S., Celik, G., Topcuoglu, S., Karatekin, G., Kirci, P., & Okatan, A. 2019. Interpretable Machine Learning in Healthcare through Generalized Additive Model with Pairwise Interactions (GA2M): Predicting Severe Retinopathy of Prematurity. *2019 International Conference on Deep Learning and Machine Learning in Emerging Applications (Deep-ML)*, 61–66.

Khamis, A.-A. 2019. Overcoming the health system challenges in the 21st century and beyond? *Public Health, 168*, 47–49.

Kolyshkina, I., & Simoff, S. 2021. Interpretability of machine learning solutions in public healthcare: The CRISP-ML approach. *Frontiers in Big Data, 4*. 10.3389/fdata.2021.660206

Krishnan, M. 2020. Against Interpretability: A critical examination of the interpretability problem in machine learning. *Philosophy & Technology, 33*. 10.1007/s13347-019-00372-9

Kruppa, J., Liu, Y., Diener, H.-C., Holste, T., Weimar, C., König, I. R., & Ziegler, A. 2014. Probability estimation with machine learning methods for dichotomous and multicategory outcome: Applications. *Biometrical Journal. Biometrische Zeitschrift*, *56*(4), 564–583.

Kundu, S. 2021. AI in medicine must be explainable. *Nature Medicine*, *27*(8), 1328–1328.

Kwon, B. C., Choi, M.-J., Kim, J. T., Choi, E., Kim, Y. B., Kwon, S., Sun, J., & Choo, J. 2019. RetainVis: Visual analytics with interpretable and interactive recurrent neural networks on electronic medical records. *IEEE Transactions on Visualization and Computer Graphics*, *25*(1), 299–309.

Linardatos, P., Papastefanopoulos, V., & Kotsiantis, S. 2020. Explainable AI: A review of machine learning interpretability methods. *Entropy*, *23*(1), 18.

Lipton, Z. C. 2018. The mythos of model interpretability. *Queueing Systems. Theory and Applications*, *16*(3), 31–57.

Logg, J. M., Minson, J. A., & Moore, D. A. 2019. Algorithm appreciation: People prefer algorithmic to human judgment. *Organizational Behavior and Human Decision Processes*, *151*, 90–103.

Loyola-Gonzalez, O. 2019. Black-box vs. white-box: Understanding their advantages and weaknesses from a practical point of view. *IEEE Access*, *7*, 154096–154113.

Lundberg, S. M., Erion, G., Chen, H., DeGrave, A., Prutkin, J. M., Nair, B., Katz, R., Himmelfarb, J., Bansal, N., & Lee, S.-I. 2020. From local explanations to global understanding with explainable AI for trees. *Nature Machine Intelligence*, *2*(1), 56–67.

Margot, V., & Luta, G. 2021. A new method to compare the interpretability of rule-based algorithms. *AI*, *2*(4), 621–635.

Miotto, R., Wang, F., Wang, S., Jiang, X., & Dudley, J. T. 2017. Deep learning for healthcare: Review, opportunities and challenges. *Briefings in Bioinformatics*, *19*(6), 1236–1246.

Mishra, S., Sturm, B. L., & Dixon, S. 2017. Local Interpretable Model-Agnostic Explanations for Music Content Analysis. In S. J. Cunningham, Z. Duan, X. Hu, & D. Turnbull (Eds.), *Proceedings of the 18th International Society for Music Information Retrieval Conference, ISMIR 2017*, Suzhou, China, October 23–27, 2017 (pp. 537–543).

Montavon, G., Samek, W., & Müller, K.-R. 2018. Methods for interpreting and understanding deep neural networks. *Digital Signal Processing*, *73*, 1–15.

Murdoch, W. J., Singh, C., Kumbier, K., Abbasi-Asl, R., & Yu, B. 2019. Definitions, methods, and applications in interpretable machine learning. *Proceedings of the National Academy of Sciences*, *116*(44), 22071–22080.

Organization, W. H. 2007. *Everybody's business - strengthening health systems to improve health outcomes: WHO's framework for action.*

Ozaydin, B., Berner, E. S., & Cimino, J. J. 2021. Appropriate use of machine learning in healthcare. *Intelligence-Based Medicine*, *5*, 100041.

Pesapane, F., Volonté, C., Codari, M., & Sardanelli, F. 2018. Artificial intelligence as a medical device in radiology: ethical and regulatory issues in Europe and the United States. *Insights into Imaging*, *9*(5), 745–753.

Pramanik, M. I., Lau, R. Y. K., Azad, M. A. K., Hossain, M. S., Chowdhury, M. K. H., & Karmaker, B. K. 2020. Healthcare informatics and analytics in big data. *Expert Systems with Applications*, *152*, 113388.

Ramchandani, A., Fan, C., & Mostafavi, A. 2020. DeepCOVIDNet: An interpretable deep learning model for predictive surveillance of COVID-19 using heterogeneous features and their interactions. *IEEE Access*, *8*, 159915–159930.

Richens, J. G., Lee, C. M., & Johri, S. 2020. Improving the accuracy of medical diagnosis with causal machine learning. *Nature Communications*, *11*(1). 10.1038/s41467-020-17419-7

Roncarolo, F., Boivin, A., Denis, J.-L., Hébert, R., & Lehoux, P. 2017. What do we know about the needs and challenges of health systems? A scoping review of the international literature. *BMC Health Services Research*, *17*(1). 10.1186/s12913-017-2585-5

Rudin, C. 2019. Stop explaining black box machine learning models for high-stakes decisions and use interpretable models instead. *Nature Machine Intelligence*, *1*(5), 206–215.

Rudin, C., Chen, C., Chen, Z., Huang, H., Semenova, L., & Zhong, C. 2022. Interpretable machine learning: Fundamental principles and 10 grand challenges. *Statistics Surveys*, *16*(none). 10.1214/21-ss133

Rudin, C., & Radin, J. 2019. Why Are We Using Black Box Models in AI When We Don't Need To? A Lesson From An Explainable AI Competition. *1. 2*, *1*(2). 10.1162/99608f92.5a8a3a3d

Rumelhart, D. E., Hinton, G. E., & Williams, R. J. 1986. Learning representations by back-propagating errors. *Nature*, *323*(6088), 533–536.

Senn, N., Breton, M., Ebert, S. T., Lamoureux-Lamarche, C., & Lévesque, J.-F. 2021. Assessing primary care organization and performance: Literature synthesis and proposition of a consolidated framework. *Health Policy*, *125*(2), 160–167.

Shah, N. H., Milstein, A., & Steven C. Bagley, P. 2019. Making machine learning models clinically useful. *JAMA: The Journal of the American Medical Association*, *322*(14), 1351.

Shamshirband, S., Fathi, M., Dehzangi, A., Chronopoulos, A. T., & Alinejad-Rokny, H. 2021. A review on deep learning approaches in healthcare systems: Taxonomies, challenges, and open issues. *Journal of Biomedical Informatics*, *113*, 103627.

Shortliffe, E. H., & Buchanan, B. G. 1975. A model of inexact reasoning in medicine. *Mathematical Biosciences*, *23*(3-4), 351–379.

Simpao, A. F., Ahumada, L. M., Gálvez, J. A., & Rehman, M. A. 2014. A review of analytics and clinical informatics in health care. *Journal of Medical Systems*, *38*(4). 10.1007/s10916-014-0045-x

Stiglic, G., Kocbek, P., Fijacko, N., Zitnik, M., Verbert, K., & Cilar, L. 2020. Interpretability of machine learning-based prediction models in healthcare. *WIREs Data Mining and Knowledge Discovery*, *10*(5). 10.1002/widm.1379

Thongpeth, W., Lim, A., Wongpairin, A., Thongpeth, T., & Chaimontree, S. 2021. Comparison of linear, penalized linear and machine learning models predicting hospital visit costs from chronic disease in Thailand. *Informatics in Medicine Unlocked*, *26*, 100769.

Tomar, D. 2013. A survey on Data Mining approaches for Healthcare. *International Journal of Bio-Science and Bio-Technology*, *5*, 241–266.

Wang, J., Xu, C., Yang, X., & Zurada, J. M. 2018. A novel pruning algorithm for smoothing feedforward neural networks based on group Lasso method. *IEEE Transactions on Neural Networks and Learning Systems*, *29*(5), 2012–2024.

Wang, T., & Lin, Q. 2021. Hybrid predictive model: When an interpretable model collaborates with a black-box model. *Journal of Machine Learning Research: JMLR*, *22*(137), 1–38.

Yang, Z., Zhang, A., & Sudjianto, A. 2021. GAMI-Net: An explainable neural network based on generalized additive models with structured interactions. *Pattern Recognition*, *120*, 108192.

II

Management Perspectives

Nilmini Wickramasinghe, Freimut Bodendorf, and Mathias Kraus

Like enterprises in all sectors of the economy, healthcare providers too strive to improve the effectiveness and efficiency of their services and performances by making the right management decisions, both on a strategic as well as on an operational level. These decisions occur within healthcare companies and organisations as well as on the side of healthcare consumers, aiming at improving business as well as customer relationships and processes.

Artificial intelligence and advanced analytics help support these management decisions in order to deliver superior healthcare and foster self-care of individuals. So, artificial intelligence and advanced analytics in healthcare can take a business perspective as well as a patient-centric view. The first two chapters of this section discuss potentials and issues of data sharing and data governance in healthcare. Here, patient data is in the foreground. After the third chapter, addressing self-management of preventive care, the perspective of both subsequent chapters of this section moves towards operational and strategic decisions in healthcare companies and corresponding methods and models of supporting smart analytics.

Chapter 5: Data Ownership and Emerging Data Governance Models in Healthcare, by Pavlina Kröckel, unpacks the critical issues of data sharing and data protection within and between healthcare providers and consumers.

DOI: 10.1201/9781032699745-6

Chapter 6: Privacy-Preserving Roadmap for Medical Data-Sharing Systems, by Belal Alsinglawi et al., addresses the crucial topic of data privacy when using analytics, artificial intelligence, and machine learning to analyse data and exhibit data relationships.

Chapter 7: Comparative Review of Descriptive Process Models in Healthcare Operations Management and Analytics, by Isabella Eigner et al., focuses on operational healthcare and related artificial intelligence models for process management.

Chapter 8: AI Approaches for Managing Preventive Care in Digital Health Ecosystems, by Andreas Hamper, deals with personal self-management to prevent and better cope with chronic diseases by using artificial intelligence.

Chapter 9: Competitive Intelligence in Healthcare, by Annika Lurz, takes the perspective of a technology provider for healthcare and explores the possibilities of artificial intelligence and graph-based analytical models to support strategic decisions with mergers & acquisitions as an example.

The chapters in this section provide various insights into the wide field of operational and strategic management in healthcare and the great possibilities of decision support by artificial intelligence and advanced analytics. However, the concepts and solutions described are only a very small excerpt and show some cherry picking of scenarios. Nevertheless, the chapters depict how data-driven and intelligence-guided management in the healthcare of the future can look like. The transfer to other contexts is evident and easy to imagine.

CHAPTER 5

Data Ownership and Emerging Data Governance Models in Healthcare

Pavlina Kröckel

INTRODUCTION

The term data governance has been mentioned for almost two decades now. A quick search in Google Trends shows that the interest in data governance has been consistently increasing since 2004 (earliest date for trend search) and has peaked in 2022[1]. Following the big data trend since approximately 2012/13 and the resulting developments in data science, many interesting and valuable applications based on data analytics at their core have been adopted in various fields, including healthcare. Data are being processed with the help of machine learning, a branch of artificial intelligence (AI). There has been a lot of excitement around AI applications and the advancements they are expected to bring to the field of medicine. Some examples here are personalised medicine, drug discovery, and patient management (Reddy, Allan, Coghlan, & Cooper, 2020), to name a few.

However, following the initial excitement over the promise of AI, a more critical point of view has been gaining traction in the last few years, and has been especially exacerbated thanks to the global pandemic. There are a host of issues related to using AI for decision making, especially in sensitive domains such as healthcare or medicine. Some of

DOI: 10.1201/9781032699745-7

the most critical themes are ethics, trust, bias, accountability, privacy, and security (Reddy et al., 2020). The European Union is currently leading the way when it comes to adopting rules and regulations around these topics. Examples are the General Data Protection Regulation (GDPR) and the Data Protection Law Enforcement Directive which came into effect in 2018 (European Commission, 2023). A detailed description of the legal aspects behind these regulations can be found on the official page of the EU Commission. Both aim at protecting personal data, however, the GDPR is mostly relevant for patient data as the Data Protection Directive refers to cases when personal data is "used by criminal law enforcement authorities for law enforcement purposes" (European Commission, 2023). There is a lot more to be done in this regard and we are only at the beginning of the road when it comes to well-established government regulations for the design, use, and adoption of AI systems based on processing personal (health) data.

As the core of an AI-based system for clinical decision support is usually data, the governance of these data has consequently gained increased attention due to the mentioned factors. Data governance is seen as a prerequisite for a trustable and responsible AI in healthcare, without which health professionals cannot maintain broad public trust (Reddy et al., 2020). There are various definitions of the term in the literature and occasionally, data governance is used as a synonym for data management, which is misleading. Data governance specifically refers to any decision made over data (access, control, use, benefit) and who can make such decisions i.e., to exercise authority in data-related matters (Janssen, Brous, Estevez, Barbosa, & Janowski, 2020; Micheli, Ponti, Craglia, & Berti Suman, 2020). Data management is concerned primarily with the regular execution of data-related decisions as part of established governance policies (Abraham, Schneider, & vom Brocke, 2019). In a nutshell, the purpose of data governance is to increase the value of data, while minimising the costs and risks of data-based decisions (Abraham et al., 2019).

With data being valued at 20 to 25% of an enterprise value, according to Gartner (Couture, 2019), adequate data governance is becoming even more important, especially in healthcare where data are of the most sensitive nature. To ensure data value for all stakeholders involved (hospitals, patients, scientists) more research into data ownership is necessary – aspects of data ownership as well as workable solutions (Mirchev, Mircheva, & Kerekovska, 2020). Data are the central currency of science in the 21st century, with personal data being a new asset class (Evans, 2016; World Economic Forum, 2011). Thus, the main question is "Who will control them?" (Evans, 2016).

There are increasing calls for patients to be owners of their data. This is also a complex topic as what constitutes health data has changed over the years (see next section on health data definition). Furthermore, there are debates on making health data a public good. As it is personal data, there would be some exceptions compared to other data types – one needs to consider the right degree of openness or restriction, while at the same time reducing the potential for harm (WHO, 2021b). This is important because often, to gain value data need to be aggregated – e.g., individual genomic sequence data has limited value on its own, as well as smaller Covid clinical trials (WHO, 2021b).

Finally, privacy and security are topics closely related to ownership of data. In spite of this, in this chapter, we focus on the data ownership aspect exclusively and the emerging data governance models. The reason for this narrow focus is that privacy and security are topics that are widely discussed in the literature both in general and in healthcare, as opposed to the data ownership topic. We give an overview of these models, investigate if and how they have been used in healthcare, and identify the models that based on our literature analysis are the most applicable to health data.

DATA OWNERSHIP IN HEALTHCARE – THE ACADEMIC DISCOURSE

In this section, we review the latest research on data ownership in healthcare by looking into definitions, challenges, and future research questions on the topic. We are specifically interested in how data ownership affects the future of data governance models.

We start by first extracting articles in Google Scholar by using the following parameters:

- Timeline: From the beginning of time till January 2023
- Query: "data ownership AND health"

The results are summarised in Figure 5.1. To create a visual summary, we rely on the tool for network and text analysis by InfraNodus (Nodus Labs, author's own license).

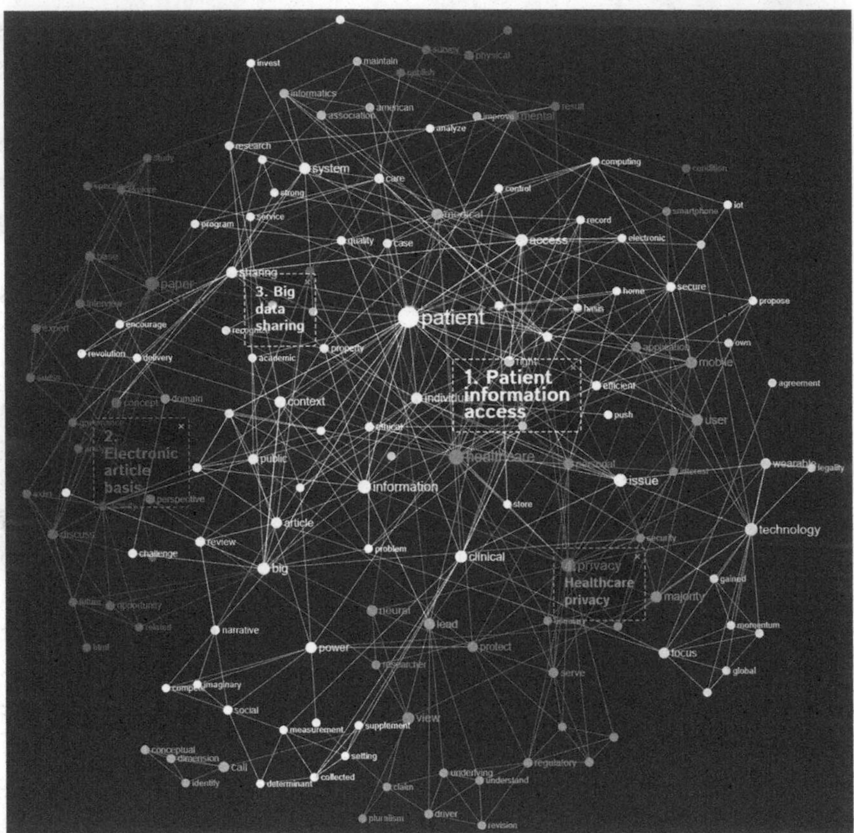

FIGURE 5.1 Key topics in the literature on "data ownership" based on results in Google Scholar. Figure by the author, generated with InfraNodus.

As seen in Figure 5.1, the latest academic discourse on data ownership in healthcare can be grouped into four topic clusters. The biggest cluster relates to the topic of "patient information access" and "big data sharing" (both in green in Figure 5.1). The fourth cluster "healthcare privacy" has gained more relevance in the last few years, as the keywords "privacy" and "patient" occur together the most in the last part of the time period analysed.

We conducted an additional extraction of full-text studies in Google Scholar, EbscoHost, and Scopus for the period 2015 – 2023 by using the queries "data ownership AND health", "data access AND health". Following an initial scan of the title and abstract, we could identify only 11 papers specifically discussing the issue of data ownership in the healthcare domain (see Table 5.1). The paper by Asswad and Gomez

TABLE 5.1 Papers on Data Ownership in Healthcare Published between 2015–2023

Authors	Year	Article Title
Scandurra et al.	2015	Is "Patient's Online Access to Health Records" a Good Reform? – Opinions from Swedish Healthcare Professionals Differ
Priisalu et al.	2017	Personal control of privacy and data: Estonian experience
Ballantyne	2020	How should we think about clinical data ownership?
Mirchev et al.	2020	The Academic Viewpoint on Patient Data Ownership in the Context of Big Data: Scoping Review
Asswad et al.	2021	Data Ownership: A Survey
Chiruvella & Guddati	2021	Ethical Issues in Patient Data Ownership
Martani et al.	2021	It's not something you can take in your hands. Swiss experts' perspectives on health data ownership: an interview-based study
Sorbie et al.	2021	Examining the power of the social imaginary through competing narratives of data ownership in health research
Liddell et al.	2021	Personal control of privacy and data: Estonian experience
Piasecki & Cheah	2022	Ownership of individual-level health data, data sharing, and data governance
Pinto et al.	2022	A System for the Promotion of Traceability and Ownership of Health Data Using Blockchain

(2021) is not specifically focused on healthcare data ownership, however, the points that the authors make are valid for the health domain as well. Thus, we included it in our review. Most articles have been published since 2020. These results are surprising, especially considering the ongoing debate on ethics, privacy, and transparency in the use of AI systems in general. Mirchev et al. (2020) conducted a scoping review and analysed the literature between 2000 and 2019 and came to a similar conclusion – the research on this important topic is surprisingly limited. One reason for this is due to the term "ownership" being ill-defined in the health domain, including debates on who is the owner and is patient ownership of the data in fact beneficial or does it create more challenges – in terms of data access for research as well as incurring more costs for organisations. Opinions, even in academia, differ greatly.

Before defining data ownership in healthcare, it is necessary to briefly define what **"health data"** are. This is important because what nowadays constitutes health-related data affects data ownership questions and consequently, data governance itself. In the past, health data were data collected as a result of health services e.g., diagnosis and treatment (Kariotis et al., 2020). Today, we also need to include health-related data or patient-generated data as part of the definition. These data have been defined by Shapiro et al., (2012, p.2) as data including "health history, symptoms, lifestyle choices created, recorded, gathered, or inferred by or from patients or their designees (i.e., care partners or those who assist them) to help address a health concern". As the authors mention, such data although not new, will increase in volume due to the technologies used that assist their collection. This makes data ownership in healthcare an inherently more complex issue and a subject of ongoing debate (Mirchev et al., 2020).

Even though the term **"data ownership"** has been mentioned in the literature since 1981, there is no standardised definition that covers all aspects of owning data (Asswad & Marx Gómez, 2021). Even the term "ownership" does not have a unified definition. What makes defining data ownership particularly challenging is the fact that data are of an intangible nature and applying ownership to immaterial objects is seen as controversial (Praduroux, 2017). However, some studies suggest that considering data and information as a product of raw data, should also not be defined as a property in the typical sense of the word. For instance, Liddell et al. (2021) argue that it is better to rely less and not more on property in this context, as a property framework would not be beneficial for the patients as data owners.

The main topic in the reviewed articles in Table 5.1 revolves around the possibility of giving patients the right to completely own their health data, decide on who has the right to access it and revoke access if and when they choose to, and finally, the possibility to sell their own data. This is a topic that is somewhat seen as controversial by health experts and researchers. However, the discussion is mostly theoretical as there is a lack of studies of a more practical nature e.g., directly with patients or health practitioners. Of the papers we review only three discuss patients owing or having access to their health data, what challenges this brings, and how they should be tackled. Scandurra et al. (2015) sent out three questionnaires to Swedish health practitioners (physicians, nurses, and licensed professionals) with the goal of finding out whether they agree that the newly introduced eHealth service in a Swedish county giving rights to patients to access their health records online, is a good reform or not. The study found that opinions differ not only between the different professions but also between those who have experience with their patients having access to their records and those who have no such experience. Interestingly, the study found that physicians are overall more negative to the reform while nurses with experience are more positive. As this was a study based on questionnaires, more depth on the reasons behind health professionals being positive or negative is lacking. Moreover, the study investigates a limited aspect of patient data ownership by considering only the patient's access to their electronic health records (EHRs).

A newer study by Martani et al. (2021) investigates the topic more specifically, by conducting interviews with Swiss experts. The findings show that experts have different opinions on who is the owner of health data (the patient or e.g., the data collector and processor) and what ownership would exactly constitute. This is an interesting and important study as it is the only one to directly investigate data ownership with health practitioners. Even though there are some suggestions in the literature that health data can be considered a public good, this study found that only two out of 48 interviewees were supportive of this idea. In addition to the question of who the data owner is, other important findings concern treating data as an asset and being able to use it as a trading commodity by e.g., patients selling their data. Finally, most participants agreed that there is a connection between labour and property, meaning that those who collect and process or manage the data also should have certain rights or privileges over said data. Obviously, this is in contradiction to patients fully owning their data.

In line with discussing health data ownership in practical terms, in Europe, we have a positive example of patients owning their health data. Estonia is leading the way in providing digital public services to its citizens – way above the average compared to the rest of Europe (European Commission, 2022). An Estonian citizen has an overview of everyone who has access to their health data and can limit that access if needed (Priisalu & Ottis, 2017).

However, data has not only an intrinsic value (although some experts claim data has no such value), but also added value as a by-product resulting from processing raw data and converting it into information and consequently knowledge (we refer to the data, information, knowledge, wisdom pyramid (Sabherwal & Becerra-Fernandez, 2011)). Data must be stored and processed (usually by a governmental organisation or a healthcare stakeholder). Thus, trust and security are topics that go hand-in-hand with data ownership. Finally, clear data ownership is important for another major principle of trustworthy AI – accountability. Since data are usually owned by different stakeholders, and the development and use of an AI system involves various stakeholders from different domains (software developers, governmental agencies, or even patient interest groups) accountability is the most challenging aspect of data governance in healthcare (Reddy et al., 2020).

From the presented academic discourse on data ownership, we can conclude that moving forward, it is imperative to solve the question of data ownership in healthcare, even more so compared to other domains due to the nature of these data. However, it is unreasonable to expect a one-size-fits-all definition or a data governance model that would be applicable in all healthcare scenarios. If we consider existing research on other AI or machine learning topics, we learn that a general approach is often an unwise solution. An example here is explainability or explainable AI (XAI). Latest findings show that any explainable algorithm is not appropriate for all use cases, and that explainability should be defined and solved on a case-by-case basis.

One way forward would be to establish more precise definitions of data ownership rights of all the stakeholders involved throughout the entire process of data collection, management, and processing (Martani et al., 2021). A good starting point is the extended definition of data ownership suggested by Asswad and Marx Gómez (2021) who specify five characteristics for addressing data ownership in general: data possession, rights, control over data, granting rights, and responsibility. The last part, responsibility, brings up an interesting point – that those who own the data are also responsible for it. If patients fully own their data, does this mean they should be responsible for e.g., data quality? This concerns cases when they monetise their data. In their study, Liddell et al. (2021) suggest a regulatory framework consisting of four components – data access (limit to how and when data can be used by considering security, transparency, accuracy, and enforceability); more guidance to describe the conditions for disclosing patient information; developing interoperable data and platforms to support health data innovations; and finally, more research on health data transactions based on a service and not a goods model.

If efforts to define data ownership and to establish an appropriate data governance framework fail, the next option would be to put forward and accept the idea that health data do not belong to anyone and are a public good, donated by patients and guarded by data processors (Martani et al., 2021).

There is a need for more research on data ownership in healthcare, as this is a complex issue entangled with topics such as data access and sharing, privacy, security, transparency, and ethics – all topics of establishing trustworthy AI-based systems. In Europe, policy debate around data governance is continually active (Micheli et al., 2020), especially concerning AI ethics. However, even though there is much debate on ethical issues around data and AI in general, there is not enough research on how to address such issues in healthcare practice (Reddy et al., 2020). Thus, in the next step, we investigate emerging data governance models that address some of the concerns mentioned so far.

EMERGING DATA GOVERNANCE MODELS

We searched the literature on new and emerging data governance models. We used the same databases as mentioned in the previous section with the query "data governance model" and the time period between 2018 and 2023, as we were interested in extracting only studies from the last five years. An overview of the emerging data governance models found in the literature is presented in Table 5.2.

TABLE 5.2 Emerging Data Governance Models Based on the Latest Research. Highlighted Models Are Overlapping – Same Model under a Different Name

Study	Governance Models	Motivation
Smichowski 2019	• **Crowdsourced data commons** • Data requisition • Collective bargaining on rights over personal data • **Data pooling**	• Insufficient data sharing between private and public actors • Avoiding the so-called "hegemonic data governance model"
Kariotis et al. 2020	• **Data trusts** • **Data marketplaces** • **Data cooperatives**	• Avoid the problem of data being in traditional data silos • Tensions between data protection and using data for the public good (e.g., research)
Micheli et al. 2020	• **Data sharing pools** • **Data cooperatives** • **Public data trusts** • **Personal data sovereignty**	• Stakeholders' competitive struggles for governing data • Civic society and public bodies are seen as key actors in democratising data governance and redistributing value produced through data

TABLE 5.3 Examples of the Emerging Data Governance Models (Based on Information from Kariotis et al., 2020; Micheli et al., 2020; Schneider, 2022; Smichowski, 2019)

Data Governance Model	Examples
Crowdsourced data commons / Data cooperatives	• MiData • Moipatient
Data requisition	/
Collective bargaining on rights over personal data	/
Data pooling	• 23andMe and pharmaceutical companies Pfizer, Genentech and GlaxoSmithKline • Google and Sanofi • Google DeepMind and Royal Free Hospital • IBM and Lombardia Region
Data trusts	• PatientsLikeMe • Health Record Banks • unforgettable.me
Data marketplaces / Personal data sovereignty	• citizenme.com • Digi.me • datacoup.com

As seen in Table 5.2 - motivation, data ownership and the resulting rights from it are at the core of the emerging data governance models. Some authors refer to the same type of model but use a different name – "Crowdsourced data commons" (Smichowski, 2019) is essentially the "Data cooperatives" model (Micheli et al., 2020). Both studies mention, for instance, the platform MiData as an example (see Table 5.3). Public data trusts are a type of data trust with a public actor taking over the role of a trustee. Data pools are mentioned by Smichowski (2019) and Micheli et al. (2020). Finally, personal data sovereignty and data marketplaces refer to the same model as well.

In Table 5.3 we give an overview of the examples we found in the literature on each identified model. All examples are from the healthcare sector. For the data requisition and collective bargaining of rights models, we did not identify health-related examples.

The data governance models identified are not exclusively focused in the healthcare domain. In the following, we define each model and review if and how it has been applied so far in healthcare.

Crowdsourced Data Commons and Data Cooperatives

Data commons or data cooperatives collect data from various sources and make them accessible and useful, usually for research. This model is also referred to as being a type of citizen research sponsorship – using people's data for projects they care about (Evans, 2016). Usually, data collected are made publicly available except in the case of health data commons, as they deal with data about persons (Smichowski, 2019). In the examples mentioned in Table 5.3, both platforms allow users to keep full access and ownership of their data and they can choose the study they want to participate in. Users can also pay for becoming a member (MiDATA) of the cooperative in which case they have a say in how data are used (Kariotis et al., 2020).

So far, there is no extensive research on this type of governance model. Some examples from research in healthcare include the study by Evans (2016) which gives an in-depth view of data commons in healthcare by viewing them as a way to give patients a voice; Jensen et al. (2017) present a genomic data commons collecting genomic and clinical data from patients with cancer with the goal of improving precision medicine; and finally, Do et al. (2019) present a similar data commons initiative in oncology but specifically for improving the care of veterans.

The overall theme in these data commons is the support for medical research and fostering innovation through collaboration and resource (data) sharing (Do et al., 2019). Thus, they are of interest to research institutions mostly including (university) hospitals. There have been some suggestions of, for instance, forming national data cooperatives which would facilitate clinical research (Hafen, Kossmann, & Brand, 2014).

Although they are meant to support a noble goal, most data commons struggle with financial stability over time, a user-friendly software is necessary to collect the data, and occasionally training to inform patients on the proper use of technology (Smichowski, 2019).

Data Requisition

This model refers to a situation when a public actor (e.g., the government) demands a private actor to share their data by either selling it or giving it for free (Smichowski, 2019). There is not much information available on such a model in the healthcare sector. Considering the nature of the requested data in this case, this would be only feasible if e.g., the government needs the patient data to prevent and control an outbreak. Thus, this model requires a significant legal change or the application of existing laws to data, which can bring difficulties (Smichowski, 2019). The legal requirements behind such a scenario are beyond the scope of this article and the differences between countries are anyways too large to cover them all here. The data requisition model is a model which can be used in extraordinary circumstances but not as part of usual, everyday scenarios concerning health data.

Collective Bargaining on Rights over Personal Data

This model refers to data that has a relational value as a result of insights that can be gained from the data of many users on a platform collectively, as opposed to using the data of a single user only (Smichowski, 2019). Some examples include huge platforms like e.g., Facebook, Airbnb, or Uber (Smichowski, 2019). Users can therefore use their collective bargaining power, as the name suggests, to demand rights over their data. This is a model that also requires significant legal changes. Smichowski (2019) writes that versions of such models are starting to emerge, and users organise themselves to collectively act against a platform. Aside from the article by Smichowski, we did not find any specific example of this model in the healthcare sector. It is related to the data commons model but in that case, patients keep their rights over their data. Thus, it could apply in the case of other types of patient platforms, where people share health-related information and receive some type of service, for example, forums, chats with other patients, data visualisation services, etc. An example of such a platform could be "Patients like me" (see under Data Trusts).

Data Pooling

Data pools have been suggested by both Smichowski (2019) and Micheli et al. (2020). Most recently, Schneider (2022) discusses health data pools under European law in detail in her book on the subject. Simply put, in this model, several stakeholders (public or private) unite their data sources to fill knowledge gaps or to gain economic benefit by producing data-driven innovations – products or services (Micheli et al., 2020). According to Smichowski (2019) we can distinguish between open and closed data pools. In the open data pools, data remain open, while closed data pools cannot make their data publicly available. In the case of healthcare, closed data pools are more appropriate as data are sensitive.

The examples in Table 5.3 show that usually, health data pools have been formed by a major tech company and a healthcare stakeholder – a hospital or pharmaceutical company. There are important advantages and positive aspects of health data pools. The most important ones are faster and more cost-effective progress in scientific research, which in turn leads to speedier release of new health-related products and services, ultimately contributing to patients enjoying better health (Schneider, 2022).

Key issues with this model are related to the difficulty of setting stable rules regarding data ownership and liability (Borgogno & Colangelo, 2019; Schneider, 2022). By aiming to get maximum value by combining different data silos, while at the same time using the same proprietary schemes used by the data silos effectively, these newly formed data pools are just a form of collaborative data silos forbidding access to anyone not part of this collaboration (Schneider, 2022). From a technical point of view, Smichowski (2019) mentions the need for technical standards to share data.

In general terms and not specifically in healthcare, according to Smichowski (2019) data pools are the most popular emerging data governance models. In healthcare, especially in terms of research, the potential for innovation is much higher when various stakeholders join forces instead of everyone relying on the data they own only. So far data pools are a governance model with high potential in healthcare. Even the World Health Organisation has acknowledged that "the isolation that often-characterised traditional health actors has become impossible to sustain" (WHO cited by Schneider, 2022, p. 48). Regarding the technical issues, a new trend in machine learning and AI, federated learning, offers several advantages to overcome not only the technical challenges of data pools but also challenges related to ownership. With federated learning, the data remains in the owner's data silo, a machine learning model is trained locally and then the insights are combined by all separate silos, without the need to move data to a new location. For more information on the potentials and challenges of federated learning in healthcare, we recommend the study by Rieke et al. (2020).

Data Trusts

The data trust model is a participatory governance model with the goal of sharing data in a secure and fair way by making trustworthy decisions on who has access to data, the conditions for such access as well as who can benefit from the data (Milne, Sorbie, & Dixon-Woods, 2022). Usually, there is at least one stakeholder who would take over the role of a trustee and is responsible for determining how data should be used i.e., who the beneficiaries are - those who provide the data along with other stakeholders (Milne et al., 2022). The trustee may or may not be a beneficiary themselves. The Open Data Institute has defined a data trust as "a legal structure that provides independent third-party stewardship of data" (Hardinges, 2018).

Public data trusts are a type of data trust in which public actors (e.g., a governmental organisation) access and use data about its citizens, including data owned by private companies with which a relationship of trust is established (Micheli et al., 2020). This is opposed to the data requisition model where a public actor, by means of an established legal framework, can demand a private company to sell or donate their data in the interest of the public. This type of trust is limited to small pilot projects (Micheli et al., 2020), and we have not found an example in the healthcare sector.

We have found two ongoing research projects specifically on healthcare data trusts. Two researchers from the University of Warwick and Melbourne are currently investigating how data trusts could be operationalised as a governance model for longitudinal health studies, especially involving children (Data Trusts Initiative, 2022). In Germany, the Fraunhofer ISST is working on a project to find the best governance model involving radiology data (Fraunhofer ISST, 2022).

For the healthcare sector, experts suggest that there are strong incentives for establishing multiple trusts, each representing the interests of a particular group of stakeholders (Element AI & Nesta, 2019). As this could either limit the value of data or make the data sharing difficult because of the potentially different trusts' terms, the establishment of "meta trusts" has also been mentioned as a possibility. In such case "a health-focused trust that would negotiate with a variety of smaller, generalist trusts to pull together a larger dataset while complying with the terms of each individual trust" (Element AI & Nesta, 2019, pp. 24–25). This model is still evolving and will benefit from a rigorous evaluation (Milne et al., 2022).

Data Marketplaces and Personal Data Sovereignty (PDS)

Both models refer to the same terms of a governance model. On the one hand, such a governance model is about giving more rights and power back into the hands of those who produce the data i.e., the patients. The goal is a fairer data economy where value is created by increasing the self-determination and knowledge of the data creators while simultaneously creating a new ecosystem of services to support them (Micheli et al., 2020).

On the other hand, this model has several important limitations related to a) people not being aware of platforms used for personal gain or simply not having the time to consider the different options offered by such platforms; b) not questioning the commodification of data i.e., they do not serve any specific public good (Micheli et al., 2020), and c) considering the examples in Table 5.3, it is not clear what rights exactly users have in terms of e.g., re-negotiating the price or who has the power to decide on how valuable data are (Kariotis et al., 2020).

Based on all the discussions presented so far around data ownership and considering the rest of the presented data governance models, a model with the sole purpose of data monetisation does not seem to be the best way forward, especially concerning health-related data. Besides, there are many indications that patients are willing to share their data for advancing research and innovation. For instance, Banner (2020) cites an advocate from a patient group as saying: "*It may not help me but may help others … . It could save future generations from suffering some of the diseases in today's world*".

DISCUSSION

According to our analysis, the most promising models of data governance in health data are data commons (cooperatives), data pools, and data trusts. In fact, Micheli et al. (2020) identify data commons as bottom-up data trusts based on their working mechanisms. To make it more understandable, we have presented an overview in Figure 5.2.

In Figure 5.2, there is a dashed line between data trusts and data pools. The reason for this is that when discussing data trusts, one makes a point of e.g., patients pooling their data together in a trust. So, one could say that theoretically, data pools are also a type of data trust. However, considering the definitions of data pools and data trusts in the previous section, it does not seem entirely correct to place data pools under data trusts, as pools have been defined as models with a major focus on economic benefit from the shared data. In contrast, trusts are formed around the idea of sharing data to advance research and innovation i.e., to provide value for the public good (Element AI & Nesta, 2019; Micheli et al., 2020). And lastly, Micheli et al., (2020) (citing Delacroix & Lawrence, 2019, p. 242) also write that there is no consensus on whether data pools can be "assimilated to actual legal trust structures or a "marketing tool" facilitating the responsible sharing of data".

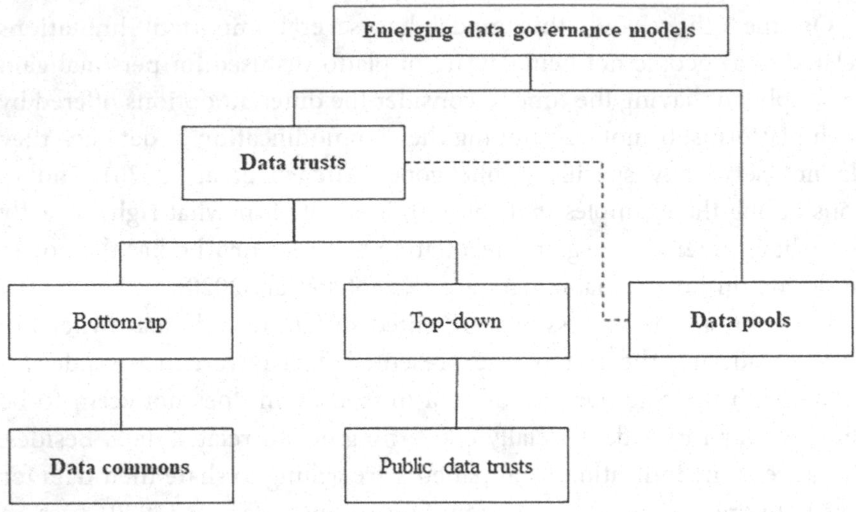

FIGURE 5.2 Relationship between the identified emerging governance models in healthcare. Figure by the author.

In terms of inner workings, as mentioned previously, trusts have a third party, the trustee, responsible for establishing trust between all parties involved and are based on an established legal framework. Thus, trusts generally seem to offer the best of both worlds – data being owned by the data providers and gaining value for all parties involved while following ethical and other human rights principles. In fact, if we consider Figure 5.2, the conclusion is that the most prominent data governance model in healthcare is data trust.

CONCLUSION AND FUTURE RESEARCH

Based on our research, there is an urgent need for new data governance models which will respect the rights of those who are providing or creating the data i.e., the patients. However, in the healthcare sector, more than in other domains, it is significantly more challenging to establish models that would give more rights to the patients but at the same time ensure security, privacy, compliance with ethics, and human rights, while driving innovation forward. There are many stakeholders each with their own interests concerning how data are handled, and complex law regulations which differ between countries. The core of all these concerns seems to be the difficulty surrounding ownership of health data. There are inherent limits to an ownership approach of data – "at most, data ownership confers the kind of access rights that are similar to water rights" (Element AI & Nesta, 2019, p. 13). Data sharing especially for research purposes is giving rise to a "free movement" of research data which is encouraged by the European Strategy for Data (Schneider, 2022).

Considering the examples in the previous section, there is an overall tendency towards models that make patients owners of their data. Our findings show that data trusts are the way forward. This type of model addresses several of the challenges around data governance – a) citizens not being consulted on their data; b) use of data systems which are seen as trustworthy by the citizens; c) one size does not fit all – governance should be flexible and adjustable to local needs; d) people and stakeholders should be brought together to discuss challenges (WHO, 2021a).

In terms of future research directions, we recommend a more in-depth exploration of the distinct types of data trusts, applied in diverse scenarios, and involving different types of stakeholders, private or public. There are several existing platforms which act as trustees even though are not specifically mentioned as such (Kariotis et al., 2020). Therefore, it would be of benefit to research them in-depth by, for instance, using a case study analysis method or a mixed method approach with interviews.

NOTE

1. Search for "data governance" with parameters: worldwide, 2004 – present, all categories on 04.01.2023.

REFERENCES

Abraham, R., Schneider, J., & vom Brocke, J. (2019). Data governance: A conceptual framework, structured review, and research agenda. *International Journal of Information Management*, 49, 424–438. 10.1016/j.ijinfomgt.2019.07.008

Asswad, J., & Marx Gómez, J. (2021). Data ownership: A survey. *Information*, 12(11), 465. 10.3390/info12110465

Banner, N. F. (2020). The human side of health data. *Nature Medicine*, 26(7), 995. 10.1038/s41591-020-0838-z

Borgogno, O., & Colangelo, G. (2019). Data sharing and interoperability: Fostering innovation and competition through APIs. *Computer Law & Security Review*, 35(5), 105314. 10.1016/j.clsr.2019.03.008

Couture, N. (2019). Data governance – Proving value: How exactly does data governance make a difference? *CIO*. Retrieved from https://www.cio.com/article/220011/data-governance-proving-value.html

Data Trusts Initiative (2022). How can legal mechanisms associated with data trusts enhance participation in healthcare research? [Press release]. Retrieved from https://datatrusts.uk/trusts-in-health-research

Delacroix, S., & Lawrence, N. D. (2019). Bottom-up Data Trusts: disturbing the 'one size fits all' approach to data governance. *International Data Privacy Law*. Advance online publication. 10.1093/idpl/ipz014

Do, N., Grossman, R., Feldman, T., Fillmore, N., Elbers, D., Tuck, D., …Brophy, M. (2019). The veterans precision oncology data commons: Transforming VA data into a national resource for research in precision oncology. *Seminars in Oncology*, 46(4-5), 314–320. 10.1053/j.seminoncol.2019.09.002

Element AI, & Nesta (2019). Data Trusts: A new tool for data governance. *White paper*.

European Commission (2022). *Estonia in the Digital Economy and Society Index [Press release]*. Retrieved from https://digital-strategy.ec.europa.eu/en/policies/desi-estonia

European Commission (2023). Data protection in the EU: The General Data Protection Regulation (GDPR), the Data Protection Law Enforcement Directive and other rules concerning the protection of personal data. [Press release]. Retrieved from https://commission.europa.eu/law/law-topic/data-protection/data-protection-eu_en

Evans, B. J. (2016). Barbarians at the gate: Consumer-driven health Data Commons and the transformation of citizen science. *American Journal of Law & Medicine*, 42(4), 651–685. 10.1177/0098858817700245

Fraunhofer ISST (2022). DaRe: Health DAta trust REallaboratory to develop and test ecosystem integration of data-driven health research [Press release]. Retrieved from https://www.isst.fraunhofer.de/en/business-units/healthcare/projects/DaRe.html

Hafen, E., Kossmann, D., & Brand, A. (2014). Health data cooperatives - citizen empowerment. *Methods of Information in Medicine*, 53(2), 82–86. 10.3414/ME13-02-0051

Hardinges, J. (2018). *Defining a 'data trust'*. Retrieved from Open Data Institute website: https://theodi.org/article/defining-a-data-trust/

Janssen, M., Brous, P., Estevez, E., Barbosa, L. S., & Janowski, T. (2020). Data governance: Organizing data for trustworthy Artificial Intelligence. *Government Information Quarterly*, 37(3), 101493. 10.1016/j.giq.2020.101493

Jensen, M. A., Ferretti, V., Grossman, R. L., & Staudt, L. M. (2017). The NCI Genomic Data Commons as an engine for precision medicine. *Blood*, 130(4), 453–459. 10.1182/blood-2017-03-735654

Kariotis, T., Ball, M. P., Greshake Tzovaras, B., Dennis, S., Sahama, T., Johnston, C., … Borda, A. (2020). Emerging health data platforms: From individual control to collective data governance. *Data & Policy*, 2. 10.1017/dap.2020.14

Liddell, K., Simon, D. A., & Lucassen, A. (2021). Patient data ownership: Who owns your health? *Journal of Law and the Biosciences*, 8(2), lsab023. 10.1093/jlb/lsab023

Martani, A., Geneviève, L. D., Elger, B., & Wangmo, T. (2021). It's not something you can take in your hands. *Swiss experts' perspectives on health data ownership: an interview-based study. BMJ Open*, 11(4), e045717. 10.1136/bmjopen-2020-045717

Micheli, M., Ponti, M., Craglia, M., & Berti Suman, A. (2020). Emerging models of data governance in the age of datafication. *Big Data & Society*, 7(2), 205395172094808. 10.1177/2053951720948087

Milne, R., Sorbie, A., & Dixon-Woods, M. (2022). What can data trusts for health research learn from participatory governance in biobanks? *Journal of Medical Ethics*, 48(5), 323. 10.1136/medethics-2020-107020

Mirchev, M., Mircheva, I., & Kerekovska, A. (2020). The academic viewpoint on patient data ownership in the context of big data: Scoping review. *Journal of Medical Internet Research*, 22(8), e22214. 10.2196/22214

Nodus Labs. *InfraNodus [Computer software]*. Retrieved from https://infranodus.com

Praduroux, S. (2017). Objects of property rights: old and new. In M. Graziadei & L. Smith (Eds.), *Comparative Property Law* (pp. 51–70). Edward Elgar Publishing. 10.4337/9781785369162.00011

Priisalu, J., & Ottis, R. (2017). Personal control of privacy and data: Estonian experience. *Health and Technology*, 7(4), 441–451. 10.1007/s12553-017-0195-1

Reddy, S., Allan, S., Coghlan, S., & Cooper, P. (2020). A governance model for the application of AI in health care. *Journal of the American Medical Informatics Association: JAMIA*, 27(3), 491–497. 10.1093/jamia/ocz192

Rieke, N., Hancox, J., Li, W., Milletarì, F., Roth, H. R., Albarqouni, S., … Cardoso, M. J. (2020). The future of digital health with federated learning. *NPJ Digital Medicine*, 3, 119. 10.1038/s41746-020-00323-1

Sabherwal, R., & Becerra-Fernandez, I. (2011). *Business intelligence: Practices, technologies, and management*. Hoboken, NJ: John Wiley & Sons Inc.

Scandurra, I., Jansson, A., Forsberg-Fransson, M.-L., & Ålander, T. (2015). Is 'patient's online access to health records' a good reform? – Opinions from Swedish healthcare professionals differ. *Procedia Computer Science*, 64, 964–968. 10.1016/j.procs.2015.08.614

Schneider, G. (2022). *Health data pools under European Data Protection and Competition Law* (Vol. 17). Cham: Springer International Publishing. 10.1007/978-3-030-95427-7

Shapiro, M., Johnston, D., Wald, J., & Mon, D. (2012). Patient-generated health data. *White paper*. Retrieved from RTI website: https://www.rti.org/publication/patient-generated-health-data-white-paper/fulltext.pdf

Smichowski, B. C. (2019). Alternative data governance models: Moving beyond one-size-fits-all solutions. *Intereconomics*, 54(4), 222–227. 10.1007/s10272-019-0828-x

WHO (2021a). Health data governance summit: Meeting report. Retrieved from https://cdn.who.int/media/docs/default-source/world-health-data-platform/events/health-data-governance-summit/summit-report_final.pdf?sfvrsn=1c6ff885_8&download=true

WHO (2021b). Health data governance summit: Pre-read: Health data as a global public good. Retrieved from https://cdn.who.int/media/docs/default-source/world-health-data-platform/events/health-data-governance-summit/preread-2-who-data-governance-summit_health-data-as-a-public-good.pdf?sfvrsn=2d1e3ad8_8

World Economic Forum (2011). Personal data: The emergence of a new asset class. Retrieved from https://www.weforum.org/reports/personal-data-emergence-new-asset-class

CHAPTER 6

Privacy-Preserving Roadmap for Medical Data-Sharing Systems

Belal Alsinglawi and Nilmini Wickramasinghe

INTRODUCTION

AI and technological innovations have revolutionised the healthcare sector by improving patient care, personalising medical care, improving diagnostics, and accelerating drug discovery. Medical imaging and diagnostics are two areas of medical computing where AI-based solutions can surpass healthcare professionals in practice. For enhanced quality and performance, AI-based medical applications such as medical imaging require a considerable amount of training data with accurate labelling, also called "ground truth". In response to this demand, medical AI researchers, research laboratories, and medical institutions specialising in data curation and annotation have started providing medical annotation for emerging AI solutions and services in medical contexts. These requirements include the privacy and security of patients, as well as the ability of AI-based predictive models to perform specific AI tasks aimed at improving patients' health outcomes and improving medical and healthcare services. (Huang et al., 2020). For sustainable AI-medical applications, however, many steps must be taken to show the potential of AI models in healthcare and medical settings. Steps must be taken to show the actual potential of AI models in healthcare and medical environments to construct sustainable AI systems. In order for AI models to be deployed in medical data-sharing systems, AI models must be trustworthy, resistant to bias and uncertainty, preserve patients' safety

DOI: 10.1201/9781032699745-8

and privacy, be secure against cybersecurity threats, accomplish justice, be able to show models' explainability, and achieve the legal, ethical, and AI-governance requirements. In medical contexts, these factors are subject to the application of artificial intelligence. (Ghallab, 2019), identifies these characteristics as "responsible AI". Before incorporating AI-based solutions into digital healthcare information systems, we must meet the privacy, security, and trust needs of individual (e.g., patient) data. This phase of responsible AI is believed to be crucial for creating sustainable AI-medical applications in healthcare, public health, and medical practice and demonstrating its potent capacity to improve well-being, healthcare decision-making, and patient health outcomes.

The availability of large-scale data for model training and optimisation is necessary for developing AI solutions that are both reproducible and practical in health situations, according to (Diaz et al., 2021). In contrast, despite the conventional acquisition of vast amounts of health and medical imaging data in healthcare settings, access to big data in medical contexts generates major hurdles between varied healthcare providers on data-sharing platforms due to patient privacy concerns (Tariq & Hackert, 2018). This is due to the fact that there are numerous health services involved (such as community hospitals, medical centres, hospital emergency departments, and pathology labs, among others). Researchers established a great interest in the medical data and medical images (e.g., CT scans, MRIs, ultrasounds, etc.) collected from a variety of health services. Given the movement of data across digital medical systems and their vulnerability to hackers and malicious activities, sharing data in decentralised medical systems while maintaining privacy presents a significant challenge for AI-mediated applications. AI models and shared data are vulnerable to online misconduct, hacking, or any other cyber-criminal act, resulting in the inseparable nature of medical resources when accessed via the internet. If cyber attackers are able to gain access to medical data-sharing systems and medical imaging data, for instance, they will be able to change, alter, or manipulate medical and imaging data, (Ali & Alyounis, 2021). As a result, the entire process in medical data-sharing systems will be jeopardised, potentially leading to an incorrect patient diagnosis or having a serious impact on the patient's health and a negative impact on healthcare medical institutes. This necessitates the investigation of research-doable, scientific, and experimental approaches to reveal the power of information technology advancement in the era of health digitisation in favour of provisioning for scalable and secure data-sharing systems to evolve as well as provide successful means for healthcare AI-based applications that are responsible, safe, trustworthy, and secure to be utilised and operated through the heterogeneous data-sharing systems within dynamic healthcare providers.

In this work, and in particular, in Section 2, we study cyber security problems that impede the scalability of medical data-sharing platforms in the interest of patient privacy, trustworthiness, and enhanced healthcare outcomes. First, we explore the state of the medical data-sharing systems by looking at the interoperability components for preserving patients' privacy and security. Then, we identify security elements and analyse cyber threats that impede medical data-sharing systems' scalability and technical interoperability. Section 3 discusses the current privacy-preserving paradigms in medical data-sharing systems. In Section 4, we discuss the research opportunities and future research directions that serve the goals for realising medical data-sharing systems. Finally, the conclusion section summarises the contribution of this study.

THE STATE OF MEDICAL DATA-SHARING SYSTEMS

The Medical Data-Sharing Systems: Interoperability Components for Preserving Patients' Privacy and Security

Technical interoperability is the cornerstone of all data-sharing systems. Technical interoperability (Figure 6.1) enables data interchange between interoperable medical data-sharing systems (Lehne et al., 2019). For instance, transferring data from medical practice to the cloud for data analytics or exchanging medical imaging results between a medical

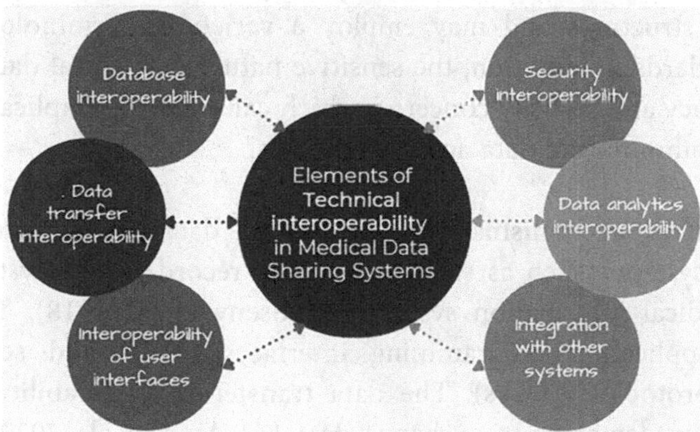

FIGURE 6.1 Interoperability components for preserving patients' privacy and security.

facility and a hospital. Data transmission involves communication channels, security, and exchange procedures. Depending on the data-sharing paradigm, attaining technical interoperability with today's digital networks and communication protocols is usually either relatively simple or complex. However, straightforwardness in transferring data from a source to a target is suboptimal. To process the data and extract useful information, it is necessary to achieve data security, and users' privacy and comprehend the technological interoperability components involved. Consequently, it is essential to evaluate technical interoperability and its associated threats. The subsequent sections examine the components of medical data-sharing systems in relation to technical interoperability and the accompanying cyber threats.

Medical data-sharing systems generally include a database for data storage, a mechanism for transferring data between systems, and a user interface for accessing and managing data. The following are the primary elements of medical data-sharing systems that contribute to the realisation of technical interoperability:

Database: This is the centralised repository for all medical data (Johnson et al., 2020). It may be hosted on a local server, edge servers, decentralised infrastructure, or in the cloud and is often arranged so that data owners manage retrieval and maintenance of the data.

- Database interoperability in medical data-sharing (Al Asad et al., 2020) systems signifies the ability of various databases to communicate and exchange information. This is a complicated task due to the fact that medical data is frequently stored in a variety of forms and structures and may employ a variety of terminologies and standards. In addition, the sensitive nature of medical data creates privacy and security concerns, which can further complicate efforts to communicate data across platforms.

Data transfer mechanisms: This is where the data is transmitted across digitised systems, such as electronic health record (EHR) systems and other medical information systems (Elhoseny et al., 2018). This may involve application programming interfaces (APIs) and secure file transfer protocols (SFTPs). The data transfer interoperability mechanisms allow databases to exchange data (Al Asad et al., 2020). By establishing a standard method for databases to communicate and share data, these techniques can help overcome the technological obstacles of interoperability. Common interoperability protocols for data transfer in medical data exchange include the following:

I. APIs (Application Programming Interfaces) are protocols and technologies that enable software programs to communicate with each other. In the context of medical data sharing (Dullabh et al., 2020), APIs can facilitate the standard interchange of information between databases.

II. HL7 (Health Level Seven) (Baskaya et al., 2019) is an international collection of standards for exchanging, integrating, and sharing electronic health information. It establishes a standard framework for the layout and formatting of medical data, as well as a standard set of terminology and codes. Using HL7, databases may communicate with one another and share data in a standard and consistent manner.

III. FHIR (Fast Healthcare Interoperability Resources) (Baskaya et al., 2019) is a more recent collection of interchange standards for electronic health information. It builds upon HL7 and employs contemporary web technology and data formats to facilitate faster and more efficient data transfer.

Therefore, interoperability strategies can aid in overcoming the technological obstacles of data sharing and enable databases to exchange information successfully. This can enhance the quality and accessibility of medical data, thereby facilitating improved decision-making and care delivery. Consequently, assessing the appropriate data transfer interoperability mechanisms while considering protocol-related challenges in the context of medical data-sharing systems and paying attention to users' privacy and security is deemed an important research task.

User interface: Medical staff utilise the interface to obtain and manage the data (Huckvale et al., 2019). Typically, it is a web-based programme that enables healthcare staff users to view, search, and alter data in a variety of ways. Also, medical data mobile apps allow patients to interact with their personal health information and further interact with medical professionals for more healthcare assistance, such as telemedicine and remote health monitoring, managing patients' appointments and bookings, and many more.

The interoperability of user interfaces (Gohar et al., 2022) ensures the capacity of multiple user interfaces (UIs) to communicate and exchange information efficiently. This is significant in the context of medical data sharing because it enables various systems to present data in a uniform and user-friendly way and allows users to access and interact with data across systems.

User interface interoperability is significant from a privacy and security standpoint since it can help ensure that only authorised personnel can access sensitive medical information.

Using standard authentication mechanisms and access controls, for instance, various user interfaces (UIs) can authenticate users' identities and guarantee that they have the proper permissions to view and interact with data. This can prevent unauthorised access to sensitive information and safeguard patients' privacy. Moreover, user interface interoperability can facilitate data communication between systems in a secure environment. Numerous UIs can ensure that data is protected during transit and cannot be intercepted or altered by unauthorised persons, for instance, by employing encryption and other security measures. Consequently, Interoperability of user interfaces is crucial for the usability and security of medical data-sharing systems. User interface interoperability can help improve the effectiveness and security of medical data-sharing by facilitating consistent and user-friendly data access and by providing secure transmission and access controls.

Security features: In some instances, medical data exchange platforms may contain security elements to protect the privacy and integrity of the data (Nguyen et al., 2019). This may involve the encryption of data in transit and at rest, as well as authentication and access control measures to restrict data access. Interoperability amongst security features (Jabbar et al., 2020) is necessary in order to prevent unauthorised access to sensitive medical information. By permitting various systems to interact and share information together, risks and vulnerabilities can be mitigated, and data can be safeguarded from prospective attackers. For instance, if one system detects a security breach, it can notify other systems and prevent the attacker from accessing data. Additionally, the compatibility of security features can facilitate the secure exchange of data between systems.

Using encryption and other security measures, for instance, various systems can ensure that data is protected during transmission and cannot be intercepted or modified by unauthorised persons. Hence, security features and interoperability are vital for safeguarding sensitive medical information in data-sharing systems. By enabling coordinated and effective security measures, security feature interoperability can assist in preserving the patient's privacy and ensure their security in medical data systems, as well as enabling the safe and effective sharing of information.

Data analytics and visualisation tools: Some systems for sharing medical data may also include tools for analysing and visualising the data (Goldman et al., 2020), quantifying the data, and curating the data. This may include statistical analysis tools, graphical data visualisations, and the ability to generate customised medical and healthcare reports for medical data-sharing system users. Data analytics and visualisation interoperability (Jin et al., 2019) in sharing medical data are essential for the privacy and security of patients; therefore, it enables healthcare organisations to govern who gets access to sensitive medical data. Only authorised employees, such as healthcare professionals and other authorised personnel, can view, analyse, annotate, curate, and visualise the data.

Data analytics interoperability can help ensure data is represented appropriately and uniformly across all systems and applications, especially in federated learning systems (discussed in section 4). This can help in preventing errors and misunderstandings, which is particularly vital in the medical field. In addition, interoperability can enable the adoption of secure protocols and encryption to prevent unauthorised access to the data. This can prohibit unauthorised parties from viewing or accessing the data, thereby protecting the privacy and security of the patients. As a result, data analytics and visualisation interoperability is a crucial part of medical data sharing and can aid in enhancing the precision and efficacy of healthcare decision-making while preserving patients' privacy and security.

Integration with other systems: In many instances, medical data-sharing systems are meant to be coupled with other systems, such as electronic health records (EHR) or information management systems with healthcare government systems, supply chain and microservices, and IoT systems (Tang et al., 2019), and other forms of integrable systems. This enables the seamless interchange of data between systems, which can enhance the overall efficiency and efficacy of the healthcare data-sharing system. Thus, compatibility with other systems Interoperability in sharing medical data (Soni & Singh, 2021) is essential for patients because it enables a more comprehensive view of their medical records. This can assist healthcare providers in making more informed decisions regarding their patient's care and help patients better understand their own health and medical situations. For instance, if a patient's medical information is maintained in various interoperable systems, such as an EHR system and a laboratory information management system, interoperability enables these systems to interchange data. This means that a healthcare provider may access all pertinent data in a single location rather than switching between several systems to obtain a comprehensive view of a patient's health. In addition, interoperability is significant in terms of the privacy and security of patients since it enables healthcare organisations to restrict access to sensitive medical data and ensure that only authorised individuals may view and evaluate the data. This can be accomplished by employing secure protocols and encryption, which prohibit unwanted data access. Integration with other systems, or interoperability, is a crucial part of medical data sharing, and it can enhance the precision and efficacy of healthcare decision-making for the benefit of patients.

Obtaining consensus on how technical interoperability may be reached amongst relevant parties and maintained within the intelligence community is one of the most challenging components in data-sharing ecosystems in the medical and healthcare context. This entails having a consistent understanding of what information is shared, how it is shared, and if its sharing is lawful. Therefore, understanding security and privacy elements and analysing cyber threats connected to interoperability challenges are deemed important research tasks in the cybersecurity information-sharing ecosystem. The following section analyses the security and privacy-related requirements and then discusses the cyber threats hindering the sustainable medical data-sharing system and, therefore, interoperable technical systems.

SECURITY ELEMENTS AND CYBER THREATS IN DATA-SHARING SYSTEMS

Cybersecurity threats and sources of cyberattacks in data-sharing systems are triggered by communication heterogeneity, mechanisms, and interactions between different data-sharing layers (Alsinglawi et al., 2022). Thus, we are motivated to investigate first the security aspects and classify cybersecurity attacks based on security issues identified in the literature. Then, we explore these potential vulnerabilities to the security of data-sharing systems and relate them to their presence in the correspondent data-sharing system layers.

The literature (Chenthara et al., 2019), (Fatima et al., 2022) and (Ghonge et al., 2023) examined the data-sharing systems from security elements. The following are unanimous that were studied in the literature:

- **Privacy:** Protecting personal information and data from unauthorised access or use is a crucial feature of data-sharing platforms. However, privacy problems may occur when exchanging sensitive data with third parties, such as cloud service providers or via connected micro-services with other organisations in the context of data-sharing platforms.
- **Trust** is an essential component of data-sharing systems since it refers to individuals' and organisations' confidence in the system's security and dependability. In the context of data-sharing systems, trust may be associated with the data's confidentiality, integrity, and availability.
- **Authenticity** is the ability to confirm that data is genuine and has not been altered. Importantly, ensuring the authenticity of data helps prevent the spread of false or misleading information and preserves the data's integrity.
- **Confidentiality** refers to the protection of sensitive or private data against unauthorised access or exposure. It is a crucial component of data security and privacy since it ensures that only authorised individuals or systems can access sensitive data.
- **Integrity** in data-sharing systems refers to the precision and exhaustiveness of the exchanged data. It is essential to preserve the integrity of data so that it may be relied upon and trusted for decision-making and other purposes.
- **Availability** entails the ability of authorised users to obtain the data they require when they require it. It is crucial to ensure data availability since it enables users to complete their tasks and make decisions using the most recent and correct information. There are numerous approaches to guaranteeing the availability of data in a system for data sharing. Utilising redundant systems and backup procedures can prevent data loss in the event of a system breakdown or other problems. Using load balancing and other techniques to distribute the workload over several systems is another method for ensuring that data is available even during peak load.
- **Non-repudiation** in data-sharing systems signifies the ability to demonstrate that a particular action or event occurred and was performed by a particular individual or system. Giving a precise

record of who did what, when, and how, can help eliminate disagreements and misunderstandings. Non-repudiation is a crucial component of data security and trust in data-sharing systems. It ensures that activities and occurrences can be precisely recorded and traced, which is essential for legal and regulatory purposes and for settling disputes or misunderstandings.

Table 6.1 presents the security aspects of data-sharing. The table below discusses the description of the aspects. Then it provides examples of cyberattacks that present a serious threat to each aspect of the data-sharing components. Finally, it describes the impact of these different types of cyberattacks and relevant studies in the scope of each security aspect.

CYBER THREATS IN DATA-SHARING SYSTEMS

Cybercriminals are increasingly focusing their attention on medical data exchange platforms, such as electronic health record (EHR) systems. These cyberattacks can have serious repercussions, including the theft of sensitive patient information and the disruption of crucial healthcare services. We pinpoint some of the most prevalent cyberattacks that threaten medical data exchange systems, as discussed below:

Ransomware attacks: an attacker gains unauthorised access to a healthcare system and encrypts data, preventing authorised users from accessing it. The attacker demands a ransom payment in exchange for the decryption key (Wazid et al., 2022). One of the main consequences of a ransomware attack on medical data-sharing systems is the disruption of ordinary data interchange between healthcare organisations. This might result in delays in the exchange of vital medical information related to vulnerable patients, which in certain situations can have dire repercussions. For instance, if a healthcare organisation's data-sharing system is compromised by ransomware, the exchange of vital patient's pathology results could be delayed, which could have severe ramifications for patient care. A ransomware attack can compromise the security of shared data in addition to disrupting the normal flow of data transmission. If the attacker has access to and can encrypt the data, it may be conceivable for them to see

TABLE 6.1 Data Sharing and Security Aspects and Their Possible Types of Attacks

Security Aspect	Description	Example of Attacks	Impact	Studies
Privacy	User protection from unauthorised access to other users' information	• The attack on healthcare physical infrastructure. • The masquerade Attack • Replay Attack	• Information leaks can provide attackers access to infrastructure and production data • Putting the privacy of the system at risk (Compromising the privacy of the system) • Vandalism or theft may result from a possible violation of privacy.	(Ferrag et al., 2020; Idoje et al., 2021)
Trust	An attacker cannot spoof another user's identity.	• Ransomware • Cyber-terrorism • Indirection Attacks • Botnets • Cloud attacks	• Data-sharing systems cannot automatically establish trust with one another.	(Melara & Bowman, 2021; Zhang & Jiang, 2021)
Authenticity	It prevents users from spoofing other identities.	• Cloud attacks • Ransomware • Cyber-terrorism • Indirection Attacks	• Data breach • loss of data • Data alteration • Service unavailability • Loss of device connectivity • Systems corruption and destruction	(Ferrag et al., 2020; Nesarani et al., 2020)
Confidentiality	It protects data from unauthorised access	• Tracing Attack • Brute Force Attack	• loss of privacy • Loss of data/information breaches	(Ametepe et al., 2019; Yu et al., 2012)

(Continued)

TABLE 6.1 (Continued) Data Sharing and Security Aspects and Their Possible Types of Attacks

Security Aspect	Description	Example of Attacks	Impact	Studies
			• the access to confidential information	
Integrity	Ensures that information will not be altered during storage or transmission.	• Man-In-The-Middle Attack (MITM) • Trojan Horse Attack • Biometric • Botnets • False Data Injection • Data Fabrication	• Lead to unreliable or inaccurate information in data-sharing systems. • Possible financial or authentication frauds.	(Chamarajnagar & Ashok, 2019; Davcev et al., 2018)
Availability	Ensures continuity of the services provided.	• Denial of Service (DoS) attacks • Attacks on devices, networks and hardware. • Attacks on Software	• Business disruption and downtimes. • Possible loss of customers/clients. • Loss of confidence and revenue. • affect business reputation.	(Bisogni et al., 2011; Ferrag et al., 2020)
Non-Repudiation	It prevents users from repudiating their actions when using the system.	• Repudiation Attack • Malicious Code • Attacks on computers and equipment.	• Granting the power to attackers, which leads to the refusal of data transmissions, authentication information or services within the systems' nodes	(Ferrag et al., 2020; Holkar et al., 2013)

or modify the healthcare patients' critical data. This could result in a loss of confidence in the data's authenticity, as there is no way to confirm that the data has not been hacked.

Ransomware attacks hinder database interoperability (Hagen et al., 2018); hence, ransomware attacks can have severe effects on databases and servers. For instance, one of the prominent reasons ransomware attacks affect databases and servers is by encrypting the stored medical data on these systems. This may prevent users from accessing the data and make it difficult or impossible for a healthcare organisation to recover the data without paying a ransom. In some instances, ransomware attacks can prohibit users from accessing information held on databases and servers. This can have serious consequences, particularly if the data is critical to the operations of healthcare and medical institutions. One of the most significant effects of ransomware attacks is the harm they inflict on healthcare systems, which can result in increased expenses and interruptions for healthcare organisation. This may include damage to hardware, software, or other system components. Last but not least, ransomware attacks can trigger a loss of trust in the healthcare system and the information it stores. This can be especially detrimental to businesses that rely on the confidence of their consumers or clients, as it can result in a loss of business or credibility.

A phishing attack is when an attacker sends a victim a fraudulent email or message while posing as a legitimate source, such as receiving a parcel in the mailbox, bank account updates, or healthcare provider notifications (Abdelhamid, 2020). Typically, the message comprises a link or file that, when clicked, downloads malware on the user's device. Phishing attacks can have serious impacts on data-sharing systems. Some of the ways that phishing attacks can affect these systems include: compromised user accounts, where phishing attacks often involve tricking users into revealing their login credentials or other sensitive information. If a user falls victim to a phishing attack, their account on a medical data-sharing system could be compromised, allowing the attacker to access the system and potentially the data stored on it. Phishing attacks can also be used to deliver malware to a user's computer or device. If a user falls victim to a phishing attack and downloads the malware, it could spread to other systems, including data-sharing systems, potentially infecting those systems as well. Disruption of operations: Phishing attacks can disrupt the normal flow of operations on data-sharing systems. This can occur if users are unable to access their accounts due to a compromised password or if the system itself is infected with malware. Loss of trust: Phishing attacks can also lead to a loss of trust in the data-sharing system. If users are concerned that their accounts have been compromised or that the system itself is not secure, they may be less likely to trust the data being shared. API-based phishing attacks (Aonzo et al., 2018) are a type of phishing attack that targets the application programming interfaces that organisations use to facilitate communication and data exchange across different systems. An API-based phishing attack involves the attacker sending a bogus request to the API in order to gain unauthorised access to sensitive data or compromise the system. API-based phishing attempts can wreak havoc on data-sharing platforms, especially when the API is used to access and exchange sensitive data. In medical data-sharing systems, API interoperability is hampered by API-based phishing attacks. As a result, healthcare organisations should implement strong cybersecurity measures, such as API security features like authentication and authorisation controls, to ensure that only authorised users can access the API.

A Denial of Service (DoS) attack (Xu et al., 2021) is a type of cyberattack in which the attacker attempts to render a network or system unavailable to its intended users by overwhelming it with traffic or requests. This can be accomplished in numerous ways, including: a) Flooding entails delivering a huge volume of traffic or requests to a network or healthcare system in an attempt to overload and prohibit its operability. b) Distributed Denial of Service (DDoS) is the use of several devices or systems to flood a network or system with traffic or requests, making it harder to defend against. Primarily, threat actors deploy botnets, which are collections of compromised, internet-connected devices (e.g., IoT health devices) to exploit device vulnerabilities and seize control. Once in control, the attacker might direct the botnet to launch a DDoS against the victim. DDoS attacks permit substantially more requests to be issued than regular DoS attacks, hence enhancing the attack's effectiveness. c) Resource depletion is the exhaustion of a network's or system's resources, such as bandwidth or processing power, to the point where they can no longer operate properly. d) Protocol attacks exploit flaws in network protocols to disrupt the normal operation of a system or network. e) Application-layer attacks target individual programmes or services, such as web or email servers, in an attempt to render them unavailable to users.

DoS attacks can have severe repercussions in the context of healthcare data-sharing networks (Latif et al., 2016), such as blocking patients from obtaining vital medical information or disrupting the ability of healthcare practitioners to interact with patients and coordinate care. The DOS and DDOS attacks result in consequences that hinder the ability of healthcare systems to interact, integrate, and share data with each other. Therefore, it is considered one of the most service disruption-related attacks (Djenna & Saïdouni, 2018) on technical healthcare infrastructure and, therefore, achieving optimal technical interoperability. To protect against these types of attacks, it is crucial that healthcare organisations establish effective security measures and implement the most effective risk evaluation and mitigation strategies.

SQL injection attacks are a kind of cyber attack encompassing malicious code into a website or healthcare service's Structured Query Language (SQL) database. SQL injection attacks can be used to access, modify, or destroy sensitive patient data, impair the operation of the medical healthcare system, and even gain unauthorised access to other components of the network in the context of healthcare data-sharing platforms. In healthcare data-sharing systems, SQL injection attacks can take a variety of forms, including:

a. Union-based injection: This sort of injection combines the results of many SELECT operations using the UNION operator, allowing the attacker to access data from multiple tables or databases.

b. Error-based injection: This sort of injection includes causing a database error in order to disclose sensitive healthcare data or overcome security restrictions.

c. Blind injection: This method of injection involves inserting a malicious payload that does not cause an instantly noticeable effect but allows the attacker to gradually gain information about the database's structure or data.

d. Second-order injection: This sort of injection involves inserting malicious code into a database, which is subsequently executed when the user retrieves and views the data. It is essential for healthcare data-sharing platforms to have stringent security measures to avoid SQL injection attacks and protect sensitive patient data. This may involve input validation, parameterised queries, and routine system upgrades and changes.

Cyberattacks on medical data-sharing systems might have serious consequences, including, as discussed above, confidentiality breaches of sensitive patient information, such as medical records and personal data, which could be used for identity theft or other fraudulent purposes. Applying the right security measures could prevent or at least mitigate a potential cyber threat to medical data-sharing systems. Several practical security measures can be applied to a healthcare organisation connected to medical data-sharing systems, such as encrypting data when exchanging medical data to make it of no use or not make any sense in the event that it falls into the hands of cyber attackers. Access control mechanisms are critical in preventing unauthorised users from accessing medical data. Firewalls and intrusion detection and prevention systems are essential for defending against external threats by blocking or alerting malicious traffic. Regular updates and patches that keep systems and software up to date with the latest patches and updates can help to fix vulnerabilities that attackers could exploit. Also, performing regular security assessments, such as penetration testing, can help identify and address vulnerabilities in the system. Last but not least, security awareness and training on cybersecurity best practices can help reduce the risk of accidental data breaches or other security incidents in healthcare organisations and medical data-sharing systems. Researchers are motivated to provide a practical research framework to put in place the appropriate security measures in order to protect medical data-sharing systems, hence, this remains an open research area in medical data-sharing systems.

CURRENT PRIVACY-PRESERVING PARADIGMS IN MEDICAL DATA-SHARING SYSTEMS

In medical sharing systems, data transactions are composed of centralised and decentralised paradigms. The privacy-preserving approaches necessitate the right data-sharing paradigm. The following discusses the right approach to privacy preservation in medical data-sharing systems.

The Centralised Approach

The centralised approach requires medical sites and healthcare providers to share data with each other in their repositories. Data repositories are commonly shared over cloud platforms or other forms of online data communication and sharing channels between healthcare providers, such as secure messaging applications (Agency). Secure messaging apps are the third component/service of data-sharing systems that are vulnerable to common cyberattacks (third-party attacks, Figure 6.2). For example, third-party vendors of medical providers may provide healthcare services for the healthcare providers sector, such as medical practice booking management apps or a third-party IT organisation that administers hospitals' electronic medical records (EMR). If cyberattacks (section 2.3) infect these third parties, their clients (e.g., hospitals or medical practices) are exposed to a high risk of a data breach due to cyber-related incidents (Figure 6.2).

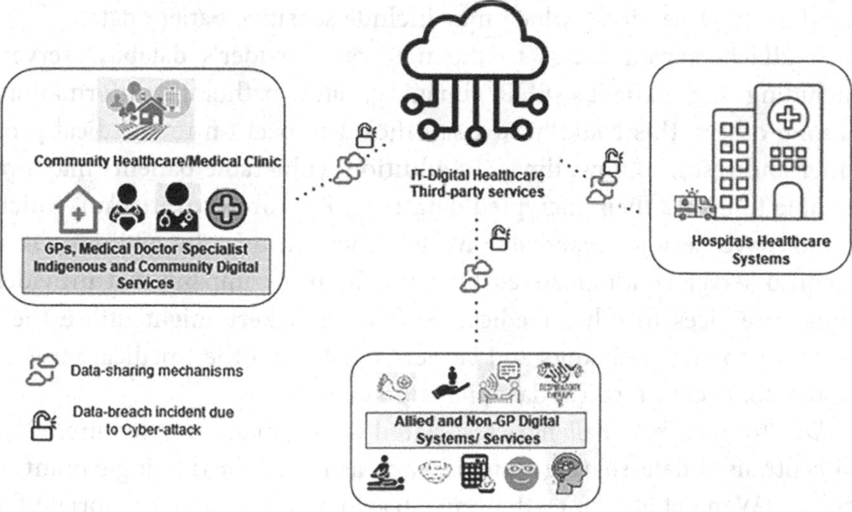

FIGURE 6.2 An illustration of a third-party data breach cyberattack in centralized medical data-sharing systems.

Throughout the history of medical systems, numerous data breaches have spurred the development of security solutions against these dangers (Sultana et al., 2020). If medical health services and third-party providers are unable to protect patients' privacy, the sensitivity of healthcare data, and the security of medical transactions, there will be severe health consequences for patients, medical results will be altered, the reputation of medical institutions will suffer, and heavy fines will be imposed by governments or federal authorities on medical providers or third-party services who do not report the accidental loss or disclosure of data (Agency). Despite the fact that a centralised database is advantageous in medical data-sharing systems, it comes with inherent risks. Recently, a ransomware criminal organisation hacked into the databases of Medibank, Australia's largest private health insurer, resulting in 10 million Australians' private health data being compromised. Sensitive medical records detailing treatments for alcoholism, drug addictions, and abortions have already been posted online (Doherty, 2022). Ransomware is a sort of malware attack in which the attacker encrypts and locks the victim's data and vital files and then asks for money (ransom) to unlock and decode the data. Extortion malware infects remote systems using phishing emails and other software vulnerabilities (Wazid et al., 2022). A member of the healthcare staff, for instance, may receive a phishing email containing an authentic-looking link. However, the phishing email will deceive recipients into installing malware on their local workstations (e.g., maintained by third-party IT services), which may include sensitive patient data.

If attackers gain access to the medical provider's database server, including the patient's EHR, imaging, and pathology information, among others, this could have a significant impact on the medical provider and result in downtimes. In addition, vulnerable patients may not be able to access their encrypted data (e.g., Ransomware attacks), which could have serious repercussions for their health. In addition, if a medical server is administered by a third-party company that provides similar services to other medical services, attackers might utilise their methods to find backdoors and launch attacks on other medical services in the connected medical data-sharing systems.

Due to the cyber challenges associated with data-sharing requirements in centralised data-sharing systems, such as DDOS or the single point of failure (Wang et al., 2021), the centralised paradigm is inappropriate for privacy-preserving and securing sensitive medical information about patients for connected medical healthcare providers that require using online shared services, such as AI applications. Therefore, this hinders achieving technical interoperability and prevents the maximum benefits for data interchange between medical data-sharing systems.

The Decentralised Approach

Decentralised data-sharing systems enable the sharing and exchange of data without a central system or server (Nguyen et al., 2021). In the context of the sharing of medical data, decentralised systems can offer various advantages (Julier & Uhlmann, 2017), such as the fact that data is stored and shared directly amongst users, as opposed to being saved on a central server, resulting in increased security and privacy. This eliminates the risk of a single point of failure or a centralised data breach and permits greater control over who has access to sensitive medical information. Another important aspect of decentralisation is increased efficiency. Hence, decentralised systems can make it easier for different systems and organisations to communicate data since they do not require a central authority to facilitate the sharing. This can enhance the overall interoperability of systems for sharing medical data. Moreover, decentralised data-sharing systems can make it easier for patients to access their own medical information because they do not need to receive it from a central authority. Eventually, this can also make it easier for healthcare practitioners to access and share patient data, resulting in enhanced patient care. As data is stored and transferred directly amongst users, decentralised systems might lower the expenses of maintaining central servers and infrastructure. Consequentially, decentralised data-sharing systems offer the potential to enhance the security, interoperability, accessibility, and cost-effectiveness of medical data sharing (Jabbar et al., 2020).

Decentralised traditional data-sharing systems are designed to allow numerous parties to share data without requiring a central authority. Nonetheless, the decentralised structure of data-sharing networks presents a number of privacy concerns, including:

Lack of control over data (Abdelhamid et al., 2017): In a decentralised system, individuals may have less control over their data due to the fact that information is shared with various parties. This may raise issues over the use and misuse of personal information. Patient privacy means having control over who has access to personal medical records and being aware that they are secure. Patients will be highly concerned about their privacy if there is a lack of oversight and they are unaware of existing safeguards in decentralised data-sharing systems. One of the main disadvantages of decentralised data sharing is the risk of patient privacy invasions and information security breaches, which are growing concerns as the volume of electronic health information transmitted increases.

Transparency: As all transactions and data on the network are transmitted over various platforms, including those where the data may be available to the public, the transparency of data-sharing systems can also pose a challenge to privacy. This can make maintaining privacy difficult, particularly for sensitive transactions or data. Transparency in medical data-sharing systems must allow the patient to foresee or control what will occur with his or her medical and personal information. Hence, transparency allows the patient to learn what happened to his or her medical and personal information (Spagnuelo & Lenzini, 2016).

Scalability: Scalability concerns in medical data-sharing systems are subjected to factors such as (Mazlan et al., 2020):

- Data volume: The volume of healthcare data can be extremely large, making it difficult to store and handle data at scale. This can be particularly difficult for systems that must manage real-time data streams or enormous amounts of data from various sources.
- Data variety: Structured data (e.g., test findings, diagnoses) and unstructured data (e.g., patient notes) are two examples of the numerous formats and types of healthcare data (e.g., notes, images). This can make it challenging to extract meaningful information from the data and include it in a system for data exchange.
- Data quality and integrity: it can be difficult to ensure the quality and integrity of data when it is derived from many sources. Data may be insufficient, inconsistent, or contain errors, which can affect the system's precision.
- Data privacy and security: Protecting the privacy and security of healthcare data is crucial, but it can be difficult when data are exchanged between many entities.
- To prevent unauthorised access and tampering, systems must be constructed with powerful security features.
- Interoperability: Ensuring that data-sharing systems are compatible with other systems and technologies can be difficult, as it necessitates compatibility with a vast array of data standards and formats.

Data Anonymisation: Data anonymisation is the process of concealing or eradicating personally identifiable information from data in order to protect individuals' privacy. It is essential to protect the privacy of patients and their personal health information in healthcare settings. This can be accomplished with data anonymisation techniques. Among these methods are the following 1) De-identification entails eliminating from the data personal health identifiers such as name, address, and social security number. 2) Pseudonymisation involves substituting personal identifiers with a pseudonym or fake name. 3) Aggregation implies grouping data and deleting personally identifiable information. 4) Data masking involves substituting sensitive data with fake data that has the same format as the original data (Scheibner et al., 2021).

Data anonymisation typically occurs on the healthcare institution's server; thus, patients generally place their trust in the data anonymization process. However, data anonymisation is subjected to linkage data attacks. In linkage data attacks (also known as re-identification attacks), patients' data are re-identified from a dataset that has been anonymised. If attackers are able to access other combined multiple datasets with the original dataset, therefore, this gives them a hint to be able to link the dataset and re-identify the patient's individual information. In re-identification attacks, the attackers may be able to use external information about the users (patients) from external sources such as social media or public records to identify patients from an anonymisation dataset (Simon et al., 2019).

Although medical data-sharing systems require strong security measures to protect the data and the potential for conflicts of interest between different stakeholders in the data-sharing systems, they have several attractive advantages that make them well suited to preserving the privacy of patients in medical data-sharing systems, from the perspectives of increased, improved privacy, increased interoperability, greater control, and reduced costs. These perceptions make decentralised data-sharing systems viable to achieve and preserve patients' privacy in medical data-sharing systems.

RESEARCH OPPORTUNITIES AND FUTURE DIRECTION IN MEDICAL DATA-SHARING SYSTEMS

This section explores the research opportunities and future direction in medical data-sharing systems. The following are important research trends and directions that require further research attention to privacy-preserving medical data-sharing systems.

Blockchain-Based Medical Data-Sharing Systems

A blockchain is a decentralised, distributed database that stores and records transactions on many computers such that the record cannot be amended retrospectively without modifying all subsequent blocks and gaining network consensus (Wang et al., 2019). The following are the primary types of blockchain technology (Morkunas et al., 2019) in healthcare/medicare care settings:

- ***Public blockchains*** are generally available to everybody and decentralised, meaning a central healthcare authority does not control them. The Bitcoin and Ethereum networks are good examples of the public blockchain.
- ***Private blockchains:*** Private blockchains are typically utilised by businesses for record-keeping purposes. They may be centralised, indicating that a single entity controls them.
- ***Hybrid blockchains:*** These are blockchains that combine characteristics of both public and private blockchains. They may be partially decentralised and have access control.
- ***Consortium blockchains*** are blockchains that are managed by a consortium of organisations as opposed to a single organisation. Common applications include the financial and supply chain industries, where several parties must collaborate and share information.

Due to its desirable characteristics, blockchain has garnered considerable interest in a variety of different fields. Various research works and projects have examined and implemented blockchain for privacy protection in medical data-sharing systems. In their literature review, for instance, the authors (Jin et al., 2019) assessed security metrics (identification, access control, data authentication, and data encryption), architecture metrics (blockchain type, data storage method), and functionality metrics (smart contract, interoperability). In addition, the authors categorised these schemes as either permissioned or permissionless blockchain-based techniques. In their survey work (Satybaldy & Nowostawski, 2020), the authors studied techniques for privacy-preserving blockchain systems and identified potential privacy issues such as transaction linkability, compliance with data protection regulations, on-chain data privacy, and malicious smart contracts. Authors (Arbabi et al., 2022) surveyed challenges related to privacy preservation based on healthcare blockchain technology related to confidentiality, anonymity and unlinkability, transparency and auditability, accountable privacy, consent management, and related Interoperability challenges.

In light of the literature analysis for privacy-preserving in medical data-sharing systems based on blockchain technology, the following are some of the directions that need further research investigation towards the realisation of interoperable medical data-sharing systems:

- ***On-chain and off-chain data storage and transactions*** *for scalable medical data-sharing systems* (Jin et al., 2019). Recent approaches to medical data sharing have chosen to store medical information off-chain. However, data query strings and hash values are stored on-chain for verification of authenticity and integrity (Jin et al., 2019). In such an architecture, medical data can be encrypted, altered, and removed as needed. On-chain or off-chain transaction approaches each have advantages and disadvantages, such as scalability and privacy preservation from technical interoperability, which remain uncharted research areas.
- ***Permissioned vs. permissionless blockchains*** (Jin et al., 2019) and (Arbabi et al., 2022). In a system for sharing medical data, both types of blockchains have advantages and disadvantages. Access to the data is restricted to authorised parties in permissioned blockchains, which may give better control and security. However, permissioned blockchains may be less versatile and permit less data sharing and collaboration than permissionless blockchains. Permissionless blockchains, on the other hand, may offer greater flexibility and data-sharing opportunities, but they may also be less secure since anyone can join the network and potentially access the data. Further research should investigate better blockchain mechanisms in the balanced need for permissioned and permissionless based solutions for medical data-sharing systems.
- ***Zero-knowledge proofs*** are cryptographic techniques that enable one party (the prover) to demonstrate to another party (the verifier) that a statement is true without revealing any extra information. In blockchain-based systems, they can be used to secure the privacy of medical data by allowing users to certify that they have access to certain data without revealing the data itself (Dwivedi et al., 2022).

- ***Homomorphic encryption (HE)*** is a type of encryption that enables data to be processed in an encrypted state without first being decrypted. This is important for sharing medical data without compromising privacy, as it permits data to be evaluated and processed without revealing the underlying data to possible attackers (Zhang et al., 2022).
- ***Differential privacy*** is a statistical technique that adds "noise" to data points in order to protect their privacy. It can be used to secure the privacy of medical data in blockchain-based systems by preventing the identification of specific individuals (Wu et al., 2022).
- *Smart contracts* are self-executing contracts with the terms of the agreement written into code. Researchers are investigating the potential of privacy-preserving smart contracts in blockchain-based medical data-sharing platforms, which would enable the automation of data-sharing agreements without disclosing sensitive data (Lee et al., 2022).

Federated Learning for Privacy Preservation

Federated learning (Li et al., 2020) enables several healthcare parties to build a machine-learning model without sharing their data. In federated learning, each participant trains a local model using their own data and then transmits a summary of the model parameters (such as weights and biases) to a central server. All model updates from all parties are aggregated by the central server and used to update a global model. The parties are then sent the updated global model, and the process is repeated until the model converges. Federated learning has the ability to enable the collaboration of data from different companies or individuals without compromising privacy, as the data is never shared. Additionally, it can be used to train models on distributed data sets, such as data from multiple hospitals or healthcare providers.

There are several varieties of federated learning, which can be categorised according to characteristics such as the number of parties engaged, the type of data utilised, and the degree of centralisation. Here are some examples of federated learning types (Patel et al., 2022):

- Single-party federated learning: In single-party federated learning, a single party (such as a hospital or healthcare provider) trains a model utilising data from several sources within the party (e.g., multiple hospitals or clinics within the same healthcare system).

- Multiple parties (e.g., multiple hospitals or healthcare providers) work together to train a model with their own data in multi-party federated learning.
- Federated transfer learning is a subtype of federated learning in which a pre-trained model is refined using data from many partners. This can be effective when the parties have relatively limited quantities of data and can benefit from the model's acquired expertise.
- Federated averaging: Federated averaging is a prominent federated learning approach that updates the global model by repeatedly averaging the model updates from several parties.
- Federated distillation is a federated learning methodology in which a "teacher" model is trained on a central dataset and then used to train "student" models on the local datasets of many parties. The student models are then pooled to provide a global model that has been updated.
- Federated stochastic gradient descent (SGD): Federated stochastic gradient descent (SGD) is a federated learning method in which model updates from different parties are aggregated using stochastic gradient descent (SGD) to update the global model.
- Federated clustering is a federated learning strategy in which the parties are first divided into clusters based on their data characteristics, and then a model is trained on each cluster. The aggregated model updates from the clusters are used to update the global model.

Federated learning is still a new and emerging topic in the literature, where the research community in medical data-sharing systems studied the federated learning potential for privacy preservings. For instance, (Xia et al., 2021) studied and proposed a new cascade vertical federated learning framework to address privacy preservation challenges associated with current vertical federated learning, such as that enables training your neural network in the scenario where features and labels are all partitioned among different parties. Federated learning approaches looked at important aspects of the number of communication rounds, and the communication consumption of each participant. For example,

(Wu et al., 2022) proposed a federated learning scheme combined with the adaptive gradient descent strategy and differential privacy mechanism, which is suitable for multi-party collaborative modelling scenarios with limited communication costs. Work by (Zhang & Li, 2022) used the federated transfer learning method to address technical challenges associated with variations in machines and operating conditions; the data distributions, which are generally different across different clients, significantly deteriorate the performance of federated learning. The approach provides a privacy-preserving means in the condition where data from different clients cannot be communicated, prior distributions.

Before constructing scalable and interoperable medical data-sharing systems, federated learning healthcare faces system and statistical challenges that must be accounted for. Hence, these challenges hinder the technical interoperability of medical information-sharing systems. These challenges are described in the subsequent sections.

- The systems challenges are associated with constrained edge devices, unreliable networks, tempered healthcare devices, fog computing infrastructure (Kasyap & Tripathy, 2021), microservices (Alsinglawi et al., 2022) and IoT healthcare systems that limit the communications between heterogeneous data-sharing interactive entities.
- Statistical challenges are related to machine learning models, and cryptographic and algorithmic issues. Researchers converged on statistical challenges as it is the system issues inherent in edge learning (Kasyap & Tripathy, 2021).

The literature identified the security issues associated with medical data-sharing systems at the clients' level, such as leakage attacks, inference attacks, positioning attacks, and knowledge-based attacks. Attacks, such as framework attacks, server attacks, and general attacks, occur on the other side (Kasyap & Tripathy, 2021). These issues must be addressed to improve machine learning performance in data-sharing-based systems and achieve technical interoperability.

The literature has highlighted study directions for preserving the privacy of medical data-sharing systems with federated learning approaches, and the following are important directions for future research:

Homomorphic encryption: privacy remains a concerning issue in three layers as security issues (edge devices, the aggregator, and the framework) in FL in medical data-sharing systems. Therefore, research attempts must consider the appropriate security measures for FL medical data-sharing systems. Homomorphic encryption started to gain much research attention for securing gradients of local models and aggregated weight from the global models (Wang et al., 2023).

Differential privacy ensures that summary statistics cannot be used to identify individual data points in a collection. This is accomplished by adding noise to outputs. A differentially private technique assures that summary statistics are not materially affected by the presence or absence of an individual's data, and hence that the individual's contribution to the data cannot be derived from the summary-level output (Khanna et al., 2022).

Quantum Federated learning: quantum federated learning (QFL) research is the most recent research trend for preserving patients' privacy. QFL trains a quantum machine learning algorithm across many decentralised servers containing non-identical and separately dispersed healthcare data without transferring them. During the quantum federated learning process, the goal is not only to conduct a thorough evaluation but also to protect the privacy of each healthcare client (Bhatia et al., 2023).

CONCLUSION

This study provided a synthesis of the technical interoperability components of medical data exchange systems. We investigated the cyber security issues that inhibit the scalability of medical data-sharing platforms in the interest of patient privacy, reliability, and improved healthcare results. We investigated the current state of medical data-sharing systems by analysing the interoperability components for preserving the privacy and security of patients. Furthermore, we identified security aspects and analysed cyber threats that hinder the scalability and technical interoperability of medical data-sharing systems. We examined the current privacy-protecting paradigms in systems for sharing medical data. Finally, we presented the research opportunities, future research roadmap, and directions that support the goals of realising medical data-sharing systems.

REFERENCES

Abdelhamid, M. (2020). The role of health concerns in phishing susceptibility: Survey design study. *Journal of Medical Internet Research*, *22*(5), e18394.

Abdelhamid, M., Gaia, J., & Sanders, G. L. (2017). Putting the focus back on the patient: How privacy concerns affect personal health information sharing intentions. *Journal of Medical Internet Research, 19*(9), e6877.

Agency, A. D. H. *Penalties for misuse of health information*. Retrieved from https://www.myhealthrecord.gov.au/about/legislation-and-governance/penalties-for-misuse-health-information

Agency, A. D. H. *Secure messaging*. Retrieved from https://www.digitalhealth.gov.au/healthcare-providers/initiatives-and-programs/secure-messaging

Al Asad, N., Elahi, M. T., Al Hasan, A., & Yousuf, M. A. (2020). Permission-based blockchain with proof of authority for secured healthcare data sharing. 2020 2nd International Conference on Advanced Information and Communication Technology (ICAICT).

Ali, K. A., & Alyounis, S. (2021). CyberSecurity in the healthcare industry. 2021 International Conference on Information Technology (ICIT).

Alsinglawi, B., Zheng, L., Kabir, M. A., Islam, M. Z., Swain, D., & Swain, W. (2022). Internet of things and microservices in supply chain: Cybersecurity challenges, and research opportunities. International Conference on Advanced Information Networking and Applications.

Alzubi, Jafar A. (2021). Blockchain-based Lamport Merkle Digital Signature: Authentication tool in IoT healthcare. *Computer Communications, 170*, 200–208, ISSN 0140-3664, https://doi.org/10.1016/j.comcom.2021.02.002. (https://www.sciencedirect.com/science/article/pii/S014036642100061X)

Ametepe, A. F.-X., Ahouandjinou, S. A. R., & Ezin, E. C. (2019). Secure encryption by combining asymmetric and symmetric cryptographic methods for data collection WSN in smart agriculture. 2019 IEEE International Smart Cities Conference (ISC2).

Aonzo, S., Merlo, A., Tavella, G., & Fratantonio, Y. (2018). Phishing attacks on modern android. Proceedings of the 2018 ACM SIGSAC Conference on Computer and Communications Security.

Arbabi, M. S., Lal, C., Veeraragavan, N. R., Marijan, D., Nygård, J. F., & Vitenberg, R. (2022). A survey on blockchain for healthcare: Challenges, benefits, and future directions. *IEEE Communications Surveys & Tutorials, 25*, 386–424.

Baskaya, M., Yuksel, M., Erturkmen, G. B. L., Cunningham, M., & Cunningham, P. M. (2019). Health4Afrika-Implementing HL7 FHIR Based Interoperability. *MedInfo*.

Bhatia, A., Kais, S., & Alam, M. (2023). Handling privacy-sensitive clinical data with federated quantum machine learning. *Bulletin of the American Physical Society, 27*(2), 790–803.

Bisogni, F., Cavallini, S., & Di Trocchio, S. (2011). Cybersecurity at European level: The role of information availability. *Communications and Strategies, 81*, 105–124.

Chamarajnagar, R., & Ashok, A. (2019). Integrity threat identification for distributed IoT in precision agriculture. 2019 16th Annual IEEE International Conference on Sensing, Communication, and Networking (SECON).

Chenthara, S., Ahmed, K., Wang, H., & Whittaker, F. (2019). Security and privacy-preserving challenges of e-health solutions in cloud computing. *IEEE Access*, *7*, 74361–74382.

Davcev, D., Mitreski, K., Trajkovic, S., Nikolovski, V., & Koteli, N. (2018). IoT agriculture system based on LoRaWAN. 2018 14th IEEE International Workshop on Factory Communication Systems (WFCS).

Diaz, O., Kushibar, K., Osuala, R., Linardos, A., Garrucho, L., Igual, L., Radeva, P., Prior, F., Gkontra, P., & Lekadir, K. (2021). Data preparation for artificial intelligence in medical imaging: A comprehensive guide to open-access platforms and tools. *Physica Medica*, *83*, 25–37.

Djenna, A., & Saïdouni, D. E. (2018). Cyber attack classification in IoT-based healthcare infrastructure. 2018 2nd Cyber Security in Networking Conference (CSNet).

Doherty, B. (2022, 6/12/2022). Medical data hacked from 10m Australians begins to appear on dark web. *TheGuardian*. https://www.theguardian.com/world/2022/nov/11/medical-data-hacked-from-10m-australians-begins-to-appear-on-dark-web

Dullabh, P., Hovey, L., Heaney-Huls, K., Rajendran, N., Wright, A., & Sittig, D. F. (2020). Application programming interfaces in health care: findings from a current-state sociotechnical assessment. *Applied Clinical Informatics*, *11*(01), 059–069.

Dwivedi, A. D., Singh, R., Ghosh, U., Mukkamala, R. R., Tolba, A., & Said, O. (2022). Privacy preserving authentication system based on non-interactive zero knowledge proof suitable for Internet of Things. *Journal of Ambient Intelligence and Humanized Computing*, *13*(10), 4639–4649.

Elhoseny, M., Ramírez-González, G., Abu-Elnasr, O. M., Shawkat, S. A., Arunkumar, N., & Farouk, A. (2018). Secure medical data transmission model for IoT-based healthcare systems. *IEEE Access*, *6*, 20596–20608.

Fatima, N., Agarwal, P., & Sohail, S. S. (2022). Security and privacy issues of blockchain technology in health care—A review. *ICT Analysis and Applications*, 193–201.

Ferrag, M. A., Shu, L., Yang, X., Derhab, A., & Maglaras, L. (2020). Security and privacy for green IoT-based agriculture: Review, blockchain solutions, and challenges. *IEEE Access*, *8*, 32031–32053.

Ghallab, M. (2019). Responsible AI: requirements and challenges. *AI Perspectives*, *1*(1), 1–7.

Ghonge, M. M., Pradeep, N., Ravi, R. V., & Mangrulkar, R. (2023). A comprehensive review of the security and privacy issues in blockchain technologies. *Research Anthology on Convergence of Blockchain, Internet of Things, and Security*, 1293–1308.

Gohar, A. N., Abdelmawgoud, S. A., & Farhan, M. S. (2022). A patient-centric healthcare framework reference architecture for better semantic interoperability based on blockchain, cloud, and IoT. *IEEE Access*, *10*, 92137–92157.

Goldman, M. J., Craft, B., Hastie, M., Repečka, K., McDade, F., Kamath, A., Banerjee, A., Luo, Y., Rogers, D., & Brooks, A. N. (2020). Visualizing and interpreting cancer genomics data via the Xena platform. *Nature Biotechnology*, *38*(6), 675–678.

Hagen, C., Dmitrienko, A., Iffländer, L., Jobst, M., & Kounev, S. (2018). Efficient and effective ransomware detection in databases. Annual Computer Security Applications Conference (ACSAC).

Holkar, A. M., Holkar, N. S., & Nitnawwre, D. (2013). Investigative analysis of repudiation attack on MANET with different routing protocols. *International Journal of Emerging Trends & Technology in Computer Science (IJETTCS)*, *2*(3), 356–359.

Huang, H., Zhu, P., Xiao, F., Sun, X., & Huang, Q. (2020). A blockchain-based scheme for privacy-preserving and secure sharing of medical data. *Computers & Security*, *99*, 102010.

Huckvale, K., Torous, J., & Larsen, M. E. (2019). Assessment of the data sharing and privacy practices of smartphone apps for depression and smoking cessation. *JAMA Network Open*, *2*(4), e192542.

Idoje, G., Dagiuklas, T., & Iqbal, M. (2021). Survey for smart farming technologies: Challenges and issues. *Computers & Electrical Engineering*, *92*, 107104.

Jabbar, R., Fetais, N., Krichen, M., & Barkaoui, K. (2020). Blockchain technology for healthcare: Enhancing shared electronic health record interoperability and integrity. 2020 IEEE International Conference on Informatics, IoT, and Enabling Technologies (ICIoT).

Jin, H., Luo, Y., Li, P., & Mathew, J. (2019). A review of secure and privacy-preserving medical data sharing. *IEEE Access*, *7*, 61656–61669.

Johnson, A., Bulgarelli, L., Pollard, T., Horng, S., Celi, L. A., & Mark, R. (2020). Mimic-iv. *PhysioNet*. Available online at: https://physionet.org/content/mimiciv/1.0/(accessed August 23, 2021).

Julier, S., & Uhlmann, J. K. (2017). General decentralized data fusion with covariance intersection. In *Handbook of Multisensor Data Fusion* (pp. 339–364). CRC Press.

Kasyap, H., & Tripathy, S. (2021). Privacy-preserving decentralized learning framework for healthcare system. *ACM Transactions on Multimedia Computing, Communications, and Applications (TOMM)*, *17*(2s), 1–24.

Khanna, A., Schaffer, V., Gürsoy, G., & Gerstein, M. (2022). Privacy-preserving model training for disease prediction using federated learning with differential privacy. 2022 44th Annual International Conference of the IEEE Engineering in Medicine & Biology Society (EMBC).

Latif, R., Abbas, H., Latif, S., & Masood, A. (2016). Distributed denial of service attack source detection using efficient traceback technique (ETT) in cloud-assisted healthcare environment. *Journal of Medical Systems*, *40*(7), 1–13.

Lee, J.-S., Chew, C.-J., Liu, J.-Y., Chen, Y.-C., & Tsai, K.-Y. (2022). Medical blockchain: Data sharing and privacy-preserving of EHR based on smart contract. *Journal of Information Security and Applications*, *65*, 103117.

Lehne, M., Sass, J., Essenwanger, A., Schepers, J., & Thun, S. (2019). Why digital medicine depends on interoperability. *NPJ Digital Medicine, 2*(1), 1–5.

Li, L., Fan, Y., Tse, M., & Lin, K.-Y. (2020). A review of applications in federated learning. *Computers & Industrial Engineering, 149*, 106854.

Mazlan, A. A., Daud, S. M., Sam, S. M., Abas, H., Rasid, S. Z. A., & Yusof, M. F. (2020). Scalability challenges in healthcare blockchain system—a systematic review. *IEEE Access, 8*, 23663–23673.

Melara, M. S., & Bowman, M. (2021). Enabling Security-Oriented Orchestration of Microservices. *arXiv preprint arXiv:2106.09841.*

Morkunas, V. J., Paschen, J., & Boon, E. (2019). How blockchain technologies impact your business model. *Business Horizons, 62*(3), 295–306.

Nesarani, A., Ramar, R., & Pandian, S. (2020). An efficient approach for rice prediction from authenticated Blockchain node using machine learning technique. *Environmental Technology & Innovation, 20*, 101064.

Nguyen, D. C., Pathirana, P. N., Ding, M., & Seneviratne, A. (2019). Blockchain for secure ehrs sharing of mobile cloud-based e-health systems. *IEEE Access, 7*, 66792–66806.

Nguyen, D. C., Pathirana, P. N., Ding, M., & Seneviratne, A. (2021). BEdgeHealth: A decentralized architecture for edge-based IoMT networks using blockchain. *IEEE Internet of Things Journal, 8*(14), 11743–11757.

Patel, V. A., Bhattacharya, P., Tanwar, S., Gupta, R., Sharma, G., Bokoro, P. N., & Sharma, R. (2022). Adoption of federated learning for healthcare informatics: Emerging applications and future directions. *IEEE Access, 10*, 90792–90826.

Satybaldy, A., & Nowostawski, M. (2020). Review of techniques for privacy-preserving blockchain systems. Proceedings of the 2nd ACM International Symposium on Blockchain and Secure Critical Infrastructure.

Scheibner, J., Raisaro, J. L., Troncoso-Pastoriza, J. R., Ienca, M., Fellay, J., Vayena, E.,& Hubaux, J.-P. (2021). Revolutionizing medical data sharing using advanced privacy-enhancing technologies: Technical, legal, and ethical synthesis. *Journal of Medical Internet Research, 23*(2), e25120.

Simon, G. E., Shortreed, S. M., Coley, R. Y., Penfold, R. B., Rossom, R. C., Waitzfelder, B. E., Sanchez, K., & Lynch, F. L. (2019). Assessing and minimizing re-identification risk in research data derived from health care records. *EGEMS (Wash DC)*, Mar 29; *7*(1), 6. doi: 10.5334/egems.270. PMID: 30972355; PMCID: PMC6450246. available at https://pubmed.ncbi.nlm.nih.gov/30972355/

Soni, M., & Singh, D. K. (2021). Blockchain-based security & privacy for biomedical and healthcare information exchange systems. *Materials Today: Proceedings.*

Spagnuelo, D., & Lenzini, G. (2016). Patient-centred transparency requirements for medical data sharing systems. In *New Advances in Information Systems and Technologies* (pp. 1073–1083). Springer.

Sultana, M., Hossain, A., Laila, F., Taher, K. A., & Islam, M. N. (2020). Towards developing a secure medical image-sharing system based on zero-trust principles and blockchain technology. *BMC Medical Informatics and Decision Making*, *20*(1), 1–10.

Tang, S., Shelden, D. R., Eastman, C. M., Pishdad-Bozorgi, P., & Gao, X. (2019). A review of building information modelling (BIM) and the Internet of Things (IoT) devices integration: Present status and future trends. *Automation in Construction*, *101*, 127–139.

Tariq, R. A., & Hackert, P. B. (2018). Patient confidentiality. Available at: https://europepmc.org/article/nbk/nbk519540

Wang, M., Guo, Y., Zhang, C., Wang, C., Huang, H., & Jia, X. (2021). MedShare: A privacy-preserving medical data-sharing system by using blockchain. *IEEE Transactions on Services Computing*.

Wang, W., Hoang, D. T., Hu, P., Xiong, Z., Niyato, D., Wang, P., Wen, Y., & Kim, D. I. (2019). A survey on consensus mechanisms and mining strategy management in blockchain networks. *IEEE Access*, *7*, 22328–22370.

Wang, W., Li, X., Qiu, X., Zhang, X., Zhao, J., & Brusic, V. (2023). A privacy-preserving framework for federated learning in smart healthcare systems. *Information Processing & Management*, *60*(1), 103167.

Wazid, M., Das, A. K., & Shetty, S. (2022). BSFR-SH: Blockchain-enabled security framework against ransomware attacks for smart healthcare. *IEEE Transactions on Consumer Electronics*, *69*(1), 18–28.

Wu, X., Zhang, Y., Shi, M., Li, P., Li, R., & Xiong, N. N. (2022). An adaptive federated learning scheme with differential privacy-preserving. *Future Generation Computer Systems*, *127*, 362–372.

Xia, W., Li, Y., Zhang, L., Wu, Z., & Yuan, X. (2021). A vertical federated learning framework for horizontally partitioned labels. *arXiv preprint arXiv:2106.10056*.

Xu, Y., Fang, M., Pan, Y. J., Shi, K., & Wu, Z. G. (2021). Event-triggered output synchronization for nonhomogeneous agent systems with periodic denial-of-service attacks. *International Journal of Robust and Nonlinear Control*, *31*(6), 1851–1865.

Yu, S., Lou, W., & Ren, K. (2012). Data security in cloud computing. *Morgan Kaufmann/Elsevier, Book Section*, *15*, 389–410.

Zhang, F., & Jiang, X. (2021). The zero trust security platform for data trusteeship. 2021 4th International Conference on Advanced Electronic Materials, Computers and Software Engineering (AEMCSE).

Zhang, L., Xu, J., Vijayakumar, P., Sharma, P. K., & Ghosh, U. (2022). Homomorphic encryption-based privacy-preserving federated learning in IoT-enabled healthcare system. *IEEE Transactions on Network Science and Engineering*, *10*(5), 2864–2880. https://ieeexplore.ieee.org/abstract/document/9812492

Zhang, W., & Li, X. (2022). Data privacy preserving federated transfer learning in machinery fault diagnostics using prior distributions. *Structural Health Monitoring*, *21*(4), 1329–1344.

CHAPTER 7

A Comparative Review of Descriptive Process Models in Healthcare Operations Management and Analytics

Isabella Eigner, Maximilian Harl, and Daniel Neumann

INTRODUCTION

Healthcare, especially healthcare operations management, is a strongly researched environment with constantly adjusting requirements for the quality of diagnosis, novel pharmaceuticals, and new approaches demanding perpetual changes in standards and operating procedures. This makes the healthcare sector a highly dynamic domain with rising importance due to the societal awareness of health on a socio-economic and individual level. While patients are no longer seen as passive service recipients, but as actively involved entities and data providers of their healthcare service, they influence the defined procedures and demand deviation from the elaborated standards to improve their experience and outcome along their journey (Hartzband and Groopman 2011). The question arises of how to keep track and manage all these medical services, allow for more precise and individualistic procedures, and be profitable at the same time to ensure the longevity of service.

DOI: 10.1201/9781032699745-9

The primary goal and benefit of patient-centered care is to improve individual health outcomes, not just population-level health outcomes. This not only increases patient satisfaction but also benefits providers and entire healthcare systems through an enhanced reputation among healthcare consumers, better morale and productivity among clinicians and ancillary staff, improved resource allocation, as well as reduced expenses and increased financial margins throughout the continuum of care. This hypothesis raises the complexity of managing healthcare operations with engaged patients and precision medicine to an unmet extent (Habicht et al. 2012).

Currently, neither operations management nor healthcare policies offer the necessary methodologies to match the required resources to manage patient needs as soon as they require more active collaboration and shared decision-making - by means of leaving predetermined standard paths. This is reflected by clinical pathways holding only significantly proven decisions. From an operations perspective, the healthcare service as an optimization problem consists of various entities: the health carrier (the individual patient) and various consumers of the health of an individual, i.e., families, health insurance, colleagues, and employers among others, and the health establishing proxies, i.e., all healthcare service providers (Zweifel et al. 2009). This complexity in interactions of multiple entities and the incorporation of their behaviour, described by their incentives and policy environments, raises issues on multiple levels, i.e., decisions as responses to certain stimuli, incentives produced by stimuli, policies to guide interactions among entities and incentives on the health delivery (Dai and Tayur 2019a). We want to leverage operations management and decision science paired with data science to tackle this kind of complex description. To this goal, we review existing major process models used in clinical and operations research in the healthcare sector.

From a clinical and patient perspective, the stronger integration of patient engagement stresses the field of healthcare operations research to an unmet extent. To understand this holistic viewpoint, the term "patient journey" has been presented in research. This concept stems from the marketing research field, investigating a customer's "journey" with a firm over time during the purchase cycle across multiple touchpoints" (Lemon and Verhoef 2016). In healthcare, a patient's journey includes the transitions across the clinical decision time span (e.g., from screening, diagnosis to medication, treatment), life cycle (such as pediatric to adult), care units or organizations (clinic to hospital, between hospital departments such as emergency room to ward, and hospital to nursing facility or home care), and space (remote or distance care, such as telehealth). The goal is to ensure a safe and seamless transition at all stages of the patient journey. Expertise and knowledge from multiple disciplines (e.g., systems engineering, electrical engineering, health informatics, computer science, psychology) need to be integrated. The amount of research in this area is still quite sparse and mainly investigated by qualitative studies. Quantitative approaches to improve the patient journey are still limited and mostly focus on an individual transition only (Zhong et al. 2017; Bhattacharjee and Ray 2014a). An alignment of clinical knowledge and organizational workflow models presented in Gooch and Roudsari (2011) is taken as a basic idea for our studies. In this alignment, the patient perspective is not represented yet. Here, we concentrate on four major concepts in the healthcare sector:

- Patient flow as a representation of organizational workflow models.
- Clinical pathways as a representation of clinical knowledge derived from clinical guidelines.
- Clinical algorithms, clinical protocols, activity roles (Luc and Todd 2020).
- Patient journeys as a representation of the patient's set of services through the healthcare services.
- Care maps as a representation of the care process of patients.

Subsequently, a literature review on the main workflow and knowledge-representation concepts in healthcare is carried out. To take the patient's perspective into account, the patient journey models that arose from the concepts of service-oriented healthcare and patient-as-a-customer will be analyzed as well. With this paper, we want to determine a baseline of existing methodologies that are capable of covering the multitude of decisions along a patient's journey and describe the events along a journey to cover the decisions that take place when providing healthcare services. Considering that hospitals are complex organizations that interact very intensely with a broad set of conditions, we want to focus on encounters of patients in a hospital. Each encounter has to be considered in operations to understand the decision-makers along one's journey better. For that, a baseline needs to be established on how to identify decision points, interpret and understand why decisions happen to be able to model decisions and establish methods on how to manage these decisions.

DEFINITIONS

Changes in Healthcare Operations Management

Today's healthcare system can be characterized as being a profession-centric and reactive system where both responsibilities and information flow are fragmented (Bayliss et al. 2008). "Healthcare centers operate as a system of interacting departments that are coordinated by the flow of patients, specimens, employees, information, materials and pharmaceuticals" (Hall 2006). As the attention on patient-centric healthcare, including personalized medicine (Schleidgen et al. 2013) and value-based healthcare (Brown et al. 2005), grows, patients often become the coordinators of a combination of specific sets of care steps provided by individual professionals. The industrialization and the focus towards precision medicine and patients as innovators require healthcare operations to be more agile in terms of resource demand determination and resource allocation. A stringent and proactive resource allocation requires knowledge about the problems to solve - the resources themselves as a sender and recipient of clinical and operational actions, the surroundings framing the possible actions to take, and necessary influences to consider.

In the recent past, healthcare operations management (HOM) has shifted from investigating individual healthcare organizations to analyzing interactions of multiple entities in a holistic healthcare ecosystem. This includes research on the decision-making behaviour of different stakeholders in this ecosystem, operating environments that foster incentives for these decisions, and policy environments as the underlying foundation (Dai and Tayur 2019a). To ensure a high quality of care within this complex ecosystem, the World Health Organization emphasizes the relevance of "transparency, people-centeredness, measurement and generation of information, and investing in the workplace, all underpinned by leadership and a supportive culture". Based on these insights, this article aims to align the "real" process connected to existent methodologies/technologies to identify and evaluate the processes with respect to promoting health, considering economic constraints.

The greatest difficulty in this context is the alignment of standardization and optimization of best practices and treatment pathways while individualizing them to individual patients. A high number of influencing factors, resource-based constraints, and involved stakeholders in the healthcare ecosystem massively increase the complexity of this task. In this context, two research streams emerge. First, the streamlining and optimization of hospital processes, e.g., with the help of lean management, attempts to find holistic solutions for increasing the efficiency of the treatment of patient groups, special departments, or the entire hospital. These neglect the patient as an individual and his or her needs and usually focus on the time, personnel, and resource constraints in the hospital. Besides the holistic optimization of patient flows in general, the treatment of individual patients is investigated with the help of so-called patient journeys. Here, qualitative factors, such as patient satisfaction or individualized treatment strategies, play a key role, while standardization and resource constraints are mostly neglected. The resulting gap in the individualized planning of patient journeys in the context of holistic hospital processes represents an exciting challenge for HOM research.

The solution to address this gap lies in clinical decision support systems (CDS). Clinical decision support is any tool that provides clinicians, administrative staff, patients, caregivers, or other members of the care team with information that is filtered or targeted to a specific person or situation. CDS tools are often integrated into the electronic health record (EHR) to streamline workflows and take advantage of existing data sets. However, many organizations are still facing significant challenges when creating intuitive, user-friendly, and effective protocols for decision-making pathways (Hitzig et al. 2020; Jarvie et al. 2019; McHugh et al. 2019; Husbands et al. 2018; Yu et al. 2019). To effectively feed CDS, descriptive models are necessary so that the machine interpretation and methodological algorithms can be made to value.

PATIENT FLOW

Definition

The concept of patient flow is a long-term analysis of a healthcare system. Patient flow is the movement of patients through a healthcare facility. It involves the medical care, physical resources, and internal systems needed to get patients from the point of admission to the point of discharge while maintaining quality and patient/provider satisfaction (Catalyst 2018). Bhattacharjee and Ray (2014b) describe patient flow as the "movement of patients through the whole process of care", which has been a primary topic in the emergency department (ED) of hospitals (De Freitas et al. 2018). Hendrich et al. (2004) further emphasize that patient flow "is influenced by the levels of care required and the severity of patients' conditions. Coté (1999) identified two viewpoints from which patient flow has been understood: an operational perspective and, less commonly, a clinical perspective. From an operational perspective, the states that patients enter, leave, and move between are defined by clinical and administrative activities and interactions with the care system, such as consulting a physician or being on the waiting list for surgery. Such states may be each associated with a specific care setting or some other form of resource. In the clinical perspective of patient flow, these states are defined by some aspect of the patient's health, for instance, whether the patient has symptomatic heart disease or the clinical stage of a patient's tumor (Coté 1999). From an operational perspective, patient flows are used to improve the delivery process and provide holistic monitoring of movements across a healthcare centre in hospitals. Healthcare is hereby similar to other forms of services in these respects (Hall 2006):

- Service demand: The demand for service is partially predictable and partially random. The assumption is made that as soon as the clinical diagnosis is done, necessary actions are known while the decision at decision points on clinical pathways as well as the times required are rather random.
- Coordination: Healthcare centres hereby operate as a system of interacting departments that must be coordinated through the flow of patients, specimens, employees, information, materials, and pharmaceuticals.

Challenges

Health services require the coordination of multiple resources, such as physicians, medications, and equipment. The department system represents the performing entities of single or closely related functions, such as the ED, surgery, or radiology. Departments must support the mission of the centres through effective coordination and be effective on their own to not become a bottleneck in the entire ecosystem. Patient flow thereby relies on queuing theory to solve the problem of identifying bottlenecks, reducing delays and, thereby, increasing efficiency.

Approaches

In patient flow management, various areas of healthcare scheduling, such as capacity planning, nurse scheduling, appointment planning, and bed management, have been addressed in the past (Hall 2012a). In this context, different types of resources play a part in healthcare operations (Hall 2012b). These include resources with dynamic behaviour and time availability and consumption (e.g., doctors and other health professionals, patients and their support system), resources that are only dependent on the surroundings and their usage by a patient and doctor (e.g., rooms, equipment, supplies), and resources that are perishable in the sense that the resources have a limited time window of usage (e.g., implantable devices and organs, instruments). Finally, resources that hold information about the patient, the clinical condition, clinical guidelines, as well as best practices on treatments can also impact the design of healthcare processes.

Ideally, the events per patient with their timestamps are available to perform process analysis on patient flow throughout the hospital. The hypothesis is that if a patient can be mapped to an individual clinical pathway by this means, forecasting for each patient can be done, and reaction time on starting or pushing action events can be accelerated. It seems obvious that patient flow concentrates on the utilization and the waiting times of the system. But considering the patient as a health innovator, and experience being of value to the patient, this is only a very small area of operations to consider. To determine patient-related problems as lot-size one problems - meaning that no patient is equal to another and cannot be bundled - make each patient a (sort of) unique project.

Design and Modelling

Patient flow is usually represented as a flow diagram or, more specifically, a Sankey diagram. While Sankey diagrams were originally used to discover energy production and utilization in natural sciences, the basic idea is to track the most important contributions along a set of action steps, which has been adopted in healthcare. One major goal is to determine systemic bottlenecks and to streamline the process and maximize patient throughput under the constraint of conforming to underlying clinical pathways and guidelines. This way, relevant resources, such as staff, patients, equipment, and assets can be visualized and tracked to mimic patient flow without distortions.

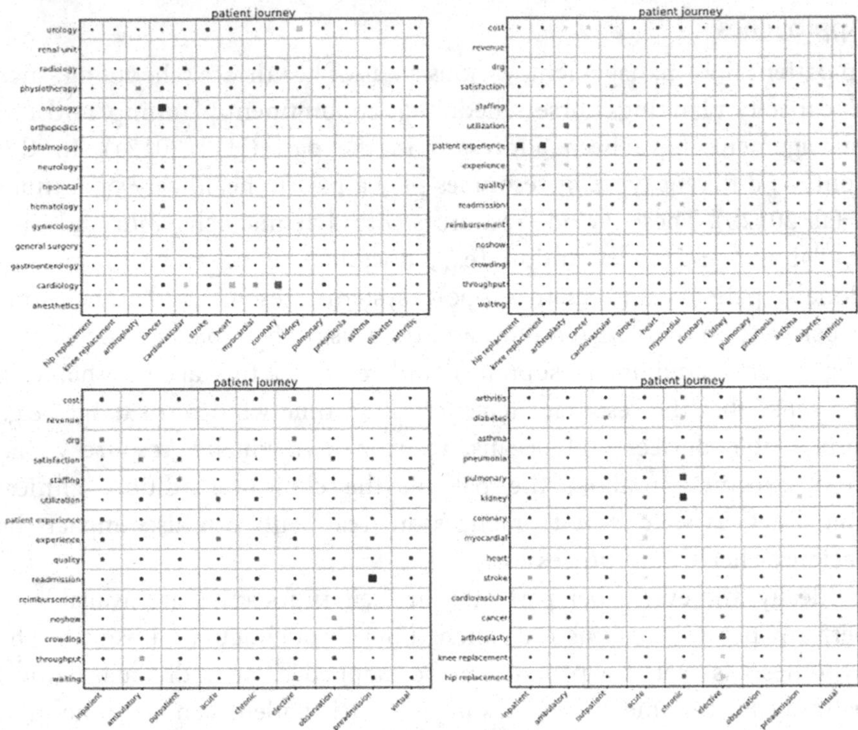

FIGURE 7.1 A patient flow diagram with operational parameters.

On a more detailed level, a typical patient flow can also be modelled for specific departments instead of the hospital level. Figure 7.1 shows a flow diagram through a surgical suite including more detailed steps and resources in this process. Finally, the patient flow can also relate to a specific patient group that follows common touchpoints, for example, as presented in Bussel et al. (2013). This focus on specific diseases or treatment groups is the most similar to the concept of clinical pathways but still has distinct differences as there are no clinical details included.

CLINICAL PATHWAY

Definition

A clinical pathway (CP), or critical pathway (Kathryn de Luc et al. 2018), care pathway, care map, or integrated care pathway, is a descriptive model that maps a course of events based on evidence-based practice. According to Peleg (2013), clinical practice guidelines are described as document models, decision trees, and probabilistic models or task network models. These guidelines contain quality indicators that are measured and directly influence the alternatives to select. A pathway is for a specific group of patients with a predictable and defined clinical course, in which the different interventions by the professionals involved in the patient's care are defined, optimized, and sequenced. Trebble et al. (2010) describe clinical pathways as the sequence of events between different activities in the process of care. The European Pathway Association further details this definition, describing a clinical pathway as a complex intervention for the mutual decision-making and organization of care processes for a well-defined group of patients during a well-defined period (Association EP 2021).

Goals

CPs are used in the clinical routine as a method for quality assurance, workflow control, workflow planning, and to identify and forecast resource expenses. Studies (Kathryn de Luc et al. 2018) indicate that a reduction of complications, readmission, or length of stay might be achieved. On the other hand, the improvement of the quality of care and the maximization of outcomes for specific groups of patients were proposed results (Lawal et al. 2016). The aim of a care pathway is to enhance the quality of care across the continuum by improving risk-adjusted patient outcomes, promoting patient safety, increasing patient satisfaction, and optimizing the use of resources.

Approaches

A subset of clinical pathways is standard operating procedures where decision points and intersections are eliminated. The biggest problem is the intense abstraction to ensure universal applicability. This is especially interesting for eliminating the assessment of side effects during clinical studies or for triaging with limited resource availability. A superset is the care map. A care map represents a sequence of care activities as part of the patient's treatment by a multidisciplinary team to produce identified outcomes. A care map can, therefore, contain multiple clinical pathways along the patient treatment (Marr and Reid 1992; D. Hampton 1993; Ogilvie-Harris et al. 1993; Blegen et al. 1995; Wilson 1995).

Design and Modelling

Clinical pathways have many similar characteristics to business processes but can also be expressed through, e.g., queuing networks (Bhattacharjee and Ray

2014b). Clinical pathways can be derived from patient journeys of a defined and representative population with a defined and statistically significant measured outcome. Hence, clinical pathways are designed after the principle of the "most effective" therapy. When two therapies have similar efficacy, the one less harmful is preferred. If harmfulness e.g., toxicity and efficacy are similar, the treatment with lower cost should be recommended (Nabhan et al. 2017). The cost prediction alone is difficult as even though the clinical pathway might be straightforward there is no direct indication of repetition or duration forecastable to determine the real costs for a patient. The efficacy is compared to randomized studies, and the comparison to commonly utilized standard procedures might or might not be mature. Data about the harmfulness might not cover post-study side effects in the community, especially not regarding precision medicine, the individual harmfulness. While industrialization and standardization are seen critically (Hartzband and Groopman 2011) this also shows that abstractions and groups lack the individual settings of patients and in hospitals. Additionally, the design and creation of clinical pathways do not follow a methodology which results in multiple variations depending on the scope, the setting and the goal to achieve with the pathway. In principle, it gives clinical personnel guidance or a task list of actions to consider paired with process flow charts (Mammen et al. 2014).

A major preliminary in setting up clinical pathways are known paths, possible decision points, the values of decisive parameters and the expected outcome. All of this has to be founded on a statistically relevant basis or on normative decisions as shown in Figure 7.2 for AML patients (de Witte et al. 2017).

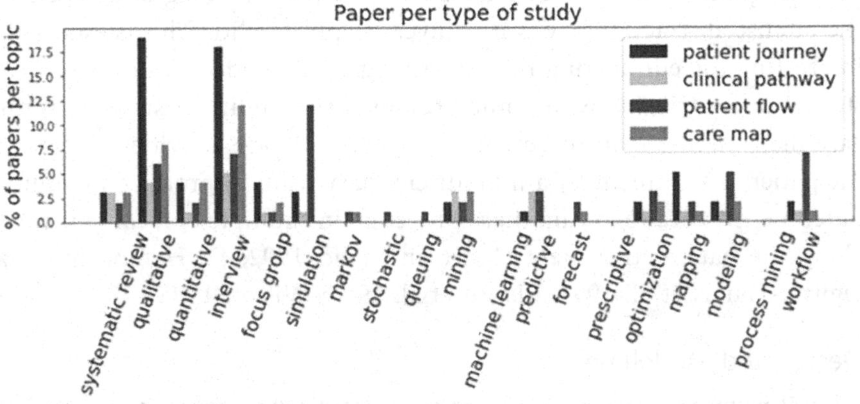

FIGURE 7.2 A clinical pathway on acute myeloma leukemia.

PATIENT JOURNEY

Definition

A clear definition of the patient journey is still absent in scientific literature, where the term is often interchangeably used with patient flow or patient pathways. Therefore, various definitions, goals, techniques, and challenges addressed in the literature are derived for each of these topics to identify distinct characteristics and overlaps. According to Gualandi et al. (2019), the patient journey is "a key cross-functional business process where patients and providers share action and information flows between people and systems across various touchpoints." These flows consist of a series of interrelated activities (Al-Hakim and Gong 2012) involving multiple stakeholders, such as doctors, nurses, and administrative staff. While this narrow definition focuses mainly on measurable interactions, other descriptions, for example by Boyd et al. (2012), also include intangible factors, such as the emotions they experience during their journey or suggested improvement ideas.

In general, the aim of the patient journey is to make the interactions between patients and all health influencers transparent to improve patients' satisfaction (Al-Hakim and Gong 2012). Trbovich and Vincent (2019) emphasize that the analysis of the entire patient journey is especially critical if "we wish to go beyond the confines of the hospital and examine healthcare in the context of people's lives" (Trbovich and Vincent 2019, p. 170).

The Patient Journey can be understood as the ongoing sequence of care events that a patient follows from the point of access into the health system, continuing towards diagnosis and care, and ending in outpatient care (Curry et al. 2006). This journey includes many activities from scheduling appointments to simply friendliness, timeliness, and quality of the outcome during the engagement. Mainly for chronic or multi-stage treatment, the patient journey can also be seen wider than just an encounter at the hospital. As Halvorsrud et al. (2019) point out, there are different interpretations of patient journeys and various practices for documenting, managing, and verifying quality assurance during patient journeys. Without a common standard for patient journeys, it is left to each institution to define the format, level of detail, and overall modelling approach.

Goals

As every health system wants to encourage patient engagement, the health provider must understand that patient engagement strongly depends on the patient's past, present, and future activities. A patient engagement journey is described in six phases (Unknown 2019):

1. Self-assessment of conditions and symptoms (Awareness).
2. Initiate contact with the health system (Help).
3. Assess health conditions in a medical facility (Care).
4. On-site and follow-up care (Treatment).
5. Changes to reduce readmissions and promote proactive health (Behavioral Change).
6. Ongoing care management between patient visits, fostering engagement between patient & physician (Proactive Health).

Approaches

A method for capturing the overall patient journey is patient journey mapping, which describes a summary of the service experiences patients have over time (Boyd et al. 2012). They can be used to depict the healthcare service from the perspective of the patient). According to Trebble et al. (2010), the patient journey process can be used to "identify and characterize value and non-value steps in the patient pathway". It "enables the reconfiguring of the patient journey from the patient's perspective in order to improve quality of care and release resources" (Trebble et al. 2010). Process mapping requires a planned approach, as even apparently straightforward patient journeys can be complex, with many interdependent steps (Trebble et al. 2010).

Design and Modelling

The mapping approach takes relevant perspectives into scope and structures events and interactions to the selected perspectives, as shown in Figure 7.3 (Boekemeyer 2016).

Meyer (2019) tries to enhance the scope across the continuum of care on patient journey maps and identifies core topics to address:

1. Shared decision-making and care planning and

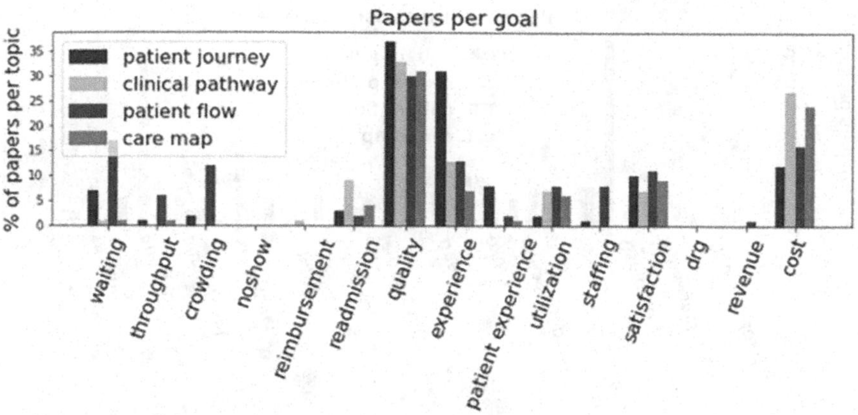

FIGURE 7.3 A patient journey map.

2. Information exchange, visibility and
3. The interdependence of experience/emotions along the path and
4. The complex handling of interactions and communications between all stakeholders.

All of the above-mentioned topics are the core topics of operations management which close the circle towards a deeper analysis of what process model concept is used to determine how they can contribute to these topics.

Conclusion and Current Gaps

The concept of patient flow differs from that of the patient journey, even if it is deeply integrated with it. This differentiation is shown as a simplification in Figure 7.4 (Gualandi et al. 2019). From a provider perspective, patient flow aims to manage the flow of patients on their clinical path, often defined in clinical pathways. The focus is on the integration of services and on the efficiency of resources that have to result in a timely care response with respect to the demand for care and by "pushing patients forward" along the route. Each service includes an operational step of a series of patients, and it must be able to respond on time and by integrating with the other services (Gualandi et al. 2019). The patient perspective, or patient journey, is the perspective of

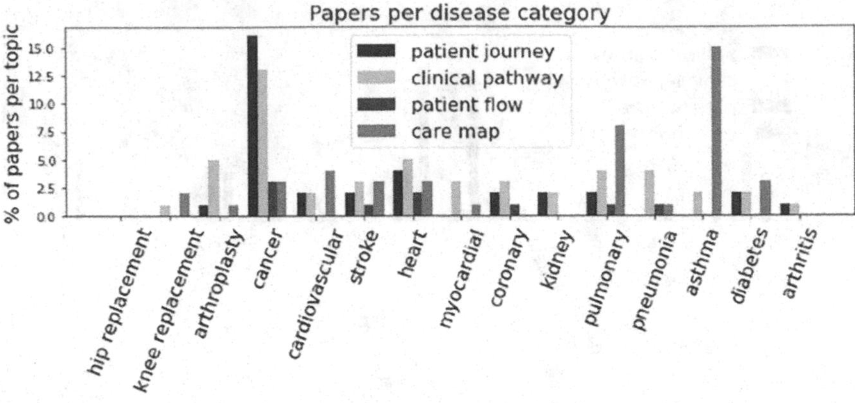

FIGURE 7.4 Provider vs. patient perspective on flows of two encounter.

the individual patient crossing the various services. The patient comes into contact with the "final result" of the services through a progressive succession of steps represented by taking charge of the individual professionals with whom he comes into contact. The service is delivered at the intersection of these two perspectives, through touchpoints that most characterize the quality of the service provided (Gualandi et al. 2019). Lastly, the clinical perspective (or functional perspective) describes the lab and examination results and their relation to action alternatives.

What is missing in patient flows:

- The division of tasks between workforces and their interdependence is not covered.
- Information exchange and interdependencies between resources are not covered.
- Patient as an innovator and patient support system as help are not covered nor implementable.
- Swimlanes and collaboration between clinical and operational resources are not covered.
- Clinical decisions are not implemented in patient flow or patient journey.

- Only the patient journey covers individualization as a descriptive model.
- Clinical pathways should not be viewed as prescriptive step-by-step instructions.

What is missing in patient journey maps:

- No defined link to clinical processes.
- No defined data points to measure or check conformance which makes it very hard.
- to move this to an individual patient-centric operations model.

QUANTITATIVE ANALYSIS

Even though several concepts on modelling the process around the operational and clinical tasks and decisions of a patient exist, it remains unclear what the distinguished use case of each concept is and how the interaction of operational and clinical tasks decisions can be mapped onto them.

Research Approach

To close this gap, a literature search is carried out in journals in the areas of healthcare management, production management, operations research, and information systems that are ranked in VHB-JOURQUAL 3 with at least B or higher to cover the aspects of operations management within healthcare. The number of considered journals (86 in total) in these departments is listed in Table 7.1, and the detailed list is provided on vhbonline. Within these journals, the keywords "Patient Journey," "Patient Flow," "Clinical Pathway," "Patient Pathway," and "Care Map" are used for an exact search for English publications on title, abstract, and keywords (Table 7.2).

To get a better understanding of the distribution and importance of the topics from the VHB journals and to include the clinical perspective, we extend the search to the medical library "PubMed." The hypothesis is to get an understanding of what might be relevant in medical science in comparison to operations and analytics science. The search[1] covers the exact same keywords for articles in English without restrictions on the year of publication. As a result, 5,750 papers are found. To explore the large

TABLE 7.1 Comparison of the Concepts

Concept	Purpose	Providing	Missing
Clinical Pathway	Purpose of structuring decisions that have been proven significantly effective or that require some sort of standardization as decisions are delicate by nature	Patients well-being and structured set of decisions to make	No focus on resources, and patients can not intervene which makes them prone to errors integrating them directly into a CDS
Patient Flow	Representing flow metrics between departments to identify information flows, the impact of eventually occurring bottlenecks as well as to determine transportation and resource allocation dependencies and constraint weights	Patients improved time-to-service but mainly the organisation's utilization and efficiency	Even though it gives an overview of the flow of patients between the units in a hospital, usually no information about the decisions nor the reason for the decisions is given which in turn makes it difficult to find control parameters to influence or understand the reason for this kind of flow as PF is representing aggregated data.
Patient Journey	The journey of a patient is usually for an encounter or a set of encounters linked to a disease. The purpose is to understand the feelings of the patient along their journey through the healthcare system	Insights on patient-clinician interactions as well as emotions and satisfaction changes along the journey for all major touchpoints	Due to the very individual journeys, such models are expensive to set up and due to their individuality patient journey models are hard to compare to each other and cannot build a basis for CDS by themselves. Even though patient-clinician interaction is considered, only the patient perspective is reviewed for these kinds of descriptive models.

TABLE 7.2 List of Journals Selected from VHB

	Healthcare Management	Production Management	Operations Research	Information Systems
A+ Journals	-	1	3	2
A Journals	6	6	13	10
B Journals	6	14	23	27

number of papers, we apply a semi-automated text mining approach. According to Feng et al. (2017), text mining can be used for various purposes in systematic literature reviews, including visualization (e.g., paper hierarchies and networks), automated querying, document classification, and summarization. To capture the status quo of the current literature, we first aim to identify key publications within the presented concepts. While the overall number of citations is a good initial indicator of a paper's relevance, its impact on a certain research topic cannot be interpreted. To extend this view, we build a citation network of all papers from our VHB search result. This way, we can capture both incoming citations (i.e., how often a paper was cited in the network) as well as outgoing citations (i.e., how many papers in the network were cited). While the incoming citations present the impact and relevance of a paper in the network, the outgoing citations can help identify recent meta-analyses that have not gained high visibility yet. Furthermore, the citation network can be used to derive publication clusters, for example, dealing with common topics or from similar outlets (see Figure 7.2). Next, exploratory data analysis and topic analysis are performed to investigate common themes across the vast amount of papers. This allows for a more comprehensive understanding of the discussed topics and helps to guide the further classification of the papers. This information is then used to dive deeper into the area of the process management of patient-centred healthcare service and filter papers according to relevant keywords identified in the previous step. Finally, this subset of papers is analyzed using both quantitative measures from text analysis as well as manual screening by the authors.

Our approach, therefore, consists of four steps: (1) Identify and analyze key papers, (2) derive common topics, (3) identify relevant keywords in patient journey management, and (4) analyze papers on patient journey management (see Figure 7.5).

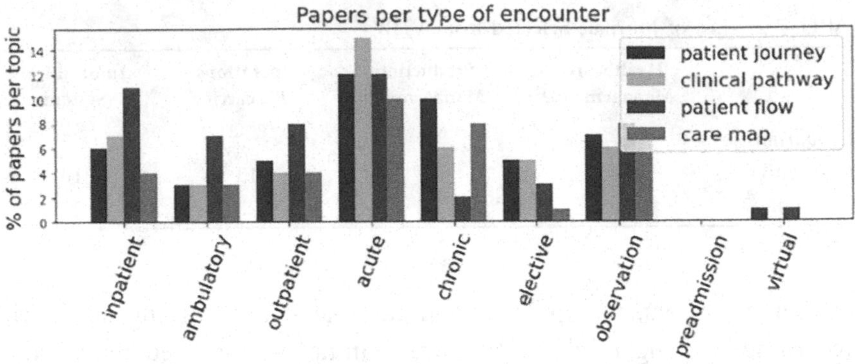

FIGURE 7.5 Semi-automated text analysis approach.

QUANTITATIVE ANALYSIS

Key Publications

To identify the core publications for the presented topics and potential publication clusters, we analyze the citation network between the VHB+ publications using CitNet Explorer 2[2]. Three distinct groups can be identified in the network, with only one group showing strong citation connections between the publications. We further investigate this group to find key papers and clusters (see Figure 7.6). Four clusters can be identified that are connected mainly by 16 identified key papers. Cluster 1 includes papers focusing on scheduling issues and capacity planning in the hospital. Cluster 2 is mainly concerned with approaches to model and optimize patient flow, utilizing methods such as discrete-event simulation and mathematical modelling. Cluster 4 especially focuses on

Abstract							
Patient Journey		Patient flow		Clinical pathway		Care map	
Keyword	*TF-IDF*	*Keyword*	*TF-IDF*	*Keyword*	*TF-IDF*	*Keyword*	*TF-IDF*
emergency department	16.48	length stay	73.36	emergency department	37.26	best practice	0.77
quality life	12.82	medical center	25.11	implementation pathway	29.56	asthma map	0.70
length stay	9.89	operating room	23.76	pathway implementation	24.74	next kin	0.64
best practice	8.47	intensive unit	22.58	outcome measure	22.36	post post	0.63
stage journey	7.96	stay los	19.99	control group	20.93	control group	0.57
outcome measure	7.69	reduce wait	19.41	significant difference	20.88	admission rate	0.57
service delivery	7.63	result total	18.42	breast cancer	20.69	potentially well	0.57
diagnosis treatment	7.49	department ed	16.89	hip fracture	20.31	well practice	0.57
focus group	7.17	outcome measure	16.13	multidisciplinary team	19.98	experimental group	0.56

FIGURE 7.6 Publication custers.

the development of network models. The papers in Cluster 3 are not as distinct as the other groups but cover meta-studies of multiple topics.

From the 16 identified key publications, seven papers are literature reviews or state-of-the-art analyses of common issues and approaches for specific departments (e.g., OR, ED), while the remaining publications present the development and evaluation of individual analyses or simulation models. The results also show that, while the importance of understanding the patient journey more holistically is apparent (Zhong et al. 2017), it has not yet been the focus of any of the key studies, resulting in a lack of common understanding and best practices thereof for decision-makers on an operational level. This may be due to the novelty of the topic of the patient journey and why it has not been thoroughly addressed in literature yet.

To investigate whether any meta-analyses on patient journey management have been published in the more recent past, we specifically search for reviews or state-of-the-art papers in PubMed to unveil promising publications on the patient journey specifically. Here, only three papers are identified. However, all of these papers show very low visibility (citation scores/h-index), which may stem from their focus on very specific application areas (influenza (Beyer et al. 2013), hearing aids (Paglialonga et al. 2018), and knowledge management (Berler et al. 2005)). Thus, no paper could be identified that deals with the systematic structure of methods, decisions, and approaches in the patient journey. Even though patient-centred care has no match in other operations management research, we widen the research to other well-applied process models – patient flow, clinical pathway, care maps – to account for a lack of naming and term conventions.

Publication History

In the next step, we perform exploratory data analysis on the titles, abstracts, and tags of the entire paper database to investigate the publication history across each concept to subsequently derive common topics and determine their relevance for patient journey management. Both PubMed and VHB articles showed more focus on clinical pathways and patient flow than patient journeys and care maps (see Figure 7.7). For care maps, this can be explained by terminological disagreements on whether a care map is another term for clinical pathways, and for its evolution towards graphical representations, which further confuses the terminology. The timeline in Figure 7.7 shows that research on patient

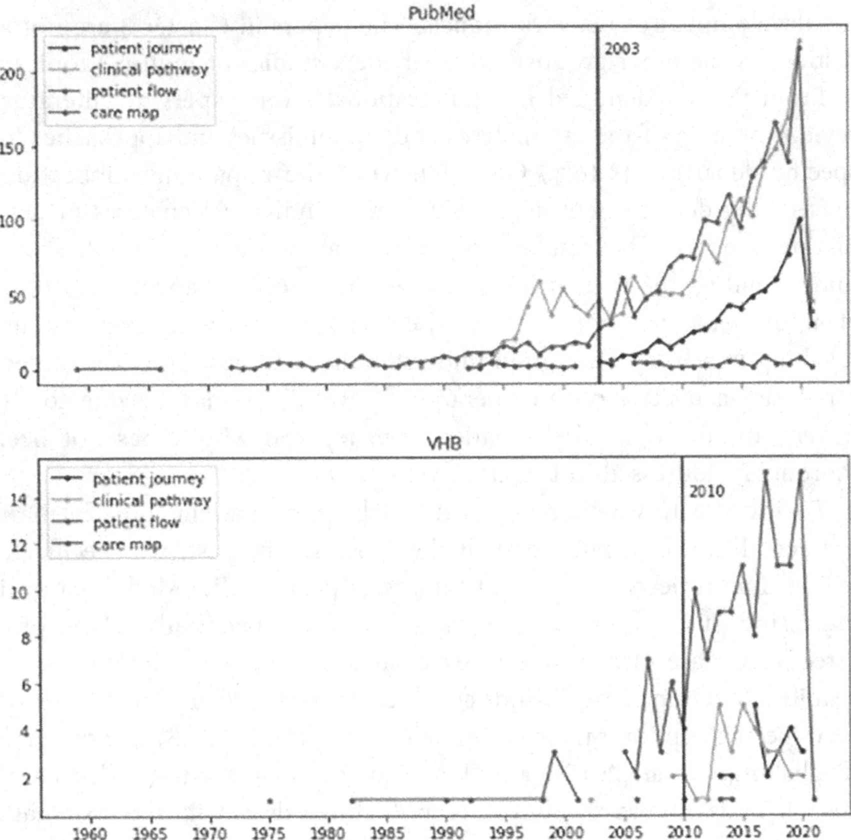

FIGURE 7.7 Increasing interest in papers.

flow already started in the early sixties, whereas papers on clinical pathways and care maps were published much later in the nineties. Patient journey is the most recently discussed topic in literature, with the first publication on PubMed in 2003 and in the VHB+ journals only in 2010. Since then, the number of publications considering patient journeys has rapidly increased. This may reflect the growing demand for the patient journey, and thus more in-depth research is needed.

Next, each concept is investigated in more detail by analyzing the papers related to each concept. This is done by filtering the publications where the title, abstract, or tags contain the concept phrase (i.e., patient journey, patient flow, clinical pathway, or care map). Some papers may cover multiple concepts, but overall, a rather clear distinction between the four concepts can be made, which supports our choice in the investigated topics.

To investigate common themes for each concept, both a keyword and topic analysis are performed using the Python library Gensim (Řehůřek and Sojka 2010). As a first step, the most relevant keywords for each concept are derived based on the term frequency-inverse document frequency (TF-IDF) value for each keyword. This way, words that appear frequently in one paper but not necessarily in other papers are weighted higher than words that are common among all papers. This is done separately based on bigrams from the title, keywords, and tags of the papers related to each concept to capture different types of information from the textual data. While the title focuses mostly on the investigated disease, the tags include information on the type of study and overall goal. The abstract includes both the information presented in the title and tags and doesn't give as clear results as the other textual data sources. However, to investigate the overall occurrence of different keywords in a paper, the abstracts present a richer source of information and will, therefore, be used in the subsequent steps.

Figure 7.8 shows the top 10 most relevant keywords for each of the presented concepts with their corresponding TF-IDF value based on the title, tags, and abstracts of the corresponding papers. While a simple keyword count would also be applicable for the short input of the titles and tags, the use of TF-IDF ensures that irrelevant keywords that may appear in most papers (e.g., hospital, healthcare) are excluded. The keywords are highlighted based on whether they refer to a specific disease, department, type of study, or optimization goal.

Next, for each concept, eight topics are modelled based on the abstracts of papers that contain the concept phrase (i.e., patient journey, patient flow, clinical pathway, or care map). Based on the identified

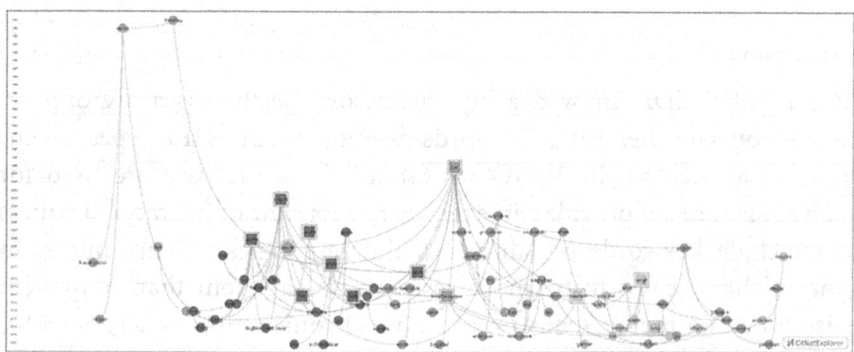

FIGURE 7.8 Keyword analysis of abstracts.

topics and keywords, various themes can be distinguished for each concept that is either centred around a specific disease (e.g., cancer, stroke), department (e.g., emergency department), or optimization goal (e.g., length of stay, cost, quality), utilizing different types of study (e.g., systematic reviews, simulation). To further investigate this phenomenon, in the next step, papers from each concept are analyzed along five dimensions to determine whether there exist specific focus areas for the different concepts. In addition to the investigated disease, department, and optimization goal, the type of study and type of encounter (e.g., inpatient vs. outpatient) are included in the analysis.

RESULTS AND INTERPRETATION

Based on the insights from the EDA, we analyze the identified literature for each concept based on five criteria:

- Which types of encounters are investigated?
- Which disease groups are primarily addressed?
- What issues and goals are addressed?
- Which departments are focused on?
- What types of studies and methods are applied?

To answer these questions, we quantify both the total and relative occurrence of relevant keywords in publications pertaining to our four concepts to derive distinct characteristics of research in each area. This reveals which topics are already covered well and which areas of research are not yet investigated.

Encounters

As the initial EDA showed a high focus on specific disease groups in patient journey literature, keywords relating to the HL7 types of encounters as well as the WHO definitions for acute care are used for analysis. Figure 7.9 provides an exemplary overview of the ratio of papers that include keywords pertaining to different types of encounters. In general, there seems to be more research on inpatient than outpatient episodes and a higher focus on acute vs. chronic episodes across all topics. However, chronic episodes and elective procedures seem to have a much higher relevance in research on patient journeys compared to

	Key papers	Research topics	Keywords	Framework
Input	VHB papers	Abstract	Title + Tags	Full Papers
Method	Network analysis	Topic modeling	TFIDF Analysis	Manual screening
Goal	*Goal: Status Quo*	*Goal: Paper categorization*	*Goal: Keyword analysis*	*Goal: Structure and analyse PJM papers*
Output	List of key papers	List of topics and paper clusters	Relevant keywords for patient journey management	Framework on patient journey management

FIGURE 7.9 No. of papers per type of encounter.

papers on patient flow. Furthermore, pre-hospital care and emergency care mostly play a role in research on patient journeys and patient flow, whereas research on clinical pathways and care maps can mostly be found in trauma and critical care.

Disease Groups and Procedures

To drill down further, the most common disease groups in acute and chronic care are investigated. We, therefore, analyze keywords based on the most common acute procedures by the OECD, as well as the major non-communicable (chronic) diseases listed by the WHO, such as cardiovascular diseases, cancers, chronic respiratory diseases, and diabetes. The relative occurrence of the keywords emphasizes multiple interesting insights. First, papers on patient flow don't seem to have a specific disease or procedure focus but rather investigate hospital processes in general. Papers investigating care maps show a higher interest in pulmonary and cardiovascular diseases, while studies on patient journeys clearly favour cancer-related episodes. Research on clinical pathways can be found across all disease groups and multiple procedures, which indicates that such pathways are investigated both for acute as well as chronic conditions (see Figure 7.10).

To also include papers that utilize a more technical language, the PyMedTermino Lamy et al. (2015) library is used that provides an API to query ICD-10 codes. Two main insights become apparent from the ratio of papers containing ICD-10 categories. First, papers including care maps seem to have a higher focus on specific diseases compared to all other concepts. Second, neoplasms play a major role across all four concepts with an even larger focus in the literature on patient journey and clinical

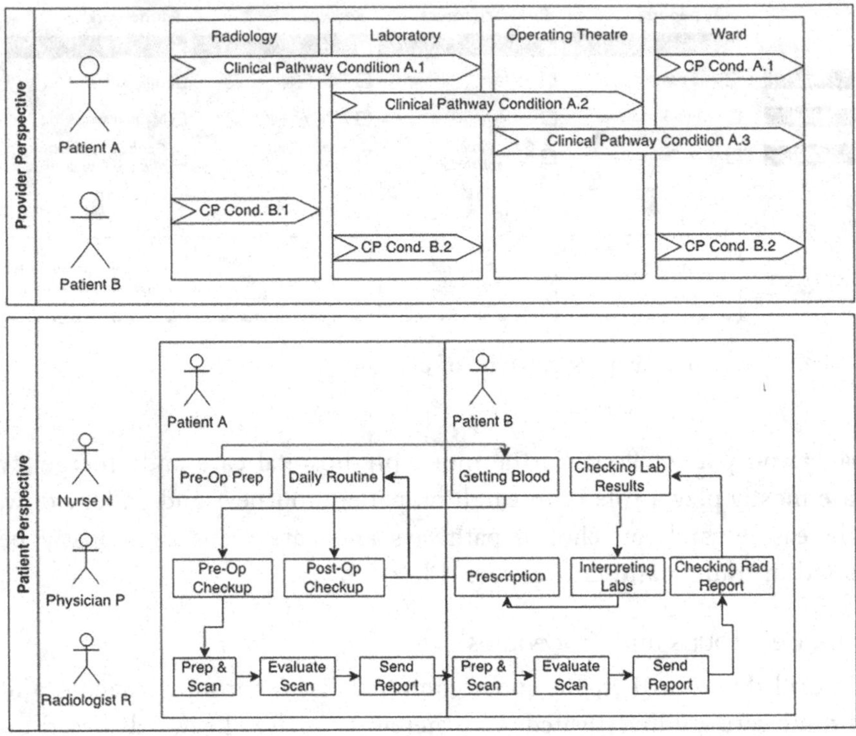

FIGURE 7.10 No. of papers per disease category.

pathways. For patient journey, chronic diseases, such as kidney diseases or diabetes, are investigated more often than acute diseases.

Goals

The optimization goals refer to the identified influences from operations management that include both financial factors (e.g., costs and revenue) as well as quality indicators (e.g., experience, waiting). The high number of papers from patient journey research dealing with patient experience and satisfaction supports the overall view of the patient as an involved customer in the healthcare delivery process instead of a passive recipient. Strictly quantitative optimization factors, such as waiting, crowding, and staffing, are typically related to patient flow that aims to increase hospital efficiency rather than patient experience (see Figure 7.11). Even though no clear distinction can be made, the assumption from the definition section glimpses through the histogram. Patient Flow concentrates on moving patients as quickly as possible to ensure high resource utilization. Clinical pathway is strongly used for qualitative measures in terms of

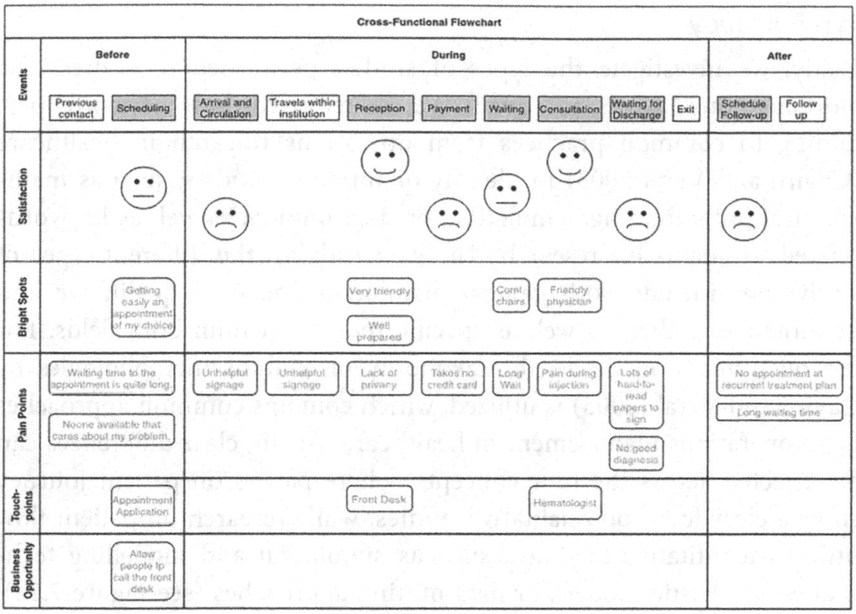

FIGURE 7.11 No. of papers per optimization goal.

quality of care and with standard procedural maps given to reduce costs and search for treatment options. Articles around patient journey focus on the quality and experience of the patient at the touchpoints between health service professionals with adjacent topics to patient flow with respect to waiting times and scheduling, and to clinical pathway with respect to treatment quality and outcome. Care map has a very similar distribution as the clinical pathway, which supports the assumption that a care map and clinical pathway have similar purposes but with different scopes.

Departments

Next, the types of departments are investigated, both based on medical specialty departments as well as acute service wards. While research on patient flow doesn't involve many medical specialty departments, a high focus on the emergency department and ICU can be detected. On the other hand, papers on patient journey and asthma prominently focus on specific departments, such as neonatal and physiotherapy for care map research, and oncology and the renal unit for patient journey. This coincides with the results from the disease groups, where both cancer and chronic kidney disease are common groups in patient journey research.

Type of Study

Lastly, we investigate the types of studies performed to address the aforementioned issues and goals. We, therefore, include keywords pertaining to common practices from operations research in healthcare (Cayirli and Veral 2003) to identify quantitative studies, such as mathematical programming, simulation, or data mining, as well as keywords related to qualitative research. The keywords on the different types of study thus include both general distinctions, such as qualitative and quantitative studies, as well as specific methods within both fields. For the quantitative methods, the taxonomy of analysis methodologies by Cayirli and Veral (2003) is utilized, which contains common approaches from operations management in healthcare. Again, clear differences can be detected across the four concepts, where papers on patient journey show a clear focus on qualitative studies, while research on patient flow utilizes quantitative methods, such as simulation and modelling techniques, stochastic models, or data mining approaches (see Figure 7.12).

Interactions

Following the one-dimensional view of the five aforementioned areas, these areas are also analyzed jointly to determine correlations and gaps in the current literature. This is done for each of the four concepts, and the results are visualized by an example of the results from patient journey research (see Figure 7.13). The most important insights are summarized in

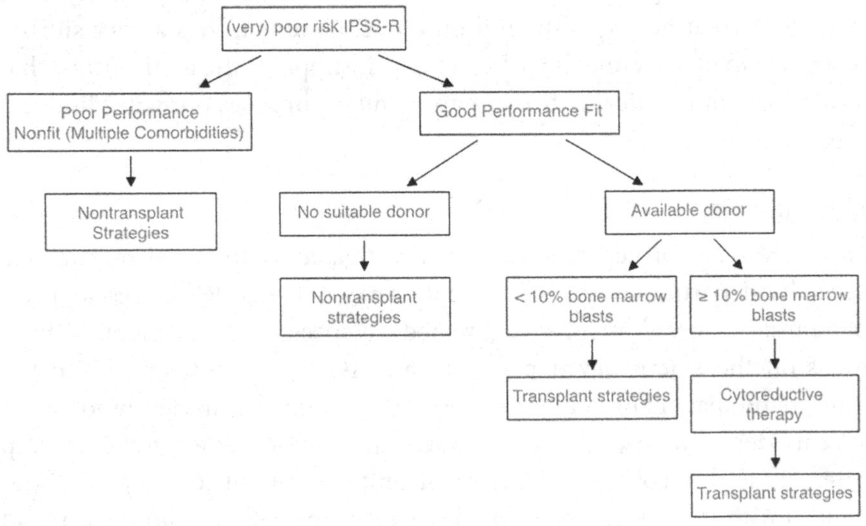

FIGURE 7.12 No. of papers per type of study.

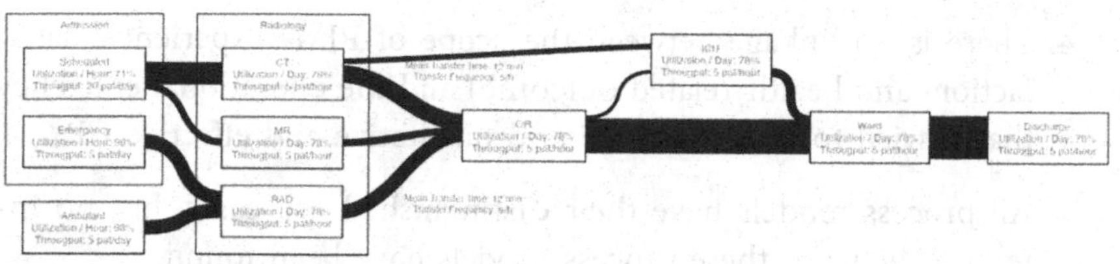

FIGURE 7.13 Correlations between topics.

TABLE 7.3 Insights from Keyword Analysis

Concept	Interactions	Insights
Overall	Department/Disease	There exist apparent department-dependent diseases (e.g., neoplasms and oncology; cardiac arrest and intensive care unit
PJ	Department/Disease	Cardiac arrests that highly relate to the intensive care unit are only highlighted in PJ
PJ	Disease/Goal	Patient experience with hip and knee procedures are commonly discussed
CP	Disease/Goal	Readmission plays an important role, especially with pulmonary diseases and asthma
CP	Encounter/Goal	Readmissions are of particular interest for elective procedures
PF	Disease/Goal	Similar to PJ, patient experience is focused on hip and knee procedures. No-shows play a key role in cancer patients
CM	Department/Disease	Obesity plays an important role in the OR
CM	Disease/Goal	Readmissions and healthcare utilization are investigated mainly for cardiac diseases. Costs play a bigger role in arthroplasty
CM	Encounter/Goal	Resource utilization and costs mainly focus on inpatient episodes with a focus on acute care. Patient experience focuses more on chronic diseases

Table 7.3. From the correlation plots, five key insights into patient journey management can be gained:

1. Patient experience is a major concern in patient journey management.
2. The focus of PJM research lies on patients who return to the hospital multiple times, i.e., with chronic diseases or a longer rehab time.
3. Qualitative research is conducted more frequently in PJM studies compared to the quantitative approach, such as simulation and modelling, in PF or CP literature.

4. There is no linkage between the scope of PJM (experience, satisfaction, and health-related outcome) and the operational efficiency that is tried to cover with PF and qualitative and effective CP.
5. All process models have their distinguished use cases, but no interfaces between these process models have been found.

From that, we are focusing on bridging the gap between operations and analytics science towards patients with individual requirements to the healthcare system with all its stakeholders, as well as the medical science that tries to map clinical sciences and patients' needs to statistically significant guidelines. The following hypotheses can be made:

1. A major open topic is the harmonization of patient-centric data-driven management.
2. Cluster 1 includes papers focusing on scheduling issues and capacity planning in the hospital. Cluster 2 is mainly concerned with approaches to model and optimize patient flow utilizing methods such as discrete-event simulation and mathematical modelling. Cluster 3 especially focuses on the development of network models.

DISCUSSION

In this literature review, a variety of process modelling methodologies are reviewed that are mainly applied within the healthcare sector. Process models are a suitable way to model behaviour, analyze inter-dependencies, and understand commonalities and variations. From six core concepts to describe processes and decisions in healthcare (clinical pathways, clinical algorithms, standard operating procedures, patient flows, care maps, and patient journeys), the research of the paper focuses on known models in healthcare service and operations research as we assume that these consider patients from a more individual, service-oriented perspective rather than as a set of clinical measures. For operational processes within healthcare, we consider the concepts of patient flow and patient journey, and from the clinical-operational side, we include structured guidelines in the form of clinical pathways and care maps.

Clinical pathways and care maps are strongly related to clinical activities; however, they do not consider how clinical resources are involved in each incident. Patient flows consider the utilization of clinical resources while analyzing the flow of patients along possible clinical pathways.

An additional aspect that supports this research is the increasing interest in involving the patient as a user in the healthcare service market. Therefore, to improve quality and better understand patients, market analysis techniques from the user journey can be used in value-based care and healthcare as a service approach. The descriptive model used in this context is called patient journeys. Patient journey models align the individual aspects, such as feelings and mood, with the operational circumstances, such as waiting time, time to service, and touchpoint quality, along the pre-defined clinical pathways. The goal is to improve the service- and quality orientation of healthcare providers and enhance the patient's satisfaction and experience from a system as a whole. That said, patient journeys provide a backbone for describing and interpreting patient interactions with the healthcare system. However, to date, no measures have been taken to make patient journeys computationally accessible, which, in turn, is necessary to establish the concept for each patient as a patient-individual journey model derived from data.

As the patient journey has been analyzed more from a qualitative perspective, no computational model exists that allows for healthcare operations to be mapped to a decision model. Another advantage of a patient journey is the strong focus on individuals that need to be considered. Mixing patient's descriptive properties (the concept of phenotyping (Uciteli et al. 2020)) with the touchpoints along the healthcare process that are mapped to the clinical guidelines, algorithms, and scenario-induced abilities to provide services and descriptions of the process as a whole can be made possible and result in the identification of inter-dependencies to support a more precise and better understanding of healthcare services.

Clinical pathways, patient flows, and patient journeys all have their individual scope. Our hypothesis is that patient journeys have the highest potential from the healthcare operations perspective to understand the behaviour of patients. Paired with the touchpoints and clinical decisions, this can enable a better understanding of the interface to healthcare professionals and their activities on the value-based care principles:

- Patients have lower costs & better outcomes.
- Providers have higher efficiency and satisfaction with patients.
- Payers have transparent cost controls and reduced risks of accepting outliers.

- Suppliers can align prices based on patient outcomes.
- Society can benefit from reduced healthcare spending and better overall health.

The literature is also missing approaches that consider clinical decisions. Even though clinical algorithms and guidelines are vastly available within clinical research, no approach exists that is able to facilitate events on a phenotype. This makes causal effect analysis, as well as time-dependency and sequence-dependency analysis, not possible with respect to precision medicine. This also hinders the possibility of building decision-support models that consider the patient phenotype.

To improve the existing descriptive models of healthcare processes, clinical algorithms need to be considered. Clinical algorithms and standard operating procedures within this research fall short, even though they guide clinicians to make decisions at touchpoints between patients and clinicians. It can be assumed that clinicians and caretakers influence each decision along the journey of the patient - might it be directly addressed to the patient or indirectly addressed to service providers that connect to the patient in any way. Also, decision-makers who influence other patients' journeys influence the currently focused patient journey as they might block a CT, an operating theatre, or a clinician. This paper showcases the current state of research on process modelling concepts for patient journeys in hospitals as well as potential gaps for further studies. The results of the literature synthesis present various blank spots that have not yet been sufficiently addressed in information systems, operations management, and healthcare management research. While traditional quantitative approaches, such as clinical pathways and patient flow have been thoroughly investigated in the past, the development of patient journeys has only been considered in a qualitative way, deeming it unsuitable for decision support models.

CONCLUSION

The individualization of patient care only applies to the touchpoints between the patient and clinician. However, clinical knowledge models, such as guidelines, standard operating procedures, and pathways, as well as operational workflow models, such as patient flow, do not allow for individual patient assessment and treatment. Patient Journey models are the first to consider the patient as a customer and take into account their satisfaction to enhance the capabilities of healthcare service providers in providing better services. There is still a gap between good operational service, patient satisfaction, and targeted diagnosis and treatment, as no model aligns the workflows of healthcare providers, patient data mapped to a patient journey, and clinical best practices in the form of clinical guidelines to build a descriptive model for each encounter. This gap leads to a constant battle between standardized hospital processes, clinical guidelines, resource allocation, and "real" pathways, leaving out the possibility of modelling patients' flows enriched with digital health records, fitness tracker data, and other relevant sources of data.

The increasing pressure on hospitals to provide healthcare services as efficiently as possible has resulted in a variety of methods for process optimization and lean management. Approaches such as patient flows or clinical pathways standardize individual medical decisions, treatment paths, and resource utilization of patient groups in the hospital on a higher level. However, these approaches neglect the individual characteristics and needs of a single patient. In contrast, the patient journey is a patient-centric approach that focuses on individual characteristics and needs. The patient is viewed as an individual whose "customer experience" with healthcare services must be optimized. However, this approach has been pursued purely on a qualitative level by collecting and evaluating the patient experience.

This paper bridges the gap between the two classes of approaches and demonstrates the need to create a quantitative, process-based model of treatment pathways for individual patients to improve their overall experience and satisfaction in the hospital. The current state of research from patient flow, clinical pathways, and patient journeys is reviewed to identify key themes and gaps in each area. The results show that the quantitative, process-oriented approaches are particularly concerned with resource optimization and readmissions, while patient journeys focus on special and complex disease patterns. The methods used in both areas also differ. Patient flows and clinical pathways have a strong quantitative focus, mostly dealing with simulations and modelling of hospital processes, resource allocation, and patient movement through the hospital. Patient journeys, on the other hand, focus on qualitative studies that evaluate the patient experience in the hospital (Druckenmiller 2019).

Based on the findings, gaps in current research are identified that require the linkage of all these approaches. These gaps include process modelling and optimization of patient-individual experiences throughout the entire patient journey. New analysis and modelling methods that represent the totality of all relevant input factors on the quantitative and qualitative side are required. By collecting and investigating the status quo of methods and application areas of each of these techniques, this paper offers a variety of novel research topics to enable the development of a holistic modelling approach for actionable, individual patient journey models.

NOTES

1. https://pubmed.ncbi.nlm.nih.gov/?term=%22Patient+Journey%22%5BTitle%2FAbstract%5D+OR+%22Patient+Flow%22%5BTitle%2FAbstract%5D+OR+%22Patient+Pathway%22%5BTitle%2FAbstract%5D+OR+%22Critical+Pathway%22%5BTitle%2FAbstract%5D+OR+%22Clinical+Pathway%22%5BTitle%2FAbstract%5D+OR+%22Care+map%22+%5BTitle%2FAbstract%5D&filter=lang.english&show_snippets=off&size=200
2. The visualization is limited to a maximum of 100 publications, which are automatically selected based on their citation impact and number of connections in the network.

REFERENCES

Al-Hakim L, Gong XY (2012) On the day of surgery: How long does preventable disruption prolong the patient journey? 25(4):322–342, ISSN 0952-6862, URL 10.1108/09526861211221509.

Association EP (2021) E-P-A definition of care pathway. URL (http://e-p-a.org/care-pathways/).

Bayliss EA, Edwards AE, Steiner JF, Main DS (2008) Processes of care desired by elderly patients withmultimorbidities 25(4):287–293, ISSN 0263-2136, URL 10.1093/fampra/cmn040.

Berler A, Pavlopoulos S, Koutsouris D (2005) Using key performance indicators as knowledge-management tools at a regional health-care authority level 9(2):184–192, ISSN 1089-7771, URL 10.1109/titb.2005.847196.

Beyer WEP, McElhaney J, Smith DJ, Monto AS, Nguyen-Van-Tam JS, Osterhaus ADME (2013) Cochrane re-arranged: Support for policies to vaccinate elderly people against influenza 31(50):6030–6033, ISSN 1873-2518, URL 10.1016/j.vaccine.2013.09.063.

Bhattacharjee P, Ray PK (2014a) Patient flow modelling and performance analysis of healthcare deliveryprocesses in hospitals: A review and reflections 78:299–312, ISSN 0360-8352, URL 10/f6ttvd.

Bhattacharjee P, Ray PK (2014b) Patient flow modelling and performance analysis of healthcare delivery processes in hospitals: A review and reflections 78:299–312, ISSN 0360-8352, URL 10.1016/j.cie.2014.04.016.

Blegen MA, Reiter RC, Goode CJ, Murphy RR (1995) Outcomes of hospital-based managed care: A multivariateanalysis of cost and quality 86(5):809–814, ISSN 0029-7844, URL 10.1016/0029-7844(95)00270-2.

Boekemeyer B (2016) Patient journey maps.

Boyd H, McKernon S, Mullin B, Old A (2012) Improving healthcare through the use of co-design 125(1357):76–87, ISSN 1175-8716.

Brown MM, Brown GC, Sharma S (2005) *Evidence-based to Value-based Medicine* (Chicago: AMA Press), ISBN 978-1-57947-625-0.

Bussel EFV, Jeerakathil T, Schrijvers AJ (2013) The process flow and structure of an integrated stroke strategy 13(2), ISSN 1568-4156, URL 10.5334/ijic.888.

Catalyst N (2018) What is patient flow? URL https://catalyst.nejm.org/doi/full/10.1056/CAT.18. 0289, publisher: Massachusetts Medical Society.

Cayirli T, Veral E (2003) Outpatient scheduling in health care: A review of literature 12(4):519–549, ISSN 1937-5956, URL 10.1111/j.1937-5956.2003.tb00218.x.

Curry J, McGregor C, Tracy S (2006) A communication tool to improve the patient journey modeling process 2006:4726–4730, ISSN 1557-170X, URL 10.1109/IEMBS.2006.259481.

Coté MJ (1999) Patient flow and resource utilization in an outpatient clinic 33(3):231–245, ISSN 0038-0121, URL 10.1016/S0038-0121(99)00007-5.

Dai T, Tayur S (2019a) OM forum—healthcare operations management: A snapshot of emerging research 22(5):869–887, ISSN 1523-4614, URL 10/gg5g59.

De Freitas L, Goodacre S, O'Hara R, Thokala P, Hariharan S (2018) Interventions to improve patient flow in emergency departments: An umbrella review 35(10):626–637, ISSN 1472-0213, URL 10.1136/emermed-2017-207263.

de Witte T, Bowen D, Robin M, Malcovati L, Niederwieser D, Yakoub-Agha I, Mufti GJ, Fenaux P, Sanz G, Martino R, Alessandrino EP, Onida F, Symeonidis A, Passweg J, Kobbe G, Ganser A, Platzbecker U, Finke J, van Gelder M, van de Loosdrecht AA, Ljungman P, Stauder R, Volin L, Deeg HJ, Cutler C, Saber W, Champlin R, Giralt S, Anasetti C, Kröger N (2017) Allogeneic hematopoietic stem cell transplantation for MDS and CMML: Recommendations from an international expert panel. Blood 129(13):1753–1762, ISSN 0006-4971, URL 10.1182/blood-2016-06-724500.

Druckenmiller G, (2019) The Patient Journey: What Is It and Why Is It Important? | Healthgrades. URL: https://www.mercuryhealthcare.com/blog/why-is-patient-engagement-journey-important

Feng YY, Wu IC, Chen TL (2017) Stochastic resource allocation in emergency departments with a multiobjective simulation optimization algorithm 20(1):55–75, ISSN 1572-9389, URL 10.1007/s10729-015-9335-1.

Gooch P, Roudsari A (2011) Computerization of workflows, guidelines, and care pathways: A review of implementation challenges for process-oriented health information systems 18(6):738–748, ISSN 1067-5027, URL 10.1136/amiajnl-2010-000033.

Gualandi R, Masella C, Viglione D, Tartaglini D (2019) Exploring the hospital patient journey: What does the patient experience? 14(12):e0224899, ISSN 1932-6203, URL 10.1371/journal. pone.0224899.

Habicht H, Oliveira P, Shcherbatiuk V (2012) User innovators: When patients set out to help themselves and end up helping many. SSRN Scholarly Paper ID 2144325, Social Science Research Network, URL https://papers.ssrn.com/abstract=2144325.

Hall RW (2006) Patient flow: Reducing delay in healthcare delivery. Number v. 91 in International Series in Operations Research & Management Science (Springer), ISBN 978-0-387-33635-0 978-0-387-33636-7.

Hall RW, ed. (2012a) Handbook of healthcare system scheduling. Number v. 168 in International Series in Operations Research & Management Science (Springer), ISBN 978-1-4614-1733-0, OCLC: ocn755698238.

Hall RW (2012b) Matching healthcare resources to patient needs. Hall RW, ed., Handbook of Healthcare System Scheduling, volume 168, 1–9 (Springer US), ISBN 978-1-4614-1733-0 978-1-4614-1734-7, URL 10.1007/978-1-4614-1734-7_1, series Title: International Series in Operations Research & Management Science.

Halvorsrud R, Lillegaard AL, Røhne M, Jensen AM (2019) Managing complex patient journeys in healthcare. Service Design and Service Thinking in Healthcare and Hospital Management: Theory, Concepts, Practice. In Pfannstiel, MA and Rasche, C, eds, 329–346 (Springer International Publishing), ISBN 978-3-030-00749-2, URL http://dx.doi.org/10.1007/978-3-030-00749-2_19

Hampton D (1993) Implementing a managed care framework through care maps. - abstract - europe PMC 23(5):21–27, URL https://europepmc.org/article/med/8509873.

Hartzband P, Groopman J (2011) The new language of medicine 365(15): 1372–1373, ISSN 0028-4793, URL 10.1056/NEJMp1107278, publisher: Massachusetts Medical Society. eprint: 10.1056/NEJMp1107278.

Hendrich AL, Fay J, Sorrells AK (2004) Effects of acuity-adaptable rooms on flow of patients and delivery of care. *American Journal of Critical Care* 13(1):35–45, ISSN 1062-3264, 1937-710X, URL 10.4037/ajcc2004.13.1.35.

Hitzig SL, Gotlib Conn L, Guilcher SJT, Cimino SR, Robinson LR (2020-02) Understanding the role of the physiatrist and how to improve the continuum of care for trauma patients: A qualitative study 1–8, ISSN 1464-5165, URL 10.1080/09638288.2020.1719215.

Husbands S, Jowett S, Barton P, Coast J (2018) Understanding and identifying key issues with the involvement of clinicians in the development of decision-analytic model structures: A qualitative study 36(12):1453–1462, ISSN 1179-2027, URL 10.1007/s40273-018-0705-7.

Jarvie L, Robinson C, MacTavish P, Dunn L, Quasim T, McPeake J (2019) Understanding the patient journey: A mechanism to reduce staff burnout? 28(6):396–397, ISSN 0966-0461, URL 10.12968/bjon.2019.28.6.396.

Kathryn de L, Kitchiner D, Layton A, Morris E, Murray Y, Overill S (2018) *Developing Care Pathways: The Handbook* (Routledge), ISBN 978-1-315-37916-6, URL 10.4324/9781315379166.

Lamy JB, Venot A, Duclos C (2015) PyMedTermino: An open-source generic API for advanced terminology services. 924–928, URL 10.3233/978-1-614 99-512-8-924, publisher: IOS Press.

Lawal AK, Rotter T, Kinsman L, Machotta A, Ronellenfitsch U, Scott SD, Goodridge D, Plishka C, Groot G (2016) What is a clinical pathway? refinement of an operational definition to identify clinical pathway studies for a cochrane systematic review 14:35, ISSN 1741-7015, URL 10/f8b5zx.

Lemon KN, Verhoef PC (2016) Understanding customer experience throughout the customer journey. *Journal of Marketing* 80(6):69–96, ISSN 0022-2429, 1547-7185, URL 10.1509/ jm.15.0420.

Luc Kd, Todd J (2020) *e-Pathways: Computers and the patient's journey through care* (CRC Press), ISBN 978-1-315-37616-5, URL 10.1201/9781315376165.

Mammen C, Matsell DG, Lemley KV (2014) The importance of clinical pathways and protocols in pediatric nephrology 29(10):1903–1914, ISSN 1432-198X, URL 10.1007/ s00467-013-2577-6.

Marr JA, Reid B (1992) Implementing managed care and case management: The neuroscience experience 24(5):281–285, ISSN 0888-0395, URL 10.1097/ 01376517-199210000-00010.

McHugh S, Droog E, Foley C, Boyce M, Healy O, Browne JP (2019-08) Understanding the impetus for major systems change: A multiple case study of decisions and non-decisions to reconfigure emergency and urgent care services 123(8):728–736, ISSN 0168-8510, URL 10.1016/ j.healthpol. 2019.05.018.

Meyer MA (2019) Mapping the patient journey across the continuum: Lessons learned from one patient's experience 6(2):103–107, ISSN 2374-3735, URL 10.1177/2374373518783763.

Nabhan C, Mato AR, Feinberg BA (2017) Clinical pathways in chronic lymphocytic leukemia: Challenges and solutions: Pathways for CLL 92(1):5–6, ISSN 03618609, URL 10.1002/ajh.24589.

Ogilvie-Harris DJ, Botsford DJ, Hawker RW (1993) Elderly patients with hip fractures: Improved outcome with the use of care maps with high-quality medical and nursing protocols 7(5):428–437, ISSN 0890-5339, URL 10. 1097/00005131-199310000-00005.

Paglialonga A, Cleveland Nielsen A, Ingo E, Barr C, Laplante-L´evesque A (2018) eHealth and the hearing aid adult patient journey: A state-of-the-art review 17(1):101, ISSN 1475-925X, URL 10.1186/s12938-018-0531-3.

Peleg M (2013) Computer-interpretable clinical guidelines: A methodological review. *Journal of Biomedical Informatics* 46(4):744–763, ISSN 15320464, URL 10.1016/j.jbi.2013.06.009.

Řehůřek R, Sojka P (2010) Software framework for topic modelling with large corpora. Proceedings of the LREC 2010 Workshop on New Challenges for NLP Frameworks, 45–50 (ELRA).

Schleidgen S, Klingler C, Bertram T, Rogowski WH, Marckmann G (2013) What is personalized medicine: Sharpening a vague term based on a systematic literature review 14(1):55, ISSN 1472-6939, URL 10.1186/1472-6939-14-55.

Trbovich P, Vincent C (2019) From incident reporting to the analysis of the patient journey. *BMJ Quality & Safety* 28(3):169–171, ISSN 2044-5423, URL 10.1136/bmjqs-2018-008485.

Trebble TM, Hansi N, Hydes T, Smith MA, Baker M (2010) Process mapping the patient journey: An introduction 341:c4078, ISSN 1756-1833, URL 10.1136/bmj.c4078.

Uciteli A, Beger C, Kirsten T, Meineke FA, Herre H (2020) Ontological representation, classification and data-driven computing of phenotypes. *Journal of Biomedical Semantics* 11(1):15, ISSN 2041-1480, URL 10.1186/s13326-020-00230-0.

Wilson DE (1995) Effect of managed care on selected outcomes of hospitalized surgical patients URL 10.7939/R3PV6BH38, publisher: University of Alberta Libraries.

Yu TC, Zhang X, Smiell JM, Boing E, Tan H (2019-05) Understanding patient journey in terms of healthcare resource utilization (HCRU) and cost of care among patients with thermal burns and autograft in a large managed care population 22:S215–S215, ISSN 1098-3015, URL pt10/ghz4fb, WOS:000472670102126.

Zhong X, Lee HK, Li J (2017) From production systems to health care delivery systems: A retrospective look on similarities, difficulties and opportunities. *International Journal of Production Research* 55(14):4212–4227, ISSN 0020-7543, URL 10.1080/00207543.2016.1277276.

Zweifel P, Breyer F, Kifmann M (2009) Hospital services and efficiency, 311–329 (Springer Berlin Heidelberg), ISBN 978-3-540-27804-7 978-3-540-68540-1, URL 10.1007/ 978-3-540-68540-1_9.

CHAPTER 8

AI Approaches for Managing Preventive Care in Digital Health Ecosystems

Andreas Hamper

STRUCTURAL CHANGES THAT DRIVE PREVENTIVE CARE

Over the past decade, there has been a shift in the healthcare industry towards an increased focus on preventive care. This means that instead of simply treating diseases after they have developed, healthcare systems are now focusing on helping patients manage their overall well-being and take preventive measures to avoid getting sick in the first place (RKI 2015).

One key driver of this shift has been the adoption of data-oriented and artificial intelligence (AI)-based technology in the healthcare industry (Rowe & Lester 2020). With the help of AI, it has become possible to gather and analyse vast amounts of data from personal health sensors, devices, and digital records. This data can be used to identify patterns and trends that can help predict the likelihood of someone developing a particular disease or health condition as well as supporting actions to avoid diseases as well as treatment. As a result of data- and AI-driven insight, patients are now able to take more proactive approaches to their health, such as monitoring their vital signs, following healthy lifestyle habits, and taking preventive measures like getting vaccinated or taking prescribed medications. And because these interventions can be supported by digital health

DOI: 10.1201/9781032699745-10

assistants, patients can more easily access the information and resources they need to stay healthy.

Overall, the increased availability of holistic data and AI technologies is helping to drive a paradigm shift towards preventive care in the healthcare industry, enabling patients and healthcare professionals to work together to promote better health outcomes and prevent diseases before they occur.

To enable data- and AI-driven healthcare, four main paradigm changes must be understood:

- Preventing diseases rather than curing them:
  Preventive care focuses on preventing diseases or health conditions before they occur. It involves taking proactive steps to maintain good health and reduce the risk of developing diseases or health problems. By taking proactive steps to prevent illness, individuals can improve their quality of life and reduce the costs of healthcare for society.

  Although curative treatment is still considered the central pillar of the healthcare system, prevention and health promotion are increasingly coming into focus (Altgeld et al. 2006). This is due to changes in the spectrum of diseases and is forcing those in charge to adapt healthcare (Hurrelmann et al. 2014). This will require a shift in health policy to focus on the management of chronic diseases, prevention and health promotion, and the care of older people.

  Digital health applications, such as mobile apps or online tools, can play a role in promoting this shift towards disease prevention. These applications can provide individuals with access to information and resources that can help them adopt healthy behaviours and habits, such as tracking their physical activity levels, following a healthy diet, or managing stress (Hemkens 2021).

  For healthcare professionals, digital health applications can also provide valuable data and insights that can be used to identify patterns and trends that may indicate the risk of a particular disease or health condition. This can help healthcare professionals take a more proactive approach to care, by identifying and addressing potential health issues before they develop into more serious problems.

- Patient-centred care and consumerization:
  Patient-centred care is a healthcare approach that focuses on meeting the needs and preferences of the patient. It involves treating the

patient as an active participant in their own healthcare and involving them in the decision-making process.

Since the early 2010s, quantified self movement emerged with growing capabilities of mobile and wearable devices and enabled users to have personal data and technology to track and improve various aspects of their own health and well-being. This can include tracking physical activity levels, sleep patterns, nutrition, and other health-related metrics (Barrett et al. 2013).

Similarly, consumerization refers to the trend of patients taking a more active role in their own healthcare, similar to the way consumers make choices about other products and services. This includes researching treatment options, asking questions about their care, and seeking out information about their health conditions (Knight & Sorin 2016).

The combination of patient-centred care, quantified self, and consumerization can lead to a more personalized and proactive approach to healthcare. By involving patients in their own care and empowering them to make informed decisions based on their own data and preferences, healthcare professionals can help patients to be more in control of their health and better able to manage their conditions.

- Healthcare ecosystems:
  Medical data in Germany is largely siloed. While hospitals have strong and interconnected internal IT, data exchange and sharing between institutions is still often paper-based, caused by the lack of a national digital health platform or comprehensive health record. In general, such healthcare data ecosystems are systems that involve the collection, storage, and sharing of healthcare data between stakeholders and even healthcare sectors. This can include data from various sources, such as electronic health records, personal health devices, and other healthcare-related information.

  In Europe, there are several initiatives and regulations that aim to support the development and use of personal health records, healthcare data ecosystems, medical data, and digital health platforms. One key initiative is the European Health Data Space, which is a project funded by the European Union (EU) to create a secure and interoperable environment for the exchange of healthcare data across the EU (Gallina 2023). The goal of this project is to support the development of digital health services and improve the efficiency and effectiveness of healthcare delivery. On a national level, the Telematics Infrastructure (TI) is a national IT system used in the healthcare system in Germany (Leyck Dieken 2021). It serves as a platform for the exchange of electronic health data and enables the secure and standardized exchange of health information between different actors in the healthcare system. The TI includes various components, such as central databases where health data is stored, and an electronic patient record, which provides doctors and other healthcare providers with access to important health information about a patient.

To enable data- and AI-driven applications, it is crucial to integrate data from various sources and make it accessible for authorized healthcare providers across sectors to improve the quality of care, support research, and make informed decisions about healthcare. By creating a healthcare data ecosystem and enabling medical data sharing through digital health platforms, it is possible to create a more integrated and coordinated approach to healthcare.

- AI-based technologies:
  AI has the potential to revolutionize the healthcare industry by enabling the processing and analysis of vast amounts of data in ways that were previously not possible like in the following healthcare processes:

  Big-Data analysis: AI can be used to analyze large amounts of healthcare data, especially from health insurance companies, such as electronic health records and medical research, to identify patterns and trends that may not be immediately apparent to humans. This can be used to predict the likelihood of a particular disease or health condition, identify potential risk factors, or determine the most effective treatment options.

  Medical imaging and treatment: AI can be used to assist with the diagnosis and treatment of diseases. For example, AI algorithms can be trained to recognize patterns in medical images, such as X-rays or MRIs, that may indicate the presence of a particular condition. AI can also be used to analyze medical data to recommend treatment options or identify potential side effects of medications.

  Predictive analytics: AI can be used to predict the likelihood of a particular event or outcome, such as the likelihood of a patient being readmitted to the hospital or the likelihood of a particular treatment being successful. This can be used to inform clinical decision-making and prioritize care for high-risk patients.

Virtual assistants: AI can be used to create virtual assistants that can help patients follow medical advice, adopt healthy lifestyle patterns, access information, or improve adherence and compliance.

While the potential for AI is tremendous, necessary data and regulatory structures are still lacking in many cases. Therefore, the idea-to-market process, including regulatory issues, of medical technology which uses vast amounts of data rather than human expert knowledge has to be further established.

AI AS AN ENABLER IN A DATA-DRIVEN HEALTHCARE VALUE CHAIN

To leverage the power of AI, we need to look at the infrastructure and processes that collect, integrate, analyze and apply data. A data value chain in healthcare refers to the process of creating value from healthcare data by collecting, storing, analyzing, and using data in a way that supports healthcare delivery and decision-making. While there are numerous concepts for data value chains in digitalized environments, they typically involve several steps that cover the processes shown below (Wunck & Baumann 2017).

- Data collection: This involves gathering data from various sources along the preventive care process from personal care and wearable technologies, AAL sensors, medical devices, treatments from general practitioners and hospital data in a structured and automated way.
- Data integration: This involves storing data in a secure and privacy-protecting way, such as in an electronic health record system, managing it in interoperable, federated systems like the European Health Data Space (EHDS) and making it accessible with semantic standards like HL7 FHIR (Fast Healthcare Interoperability Resources).
- Data analytics: This involves using tools and techniques to analyze data and extract insights from patient data that are useful for both healthcare patients and professionals. As described, the types of data AI operates on may vary from medical imaging to personal fitness and health data to large-scale cohorts of patient records from insurance companies.

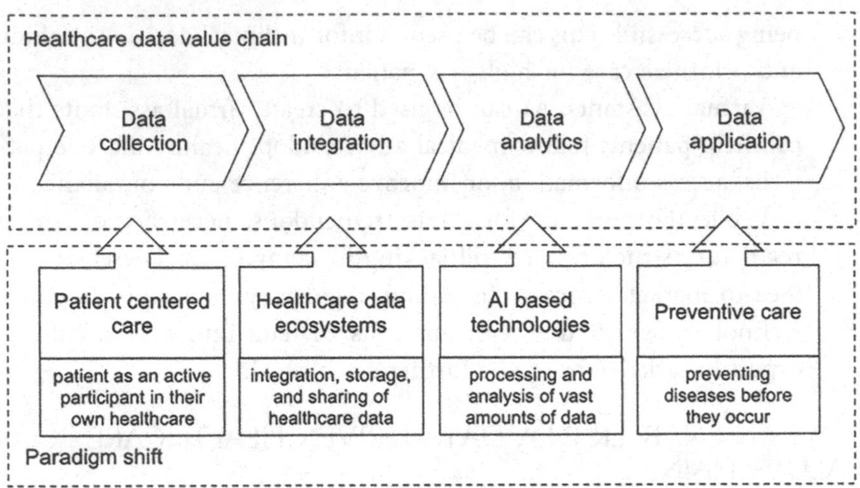

FIGURE 8.1 Fundamental shifts in preventive healthcare along the data value chain.

- Data application: This involves making data analytics available to patients and professionals in a way, that they can practically use it. While medical professionals are experts in their medical field, there is no need to understand AI and IT technologies on an engineering level. This means data provided by AI technologies must be represented in a way that is accessible for medical experts rather than AI experts. This is even more relevant for patient-centred technologies where AI is not only used to create better insights into healthcare data but also to interact with the patient and influence their behaviour.

By following a data value chain concept, the necessary infrastructure and environment for successful data- and AI-enabled approaches can be described. When looking at the paradigm changes mentioned earlier, it can be seen that each of them mainly addresses one of the elements in the healthcare data value chain (Figure 8.1).

EXEMPLARY AI USE-CASE FROM RESEARCH AND PRACTICE

To illustrate the potential for AI-based smart health solutions, four examples from research and practice are shown. Each of the examples focuses on a specific step in the data value chain and therefore emphasizes the efforts needed to meet the new challenges caused by the paradigm shifts.

Behavioural Prevention with Personal Health Devices

This example focuses on data application in the context of health and fitness promotion with mobile technology. Individual behaviour is a crucial factor for health risks that can lead to chronic diseases like diabetes, coronary heart disease or obesity. In the field of preventive care, four main risk factors are crucial to avoiding chronic diseases: Excessive consumption of alcohol and tobacco, unhealthy diets and low levels of physical activity. Behavioural prevention influences behaviour to encourage individuals to adopt a healthier lifestyle (Lengerke 2007).

Behaviour change towards more physical activity is especially challenging, as it fully depends on the individual's motivation and ability. Mobile services, like smartphone apps, can support behaviour change processes towards an active lifestyle. Existing human-to-human instruments are not suitable for carrying out behaviour change interventions to a high number of risk carriers, while mobile apps have the power to provide individualized preventative measures for broad populations in a cost-efficient manner. While today, these products are mostly used for entertainment and wellness purposes, too little is known about their mode of action to decide whether some of these apps can be used to reduce risk factors (Hamper 2018).

Preventive self-care approaches aim to involve the patient in their own medical treatment and create shared responsibility with them. This approach has been used in the treatment of chronic diseases as well as preventive measures like smoking cessation, nutrition, and physical activity. For this, understanding the process of behaviour change is essential in supporting patients in their self-care actions and preventive measures. If the cognitive and behavioural processes of the patient are well understood, AI systems can be designed to guide and support the user in this process. To maximize the impact of these AI systems, relevant behaviour change theory must be used as a foundation to guide their development.

The increase of problem awareness through information, clarification of problem behaviour and confrontation with resulting risks are identified as decisive strategies in behaviour change theory. This leads to the need for AI-based "risk calculators", which determine individual health risk factors for the user. With increasing risk and problem awareness, the user can be guided through the behaviour change process. To select risk and health indicators, we suggest relying on established standards in professional preventive care. Typically, several risks are evaluated with established medical methods e.g., for cardiovascular diseases, diabetes mellitus type II, hypertension and loss of life years caused by risk factors as they are predominant in Western societies (Hamper 2018).

To create mobile services implementing these evaluation methods from medical guidelines and research must be converted to requirement specifications for mobile AI services.

Home Care Assistance in Rural Bavaria

This example focuses on data collection from heterogeny sensors covering medical sensors and smart home/AAL technology in ambulatory care. Due to the ageing population, the average age of the rural population in Germany is steadily increasing, with a growing number of care-dependent elderly people facing a decreasing number of younger people. In typical rural regions in Germany, around 25% of the population is over 65 years old and this proportion is expected to increase (Hamper 2020).

The goal of an exemplary project is to create a holistic network, powered by integrated medical- and AAL technologies, of citizens and patients, as well as providers of health and care services. By digitally connecting the home environment with medical and nursing care, the project aims to make care and support processes more efficient and enable citizens and patients to live self-determined lives as long as possible. It comprises a set of technologies and a prototypical data integration platform to support elderly and home care patients. Systems for collecting vital data and commercial Smart Home and Ambient Assisted Living (AAL) technologies can provide a holistic view of important information in the home environment to assess the health status of citizens and patients with long-term and low thresholds. With the consent of the affected individuals and with regard to data protection, the data from different technologies from numerous manufacturers is collected, harmonized and integrated via a Home Data Gateway (HDG) and passed on to other institutions of regional care and health care via a communication platform. Patients and ambulatory care staff are able to access the patient's health data collected in the home environment. This integrated care overview makes all relevant data from care documentation, vital data trends, and data from AAL systems available digitally in the patient's home and accessible (Hamper 2020).

By having access to selected and authorized data from care documentation and the home environment, doctors receive a more holistic picture of the course of illness and the health status of the patient than by assessing the visit to the doctor's office alone.

AI-Based Polyp Detection in Colonoscopy

This example focuses on data analytics in medical imaging for polyp detection in Colonoscopy. Colorectal cancer is the third most common cancer in the world, and early detection is key to improving survival rates. Colonoscopy is a widely used diagnostic tool for the detection and prevention of colorectal cancer. During a colonoscopy, a doctor can detect and remove precancerous growths known as polyps before they have a chance to develop into cancer. This can significantly reduce the risk of developing colorectal cancer. Medical image analysis can support medical experts in the process of interpreting and analyzing visual data collected during a colonoscopy. The field of medical image analysis has been around for a while and has numerous applications within the domain of computer-assisted detection, also known as CADe (computer-assisted detection). Recent advancements in artificial intelligence and specifically deep learning have improved the automated detection of lesions (Wittenberg & Raithel 2020).

One main challenge is the availability of usable training data sets that help train AI in order to support diagnostics. Although the concept of collecting and providing medical data has existed for a long time, there was no real urgency among the community to share this valuable information. Since 2015, the number of publicly available image data collections for the development, training and evaluation of AI systems in colonoscopy-based polyp detection has grown. With more data at hand for the scientific community, the detection rate has increased in the last year and AI-assisted medical image analysis has made successful steps forward (Wittenberg & Raithel 2020).

The example shows, that the progress made by AI algorithms can substantially change the way of diagnostics and treatment in the future. While algorithms exist and become more and more usable in the field of medical image analysis, we must establish a scientific data infrastructure to make a large set of data available as well as support the regulatory processes, to bring AI technology from research into medical practice.

Big Data Integration and Analysis for Evidence-Based Treatment

This example focuses on data integration and analytics for large-scale population and patient data. Public health aims to improve the health of communities by developing and implementing interventions that target the controllable factors that contribute to poor health. To achieve this goal, it is important to accurately assess the prevalence of diseases and risk factors within the population and identify groups that are more vulnerable or at a higher risk. By doing so, public health practitioners can determine the most effective prevention and treatment strategies and evaluate their impact.

AI has become an increasingly popular tool for achieving public health goals, particularly in light of the COVID-19 pandemic. AI research has resulted in the creation of various models that can quickly and accurately analyze different types of data to provide insights and identify patterns that are relevant to public health. These models have been trained on large amounts of well-organized data, which are often labelled and structured, to achieve high accuracy rates (Baclic et al. 2020).

Due to a growing scientific community around the globe, an enormous amount of data is being produced and published at an incredible rate, including scientific literature, health records, social media posts, and surveys. This presents a challenge for public health, which seeks to use this data to make evidence-based decisions and conduct text-based research. Structured data in health records and semantic interoperability are gaining more traction with initiatives like the European Health Data Space, backed by concepts like GAIA-X and FHIR (Gallina 2023).

While there are steps towards a data infrastructure to exchange data, new methods to make unstructured knowledge available for data analytics are needed. Based on large language models, natural language processing (NLP) has emerged as a crucial tool in addressing this challenge by enabling the rapid analysis of large amounts of unstructured or partially structured text. With its ability to quickly identify populations, interventions, and outcomes of interest in publicly accessible texts, NLP is increasingly recognized as a valuable tool for disease surveillance, prevention, and health promotion (Baclic et al. 2020).

GRAND CHALLENGES AND IMPLICATIONS FOR AI-BASED SOLUTIONS IN HEALTHCARE DELIVERY

While numerous potentials for data-driven AI in preventive care can be seen, challenges across the data value chain have to be tackled. Four main challenges can be derived from the paradigm changes in the data value chain and have been identified as crucial points for practical implementation (Figure 8.2).

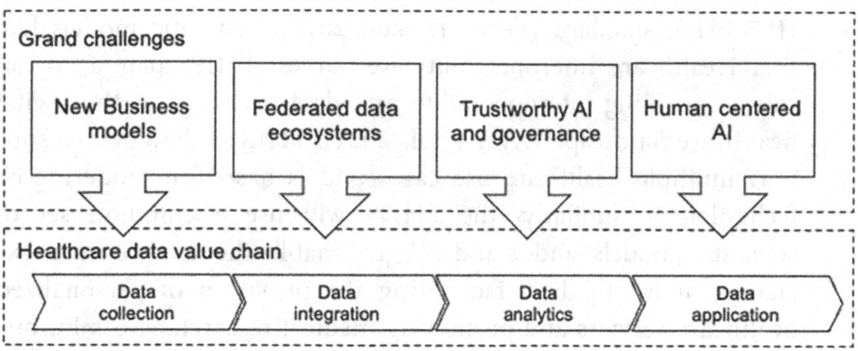

FIGURE 8.2 Grad challenges to be addressed for an AI-enabled preventive care.

These challenges can be described as follows.

- Collection: The integration of the tremendous number of medical devices, fitness apps, and smart home technologies in an interoperable and homogenous way poses several challenges. One of the primary challenges is the lack of standardization in the data format and communication protocols used by different devices and apps. While there is a certain level of standardization for medical technology, many medical devices rely on legacy interfaces which do not meet the needs for modern, IoT-based communications. This is due to the complex and costly certification process of medical technology (Ben-Menahem et al. 2020). Many vendors need to stick to implementations once they are certified. This leads to a relatively slow speed in the adoption of new IoT standards and communication systems. Looking at the consumer market of health and fitness technologies as well as smart homes and ambient assisted living, most of the large companies tried to create closed ecosystems (Miguel & Casado 2016). There are numerous restrictions on interoperability, which are largely not technical limitations but implied by the underlying business models. To leverage the potential of medical and personal health data, we need new business models for connected health and data sharing without vendor lock-in.
- Integration: In Germany, the telematic infrastructure (TI) is being developed to enable the secure and standardized exchange of electronic health data between healthcare providers. One semantic model used in the German TI healthcare system is based on the

HL7 FHIR standard (Leyck Dieken 2021). Semantic models like Fast Healthcare Interoperability Resources (FHIR) play a crucial role in enabling interoperability and data exchange in the digital healthcare landscape (Ayaz et al. 2021). FHIR is designed to support multiple healthcare use cases and is based on modern web technologies. Similarly, the EHDS will use a common set of semantic models and standards to enable the cross-border exchange of health data, facilitating the provision of personalized healthcare services and promoting medical research across Europe (Gallina 2023). It is also crucial to provide the necessary legal and ethical framework to ensure that personal health data is used and shared in a responsible and secure manner. A federated data ecosystem for semantic interoperability is needed to create accessible data sources while maintaining patient data sovereignty.

- Analytics: AI is rapidly advancing in healthcare and can potentially transform patient care, but it also presents unique regulatory challenges. The European Union's Medical Device Regulation (MDR) is a regulatory framework that establishes new rules for the manufacture, marketing, and use of medical devices within the EU (Ben-Menahem et al. 2020). The MDR imposes stricter requirements for clinical evidence, labelling, post-market surveillance, and data transparency for medical devices. The MDR acknowledges the use of AI and machine learning (ML) in medical devices and requires that these devices be safe and effective when used as intended. One of the key provisions of the MDR is the requirement for clinical evaluation and post-market clinical follow-up, which are essential for ensuring that AI-enabled medical devices are safe and effective. Manufacturers must conduct clinical investigations and demonstrate the clinical performance and safety of their AI-enabled medical devices. The MDR also emphasizes privacy and the importance of transparency and data integrity, requiring medical device manufacturers to provide detailed information about their devices, including the algorithms and data inputs used, the intended use of the device, and any limitations or risks associated with the device's use (Beckers et al. 2021).

To meet the regulatory requirements for the safe and effective use of AI-enabled medical devices in the EU, trustworthy AI and governance must be emphasized in medical technology.

- Application: When designing AI-powered technologies for preventive healthcare, the way information is presented, both for medical experts and patients, is crucial. When designing technology, it is important to consider the users' reception of information to meet the intended results. Expert systems and decision support systems are examples of technologies that can benefit from good human-computer interaction in order to guide users towards technology-supported decision-making. While human-human interaction refers to the communication and interaction between two or more human beings, computer-mediated interaction refers to communication and interaction that takes place through a computer or other digital device. With the rise of AI applications, we have seen new steps towards real human-computer interaction, as computers interact with humans without predefined actions, scripts or input from other humans. This leads to the impression of sensing, arguing and explaining machines which can merely be told apart from human actors. Therefore, the design of human-centred AI is a major challenge in the research community of HCI (Nazar et al. 2021).

This chapter provides a high-level overview of the potential and challenges for AI in preventive care. This high level is necessary to outline and understand that fundamental transformation steps towards a digital infrastructure in preventive healthcare are needed. The potential of AI largely depends on underlying data, not only for training AI on snapshots of data, but also for dynamic, connected and interoperable use of data during healthcare processes. For this real-time availability of digital data and information, it is necessary to break up silos and interconnect healthcare sectors to create digitally connected data ecosystems.

REFERENCES

Altgeld, T., Geene, R., Glaeske, G., Kolip, P. and Rosenbrock, R., 2006. "Prävention und Gesundheitsförderung: Ein Programm für eine bessere Sozial- und Gesundheitspolitik". Friedrich-Ebert-Stiftung.

Ayaz, M., Pasha, M. F., Alzahrani, M. Y., Budiarto, R., and Stiawan, D., 2021. "The Fast Health Interoperability Resources (FHIR) standard: Systematic literature review of implementations, applications, challenges and opportunities". *JMIR Medical Informatics*, 9(7), e21929.

Baclic, O., Tunis, M., Young, K., Doan, C., Swerdfeger, H. and Schonfeld, J., 2020. "Artificial intelligence in public health: Challenges and opportunities for public health made possible by advances in natural language processing". *Canada Communicable Disease Report*, 46(6), 161.

Barrett, M. A., Humblet, O., Hiatt, R. A. and Adler, N. E., 2013. "Big data and disease prevention: From quantified self to quantified communities". *Big Data*, 1(3), 168–175.

Beckers, R., Kwade, Z., and Zanca, F., 2021. "The EU medical device regulation: Implications for artificial intelligence-based medical device software in medical physics". *Physica Medica*, 83, 1–8.

Ben-Menahem, S. M., Nistor-Gallo, R., Macia, G., von Krogh, G., and Goldhahn, J., 2020. "How the new European regulation on medical devices will affect innovation". *Nature Biomedical Engineering*, 4(6), 585–590.

Gallina, S., 2023. "Preparing Europe for future health threats and crises: The European Health Union". *Eurosurveillance*, 28(5), 2.

Hamper, A., 2018. "Adaptive mobile Services zur bewegungsbezogenen Gesundheitsförderung". *Friedrich-Alexander Universität Erlangen-Nürnberg.*

Hamper, A., 2020. "Digitale Service Innovation für die Gesundheitsversorgung im vernetzten Zuhause". Mensch und Computer 2020-Workshopband.

Hurrelmann, K., Klotz, T. and Haisch, J., 2014. "Einführung: Krankheitsprävention und Gesundheitsförderung. Lehrbuch Prävention und Gesundheitsförderung". Hans Huber.

Hemkens, L. G., 2021. "Nutzenbewertung digitaler Gesundheitsanwendungen–Herausforderungen und Möglichkeiten". *Bundesgesundheitsblatt, Gesundheitsforschung, Gesundheitsschutz*, 64(10), 1269.

Knight, S., and Sorin, D., 2016. "A new healthcare alliance: Consumer engagement in the new healthcare economy". *Healthcare Transformation*, 1(3), 172–193.

Lengerke, T., 2007. "Public Health-Psychologie: Individuum und Bevölkerung zwischen Verhältnissen und Verhalten". *Juventa Verlag.*

Leyck Dieken, M., 2021. "Telematikinfrastruktur". *Telemedizin: Grundlagen und praktische Anwendung in stationären und ambulanten Einrichtungen*, 361–373.

Miguel, J. C., and Casado, M. Á., 2016. "GAFAnomy (Google, Amazon, Facebook and Apple): The big four and the b-ecosystem". *Dynamics of Big Internet Industry Groups and Future Trends: A View from Epigenetic Economics*, 127–148.

Nazar, M., Alam, M. M., Yafi, E., and Su'ud, M. M., 2021. "A systematic review of human–computer interaction and explainable artificial intelligence in healthcare with artificial intelligence techniques". *IEEE Access*, 9, 153316–153348.

RKI, 2015. "Gesundheit in Deutschland: Gesundheitsberichterstattung des Bundes", Robert Koch-Institut.

Rowe, J. P. and Lester, J. C., 2020. "Artificial intelligence for personalized preventive adolescent healthcare". *Journal of Adolescent Health*, 67(2), 53.

Wittenberg, T. and Raithel, M., 2020. "Artificial intelligence-based polyp detection in colonoscopy: Where have we been, where do we stand, and where are we headed?". *Visceral Medicine*, 36(6), 428–438.

Wunck, C. and Baumann, S., 2017. "Towards a process reference model for the information value chain in IoT applications". In *2017 IEEE European Technology and Engineering Management Summit (E-TEMS)* (pp. 1–6). IEEE.

CHAPTER 9

Competitive Intelligence in Healthcare

Annika Lurz

INTRODUCTION

"The only competitive advantage that organizations will have in the 21st century is what they know and how they use it," (Ghannay & Mamlouk 2012, p.24). In a strategic context, information about competitors' market movements is highly relevant. Among others, product launches, mergers, and acquisitions (M&A), and start-up investments can provide useful insights for top managers. Competitive intelligence (CI) describes the process of collecting data about competitors, transforming it into intelligence, and its communication (Evans 2005). This definition represents the three phases of the CI healthcare cycle: data gathering, analysis, and knowledge management (Freyn & Farley 2020). Porter can be seen as the father of CI (Ranjan & Foropon 2021). His "Five Forces" model combines rivalry, new market entrants, buyers, substitutes, and suppliers (Porter 1979). Although the model was published in 1979, it is still of great interest in literature and cited over 7,000 times. There are still various extensions of the model, e. g. by adding innovativeness, globalisation, digitalisation, (de)regulation policies, and non-governmental organisations (Isabelle et al. 2020; Khurram et al. 2020). The healthcare industry, in particular, changes rapidly due to dynamics in regulations and novel players entering the market, e.g., tech giants (Buck-Luce 2011; Sauter & Free 2005).

Additionally, those regulations for product approvals in pharmacy, medical technologies, and health insurance systems strongly differ from country to country. The Global Industry Classification Standard (GIBCS)

DOI: 10.1201/9781032699745-11

divides this industry into two business sectors: healthcare equipment & services and pharmaceuticals, biotechnology, & life sciences. Particularly in health services, data sharing is crucial to patients and therefore to providers. American healthcare policy offers incentives for hospitals to implement standards for electronic medical record exchanges, but little data sharing takes place (Botta & Cutler 2014). This also challenges CI approaches. Not only external data is not shared, but internal hospital departments also compete and therefore divisions become data hubs (Freyn & Farley 2020). Although patient data is difficult to get, there is much public data available: governmental (patent and product databases) as well as private sources (social networks and news). Open data enables CI to apply open-source intelligence (OSINT) methods (Černý & Potančok 2019).

Due to the high availability of information, artificial intelligence (AI) methods support data collection in which the relevance of sources is ranked (Silva et al. 2019). Not only data gathering, but also the analysis phase of CI is supported by AI methods that help the CI process to shift from an intuition-based intelligence of individual CI professionals to a more objective, data-driven intelligence to assist informed decision-making (Kordon 2020). AI and statistics complement executives' tasks in a strategic context and lead to consistent decisions (Kordon 2020; Krakowski, Luger, & Raisch 2022). Machine learning algorithms, e.g. Graph Neural Networks (GNN) can serve insights into evolving trends and emerging business areas. Considering the potential AI has for enhancing CI in healthcare, the academic literature on the topic is very limited.

The CI articles often deal with only one industry sector or country, e.g. US healthcare (Freyn & Farley 2020), South African pharmaceuticals (Fatti & Du Toit 2012), or hospitals in Taiwan (Sheng, Chan, Teo, & Lin 2013). Additionally, the scientific papers mostly deal with one phase of the CI cycle, e. g. data collection (Silva et al. 2019) or knowledge management (Luu 2014). In general, in CI research, there is a lack of big data methods (Ranjan & Foropon 2021).

In this chapter, the current literature is summarised within the structure of the three phases and recommendations for using AI and big data methods are given. Text mining and networks have a large presence in CI. In the following part, a theoretical background about CI and the healthcare industry is given which concludes with the research gap. Subsequently, the methodology is explained. In the fourth part, the results are divided into AI in CI in general, big data analytics in CI, requirements for successful integration, the healthcare CI cycle, and ends up with specific CI tools in the healthcare context. The discussion shows contributions, limitations of this chapter, and future research. This chapter is summarised in the conclusion.

THEORETICAL BACKGROUND

Competitive Intelligence

The management focuses on the following strategic topics described by Schwarz et al. (2019):

- Activities of competitors
- Product launches and new technologies
- New companies entering the industry
- Shifting borders of the market
- Establishing an important position in the market.

The topics concerning new competitors, their actions, their innovations, and shifting boundaries are highly interdependent. To anticipate actions (M&As and investments), patents have to be analysed and to predict new market entrants, there has to be knowledge about investments and M&As. To predict the success of innovations, awareness and information about shifting boundaries of the industry must be grounded. To have an overview of the shifting boundaries, investments, M&As, new market entrants and successful innovations have to be observed. Especially M&As, investments into start-ups which are the actions of competitors and new market entrants are two sides of the same coin. The company which is invested in is exactly the new market entrant and the investment relates to the competitor that is monitored. For the definition of a superior market position, the approach is focused on previously processed topics with a holistic view: innovations, actions, new market entrants, and shifting boundaries. After describing strategic management topics that represent a content-related perspective on CI, the question of how CI processes are conducted is answered.

Definitions in this field are inconsistent (Farley & Freyn 2022). The Society of CI Professionals describes it as "the process of ethically collecting, analyzing, and disseminating accurate, relevant, specific, timely, foresighted, and actionable intelligence regarding the implications of the business environment, competitors, and the organization itself," (Boncella 2003, p.327). In most CI definitions found, this ethical aspect is not mentioned. For future research projects, the correlation between ethics and CI should be examined (Trong Tuan 2013). From more intuition-based and manual work processes, data analytics and AI methods have been boarding the CI processes in the last decades (Ranjan & Foropon 2021). The CI process definitions are similar to business intelligence definitions: companies are using data to monitor on the one hand internal production processes (business intelligence) and on the other hand their competitors (CI) (Zheng et al. 2012). The CI process gathers data, transforms it by analysis into knowledge and communicates it to the management for optimised strategic decision-making (Evans 2005; Farley & Freyn 2022). The majority of process definitions consist of such three phases (Evans 2005; Rodriguez-Salvador & Castillo-Valdez 2021), but there are also popular CI processes that contain more stages. Dishman & Calof (2008) additionally propose the planning period before data gathering, analysis, and communication and this work is referenced over 300 times. Another fourth phase is the interpretation stage: data collection, analysis, interpretation, and communication (Archarya, Singh, Pereira, & Singh 2018). Adil, Abdelhadi, Mohamed, & Haytam (2019) propose seven steps: Adjusting the need for CI, planning, data gathering, storage, processing & analysis, dissemination, and feedback. In summary, there is no optimal path to use CI, it depends on the people involved in the tools (Maguire, Suluo, & Ojiako 2010). Even if the process and the outcome are valuable, the results are not always implemented and integrated into the strategic actions (Köseoglu, Ross, & Okumus 2016).

Healthcare and Data Sharing

This industry shows that rapid technological dynamics and research are important factors (Fatti and Du Toit, 2012; Luu 2014). The Global Industry Classification Standard (GICS) divides Healthcare into two main sectors: healthcare equipment & services and pharmaceuticals, biotechnology, & life sciences. Healthcare must handle many stakeholders: patients, doctors, lawyers, investors, regulators, management boards, and public opinion (Sauter & Free 2005). Not only patients must be served but often also business partners because a large part concerns B2B trading. In the US, hospitals and other clinical divisions (from rehabs over intensive care to emergency departments) maintain different data systems which are often handled as silos (Freyn & Farley 2020). As the healthcare industry in the US is as competitive as other industries, data sharing between such internal and external data silos is often viewed as a competitive disadvantage (Farley & Freyn 2022). Larger hospitals tend to share data internally but not externally, although successful hospitals tend to collaborate beyond conventional borders (Miller & Tucker 2014; Vaughn et al. 2014). The American government connected reimbursement to the usage of electronic medical records and rewards standardising data and adopting systems, but there are no rewards for actual data sharing (Botta & Cutler 2014; Miller & Tucker 2014), although clinical data sharing decreases morality (Miller & Tucker 2014; Spetz et al. 2014).

In Figure 9.1 the CI process in the typical US healthcare functions is represented. In step one executives plan together with CI professionals the details of the phases, step two consists of data gathering internally and externally, then the analysis is conducted, and the results are communicated to the executives again, in the end, the outcomes are disseminated to the managers of the departments (Freyn & Farley 2020).

However, overall, there is a lack of research combining CI and healthcare (Farley & Freyn 2022; Freyn & Farley 2020). In CI there are still lots of subjective, human-based approaches implemented, although systematic, objective approaches would provide informed and consistent decision-making (Kordon 2020; Sauter & Free 2005). This chapter

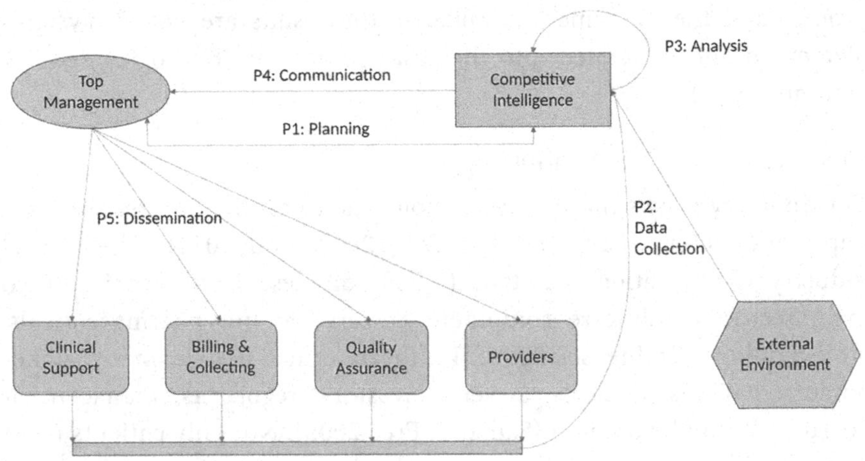

FIGURE 9.1 CI process in healthcare (based on Freyn & Farley 2020, p.10).

assembles literature on CI in healthcare (expanded by CI literature that can be adapted to the healthcare context).

METHODOLOGY

For this chapter, a literature review was conducted. Only peer-reviewed articles and papers written in English are considered. The search term consists of three parts which are connected by a logical conjunction:

> (competitive OR competition OR competitor) AND intelligence AND (healthcare OR health-care OR health care)

Since there are only a few results, the last part can be found in the whole article whereas the first and the second part must be in the title. As the results are manageable, only one screening was conducted. After the review process, backward and forward research is conducted (Webster & Watson 2002). After removing duplicates, 35 papers were analysed. Papers about other industries (He et al. 2015), and business intelligence papers (Ahmad 2015; Caya & Bourdon 2016) that cannot be transferred to healthcare are excluded. Articles on AI with valuable insights which can be adapted to the CI in a healthcare context are also included (Table 9.1).

ARTIFICIAL INTELLIGENCE FOR COMPETITIVE INTELLIGENCE

Since AI is expanding in all areas, executives have to handle such methods as a competitive threat that substitutes manual work in many businesses (Krakowski et al. 2022). Therefore, managers must understand the effects on the industry and the organisation's market position (Krakowski et al. 2022). Krakowski et al. (2022) show that excellent chess players can be substituted by an AI algorithm. Partly those results can be transferred to a business context, as chess is a competitive game that

TABLE 9.1 Results of the Literature Review

Database	*Search Results*	*After Screening*
ACM	2	1
AISeL	2	1
EBSCOhost	6	4
ieeeXplore	3	3
sciencedirect	5	5
Scopus	24	15

requires high-level strategic thinking (Krakowski et al. 2022). For decision-making contextualisation, creativity and social skills are also relevant human attributes. Nevertheless, AI can strongly support managers in informed decision-making. Non-experts assisted by AI can generate a competitive advantage in chess, therefore CI professionals with high AI knowledge are needed (Krakowski et al. 2022).

Kordon (2020) suggests that one reason for the success of AI-supported decision systems is the objectivity of machine-analysed results which leads to more consistent management. By creating solutions using statistical and machine learning algorithms, AI serves low-cost pattern recognition, and it can deal with multi-dimensional information. In contrast, human intuition-based, selective, and sometimes biased intelligence can lead to dangerous results if there is little knowledge and insufficient experience (Kordon 2020). Nevertheless, executives often trust subjective intelligence and intuition more than statistics (Sauter & Free 2005). For introducing AI management support, real business needs, data accessibility, infrastructure, and experience are necessary (Kordon 2020).

Use cases for AI in CI are predictions, e. g. in terms of business angels' investments (Blohm, Anretter, Sirén, Girchnik, & Wincent 2022), patent collaborations (Wu et al. 2013), technology knowledge (Park & Yoon 2018), and forecasting business relationships (Mori et al. 2012). There is a large potential to predict evolving trends, and emerging business fields for all market types, although practical challenges concerning few and noisy data come up (Jeong et al. 2021). The era of big data and their analytics offers huge amounts of structured, semi- and unstructured data also available for CI processes. Those methods support not only predicting and analysing but also diagnosing and prescribing scenarios in the market (Ranjan & Foropon 2021). Big data analytics enhance the detection of innovations and trends and facilitate market analysis in real-time to observe competitors' market moves (Adil et al. 2019). The following figure describes how CI can profit from big data analytics.

Although those methods offer enormous potential, they are not used for CI. There is often no real-time database and no tool to import data from competitors' public relations information, scientific papers, or government regulatory databases, but professionals use surveys of competitors and newsletters (Ranjan & Foropon 2021). The challenges of big data analytics

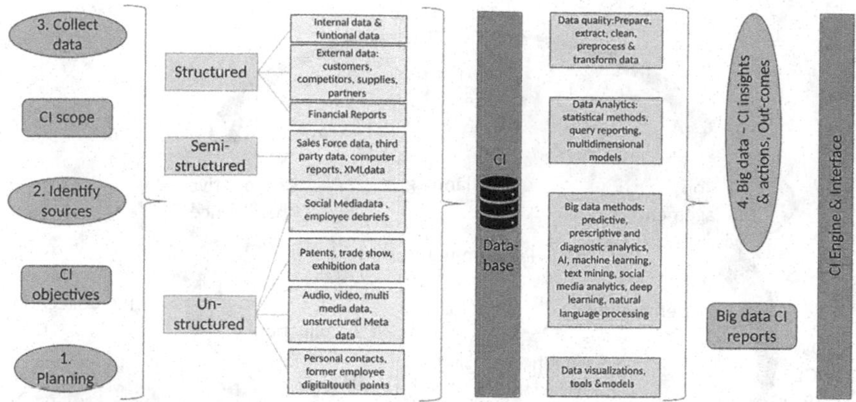

FIGURE 9.2 Framework for big data methods in CI (based on Ranjan & Foropon 2021, p.5).

can be reasons why there are few applications: missing data understanding, insufficient business and process expertise, and reliability of data (fake news) (Ranjan & Foropon 2021). Although rumours can also be valuable information for a competitive advantage, it is just important to know if your information is a rumour or a fact (Sauter & Free 2005). As CI can be seen as a subfield of business intelligence, concepts are transferable (Köseoglu et al. 2016). The most mentioned main phases for those fields are quite similar: data gathering inside and outside the company, transferring it into intelligence and communicating it to management and/or the firm (Maguire et al. 2010) (Figure 9.2).

COMPETITIVE INTELLIGENCE IN HEALTHCARE

Farley & Freyn (2022) mention very similar phases: information is collected internally and externally, and this data is analysed by CI professionals and shared with the management that manages further knowledge sharing (see Figure 9.3). In their conceptional model, the first step is a planning process between the management and the CI team, in the second step, data is gathered, the third step deals with the analysis of the data, steps 4 and 5 concern the communication and the sharing of the results to the executives and the healthcare departments. In the planning process, managers and professionals must enclose the needed information, and there are tools available to rank the relevance of sources (Freyn & Farley 2020; Silva et al. 2019). During the analysis step, the needed intelligence must be defined, and for the last step, the

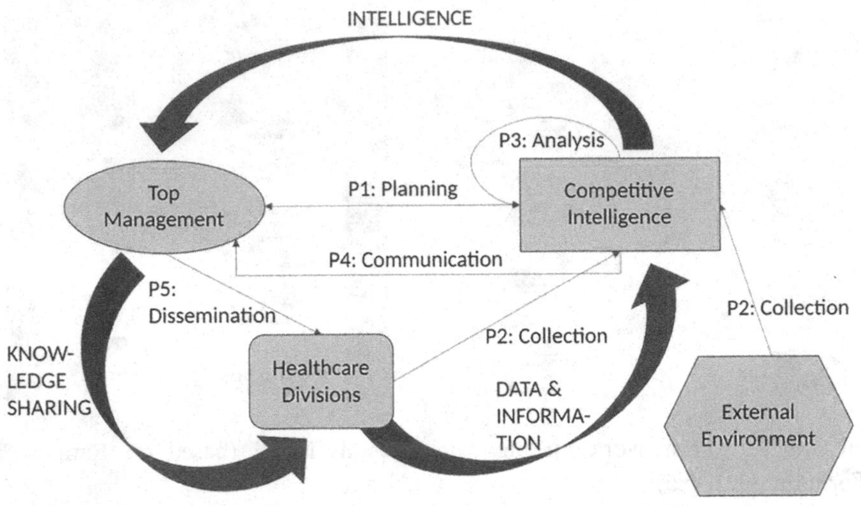

FIGURE 9.3 Conceptual CI process (based on Farley & Freyn 2022, p.5).

dissemination of knowledge within the firm and to the decision-makers and its effectiveness must be organised (Freyn & Farley 2020).

For healthcare providers five important tasks must be completed: identifying competitors and classifying them (e. g. in key, core, and landscape); estimating data information necessities; data gathering (by observation and research); information transferring, and knowledge usage (Festervand & Lumpkin 1990). Canongia (2007) does not categorise knowledge sharing and foresight into CI but differentiates between CI, knowledge dissemination/ management, and technical predictions to describe the synergies between those fields for biotechnology.

Although the literature serves formal processes, Fatti & Du Toit (2012) found that formal CI functions only arise in 42.3% of pharmaceutical organisations in South Africa, and since 2003 no real change has taken place. In general, 30% of examined companies utilise CI for management and the majority use CI continuously. CI should not be applied reactively but on an ongoing basis because of the rapid market dynamics (Fatti & Du Toit 2012; Lewis 2006). As a result, Fatti & Du Toit (2012) point out that CI came up between 2003 and 2008 and the majority of the surveyed organisations use it to increase profit, particularly for scanning the market environment with business tools and influencing strategic decisions. However, in the following sections, the academic papers concerning CI in healthcare are structured into the three dimensions of Farley's & Freyn's CI cycle (2022).

Data Collection and Sources

Most of the data collection still takes place by manual search and observation conducted by CI professionals. The analysis of articles and named sources suggests a considerable difference between potential data and actual data. In Table 9.2, sources used and recommended in the considered academic papers are summarised.

The Derwent database provides access to patents (Canongia 2007). Patent analysis is a large field in CI, but there are also use cases, e. g. services, IT, and business models which are less patentable (Jeong et al. 2021). It is also difficult to match patents with successful products, some firms hold many patents, but cannot transform them into products. Nevertheless, the attributes of patents and medical journals (author, abstract, keywords, date of publication, and country) give valuable insights (Adil et al. 2019). An early indicator for an M&A can also be the

TABLE 9.2 Sources Used for CI

Sources	*Author(s)*
Patents	Adil et al. 2019; Canongia 2007; Jeong & Yoon 2021
Scientific papers/ (medical) journals	Adil et al. 2019; Canongia 2007; Farley & Freyn 2022; Rodriguez-Salvador & Castillo-Valdez 2021
Trademarks	Jeong & Yoon 2021
(Online) news(papers)	Adil et al. 2019; Fatti & Du Toit 2012; Reyes et al. 2021
Newsletters	Ranjan & Foropon 2021
Surveys of competitors	Ranjan & Foropon 2021
Financial/ analyst reports	Fatti & Du Toit 2012; Reyes et al. 2021
Industry & market reports	Rodriguez-Salvador & Castillo-Valdez 2021
Trade shows	Ranjan & Foropon 2021
Public healthcare organisation sites	Kahlon & Tse 2013
Conferences and seminars	Fatti & Du Toit 2012
Trade literature	Fatti & Du Toit 2012
Promotional material	Fatti & Du Toit 2012
Open data: Google trends	Černý & Potančok 2019
Social media/ networks	Adil et al. 2019; Itani et al. 2017; Rodriguez-Salvador & Castillo-Valdez 2021
Not-for-profit organisations	Farley & Freyn 2022
Corporate websites	Fatti & Du Toit 2012
Regulatory & governmental agencies	Freyn & Farley 2020

sudden increase in the number of patents. This strategy is often used by possible M&A candidates to increase their value. Trademark data is not mentioned frequently, although it reflects the real business and the economic value of an organisation objectively (Jeong et al. 2021).

All types of news are important to learn about market moves of competitors, business areas, upcoming policies, partnerships, collaborations, and M&As (Reyes et al. 2021). As there is an enormous number of news published every day, an automated analysis processing of headlines, reports, and announcements can enhance informed decision-making (Reyes et al. 2021). Newsletters are ordered frequently to prefilter information about specific companies and specific business sectors (Ranjan & Foropon 2021). Not only does news provide a good source, but also people's Google search behaviour supports the prediction of upcoming health trends in a geographic region (Černý & Potančok 2019). Černý & Potančok (2019) use Google Search data to analyse antidepressant queries of the regional population. Other novel data providers are social media and social networks that have a positive impact on CI collection. Tweets, in particular, report information about political dynamics, new technologies, or product launches (Adil et al. 2019; Itani et al. 2017).

In the literature, both primary and secondary sources are mentioned. Primary sources are those which come from first-hand evidence (e. g. employees attending trade shows and conferences) while secondary sources provide information from other references. The frequency of accessing data sources ranges from daily over monthly to quarterly, whereby primary sources are accessed less rather than continuously (Fatti & Du Toit 2012). Primary or secondary information is transmitted by stakeholders in healthcare: suppliers, customers, competitors, and distributors, or more concretely: employees, insurance organisations, governments as regulators as well as payers, patients, not-for-profit organisations, hospital resources, medical technology & pharmaceutical firms, and technology & socioeconomic sectors (Farley & Freyn 2022; Fatti & Du Toit 2012; Trong Tuan 2013). If one knows if the information is a rumour or definitely true, in particular rumour that, if repeated, can act as an early warning system (Sauter & Free 2005). Most CI data is in a qualitative, unstructured format as narrative text or business patterns and many organisations do not have regular imports of such data, even in general, few companies are using standardised tools for gathering more structured information from regulatory institutions, public relations of competitors, or publications (Kahlon & Tse 2013; Ranjan & Foropon 2021). CI is an ethical process which includes data gathering, so employees in competitors' companies are not used illegally (Fatti & Du Toit 2012). Information is also exchanged while networking with business colleagues or socialising in a group (Ranjan & Foropon 2021).

Analysis: Insight and Foresight

This phase is the most important part of CI and requires high skills of the professionals and these skills must include providing objectively all relevant knowledge (Amiri et al. 2017; Lewis 2006). Executives need predigested filtered information to turn it into contextual informed decision-making (Maguire et al. 2010). CI analysis methods can be applied to predict market, technological, and scientific dynamics or to forecast competitors' activities (Rodriguez-Salvador & Castillo-Valdez 2021). Data-driven methods are used for M&A prediction and technology management (Park et al. 2013; Park & Yoon 2014). For research and development, CI analysis can support early warning systems, and reveal technology lifecycles, their impact, and potential collaborators (Rodriguez-Salvador & Castillo-Valdez 2021).

To build intelligence, metrics must be used to evaluate, explain, diagnose, and make data more understandable. Metrics provide opportunities to discover experts using a number of patents or paper citations, ranking of papers, impact factors, and collaboration networks (Rodriguez-Salvador & Castillo-Valdez 2021). Conventional metrics are the size of the business portfolio, distribution rate, competitiveness level, and market share for industry reports and more current ones for social media data: number of mentions, and number of interactions (e.g. "likes" or "shares") (Jeong et al. 2021; Rodriguez-Salvador & Castillo-Valdez 2021). In most cases, both need to be combined to represent the dynamics in technologies and science: non-traditional and traditional metrics (Staudt et al. 2018). Possible variables to form metrics are functionality and features of products and services, keywords, and social media activities (Kahlon & Tse 2013). Categories created to label firms (M&A candidates and cooperative partners) and innovation products (prevention, diagnosis, therapy) also support CI analysis (Canongia 2007; Jeong et al. 2021).

A subfield of CI is competitive technology intelligence (CTI) which deals with Scientometrics, Patentometrics, Bibliometrics, and Altmetrics (Rodriguez-Salvador & Castillo-Valdez 2021). As the names suggest Scientometrics (Bibliometrics is a subfield of Scientometrics) and

Patentometrics include methods and measurements to describe academic papers and patents. Altmetrics describe the integration of alternative, non-traditional metrics to consider scholarly activities on blogs, in the news and on social media (Rodriguez-Salvador & Castillo-Valdez 2021).

There are various general methodologies to build intelligence, starting with more manual approaches like studying article titles and abstracts to identify drugs and analysing the content of the relevant ones to identify research trends (Canongia 2007) to more machine-based methods like building decision rules from trained algorithms (Kahlon & Tse 2013). Geographic maps of research can be one part of the analysis (Adil et al. 2019) as well as visual decision-making (VDM) that points out business strategy alignments and relationships (Kahlon & Tse 2013). The challenge of machine-based approaches in practical use cases is the noise and the lack of data, therefore prediction models often gain less performance than 90% (Jeong et al. 2021). That could be one reason why advanced analysis methods are often not implemented in companies (Ranjan & Foropon 2021).

CI sources contain particularly qualitative data formats, consequently, many text-mining methodologies are applied. From sentences, semantic relationships (e.g. M&A, collaborations, or investments) between entities (e.g. organisations or institutions) are detected automatically using BERT a natural language processing model (Reyes et al. 2021). Another foundation for named entity recognition could be patents from the USPTO database and additionally extract keywords (Jeong et al. 2021). Clustering of academic articles and patents to determine activities of researchers, institutions, countries, and journals (Rodriguez-Salvador & Castillo-Valdez 2021). Adil et al. (2019) apply an unsupervised learning algorithm to cluster and sort articles and patents by topics and also identify keywords for such semantic topics. Additionally, the importance of words in the texts is ranked by using Spark Mlib API. Having identified rare important words, these could be matched with the publishing year so possible innovations can be detected. Future research could provide deep learning algorithms for such natural language processing tasks because there is enormous progress (Adil et al. 2019). Text similarities between the business portfolios can be calculated, or technology similarities to identify benchmarking targets, or text similarity measures can be used to search for strategic similarities in business descriptions (Jeong et al. 2021; Lee & Lee 2017; Park et al. 2013).

In the examined papers, not only text mining methods stand out but also networks in combination with natural language processing and only networks are highlighted in the analysis part. A co-occurrence network in trademarks is used to determine upcoming trends in business areas (Jeong et al. 2021). A correlation network of drugs is created which can be filtered by the number of citations to have a clear overview of important medications (Canongia 2007). As described in the theoretical background of CI, the topics are highly interdependent and therefore, literature often uses networks for analysis. One research field in CI concerning networks is link prediction. There are articles about recommendations for intellectual property partnerships (Wu et al. 2013), forecasting of technology information flow (Park & Yoon 2018), and predicting business relationships (Mori et al. 2012). Business proximities are also calculated and used to generate a business network (Shi, Lee, & Whinston 2016).

Jeong et al. (2021) created a deep link prediction model that analyses diversifiable business areas for target organisations. Link prediction metrics can be divided into machine-learning-based approaches which can include multiple attributes at once and are more performant and metric-based approaches (e. g. preferential attachment) which are less complex in applications. For future research, the authors recommend treating link prediction as a regression instead of a binary task to forecast the strength of a link. They propose to use semantic networks also for GNN tasks like node embedding or link prediction in the future. Additionally, network metrics are used as features for prediction tasks: certain centralities of nodes (e.g. eigenvector, cluster coefficients, and degree centrality), proximity measures (e.g. preferential attachment), and contextuality which can be calculated with NetworkX, SciPy, and PyTorch-BigGraph (Jeong et al. 2021).

Graph representations can also serve for analysis of author networks of patents and academic papers. The network can be visualised with Spark GraphX to enhance interpretations of connections between authors (Adil et al. 2019). With this tool, networks are generated from text corpus and determine teams, connections between labs, and clusters of teams with many collaborations and examine interactions between them. Semantic graphs of links between terms and concepts can also be visualised (Adil et al. 2019).

Knowledge Management and Communication

The communication phase considers the outcomes of the CI process which should be transmitted to authorities who are responsible for strategic decisions and happens in the form of mails, reports, and presentations (Freyn & Farley 2020). The format depends on the information type and how it is most interpretable to the stakeholders (Ahmad 2015). Canongia (2007) proposes knowledge maps for outcomes of data analytics. The communication style is important as well as the communication management, e. g. implementing platforms.

As knowledge sharing has a positive impact on CI scanning, internal networks or CI communities should be built (Luu 2014; Freyn & Farley 2020; Lewis 2006). As CI quality is dependent on teamwork, there exists a necessity for a CI professional network for exchange where employees can bring in their tacit and explicit knowledge (Freyn & Farley 2020; Lewis 2006). A culture that motivates people (e.g. clients and physicians) to share data with CI professionals about competitors must be established (Sauter & Free 2005) as well as the connection of experts in the business or competitive intelligence field as well as the communication path to the executives. Healthcare as a highly dynamic market with rapidly changing technologies needs to share knowledge and news immediately (Luu 2014). Ranjan & Foropon (2021) propose to employ a business unit for knowledge sharing on competitors and CI governance. The distribution phase itself should constantly give feedback to the data collection phase as well as to the analysis phase. In this way, intelligence can be optimised iteration by iteration (Lewis 2006).

TOOLS

The literature suggests architectures and tools for optimising CI tasks. Many companies still use Excel, SAP, and SAS as CI tools for their sources (newsletters, competitor surveys, and external analyst interviews) (Ranjan & Foropon 2021). The following table summarises these tools (Table 9.3).

The tools differ strongly. Adil et al. (2019) propose databases and APIs that fit the CI use cases in general. For data gathering Scrapy (a Python framework) is used to extract text from forums, blogs, patents, and websites. The Twitter API is integrated to query relevant topics by keyword creation. MongoDB and Hadoop are chosen to be capable of storing the data in raw format to not lose information in a distributed manner and deal with large datasets. Data visualisation can be realised as a dashboard by a web app which uses Spring Boot Rest API. The data can be shown by multiple graphs and charts.

TABLE 9.3 List of CI Tools

Type	*Description*	*Author(s)*
Framework/ Architecture	*Apache Spark framework, analysis and storage in Hadoop and MongoDB, further used: Spark Streaming, Spark GraphX, and Spark Mlib;* *Data collection: Scrapy, Twitter API;* *Data storage: MongoDB, Apache Hadoop;* *Data visualisation: Web app consuming Spring Boot Rest API*	Adil et al. 2019
Data ranking and filtering	*Web mining for optimised data gathering to rank the relevance of data*	Silva et al. 2019
Data extraction and analysis	*Scraping open-source data of technologies, analysis with text mining methods and data visualisation, cluster analysis and decision trees*	Wisnowski et al. 2015
Decision support system	*Constructed for strategic information sharing in hospitals*	Sauter & Free 2005

The next tool is built to support CI and technology observation for small and medium-sized enterprises. It is based on machine learning and web mining methods for optimised data gathering, particularly relevance ranking of webpages to filter out information that is less important (Silva et al. 2019). JMP extracts data from open-source information and scrapes text from different formats (PDFs, websites, etc.). Text mining based on R, data visualisation, cluster analysis, and decision trees for industry descriptions is also implemented (Wisnowski et al. 2015). Sauter & Free (2005) implement a decision support system to collect data about competitors, customers, and other important stakeholders (e. g. physicians) internally in hospitals and form monthly reports to hospital managers. The goal is to brief executives about physicians, insurance policies, and M&As from other hospitals and rumours are also traced. Monthly reports are generated including information that is inserted by five different users (Sauter & Free 2005). From a European point of view, nowadays this would be illegal due to data privacy issues and from an ethical perspective probably also very difficult. However, the success of such tools depends highly on the organisation and the users, successful systems in one company must not be successful in another, tools should be flexible for individual institutions (Maguire et al. 2010) (Figure 9.4).

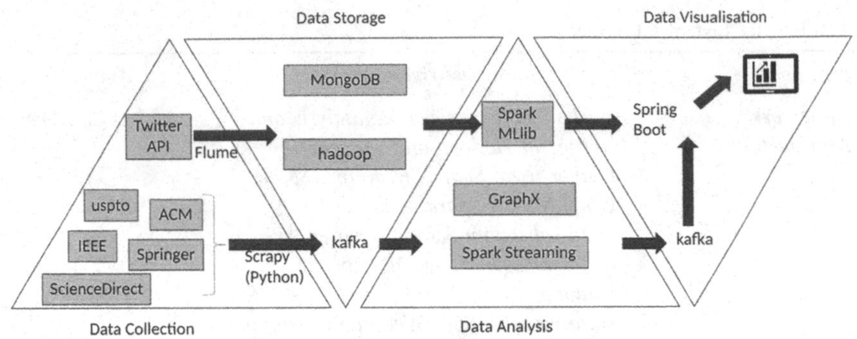

FIGURE 9.4 Proposed architecture (based on Adil et al. 2019, p.3).

REQUIREMENTS FOR A SUCCESSFUL IMPLEMENTATION OF CI

AI alone is not valuable (Krakowski et al. 2022). This is also true for CI. Successful implementation depends on people's skills which require ongoing training and continuing education (Freyn & Farley 2020). An intelligence analyst should maintain a level of objectivity, be able to familiarise themselves with new business contexts, understand them and have regular interactions with decision-makers (Lewis 2006). Competencies to approach industry information and to interpret indicators earlier than competitors are needed (Trong Tuan 2013). That applies not only on an individual level but also to team dynamics. Transition team processes that describe the processes in which groups concentrate on planning and managing a task execution, positively correlate with CI scanning (Marks et al. 2001; Trong Tuan 2013). Additionally, interpersonal and action team processes have a positive impact on CI scanning (Trong Tuan 2013). These results suggest that team spirit is an important aspect of CI. Managers take an important role in the CI process, too. They must maintain a good relationship with the CI professionals, especially with the people who provide the source information, assist collaborations, and give feedback (Farley & Freyn 2022). Executives should establish principles of ethical corporate social responsibility that relate to ethics internally and externally (Trong Tuan 2013). Politics should be avoided as far as possible; no manipulating employees or flip-flopping (Kordon 2020).

In general, a culture of sharing information and an environment of collaboration is key (Fatti & Du Toit 2012). A feedback culture with feedback in every iteration and phase represents an important consideration (Freyn & Farley 2020). Trust building in CI processes and professionals must be established (Ranjan & Foropon 2021). For building trust, data should be complete (Ahmad 2015), and text mining, deep learning, and natural language processing with open-source frameworks can help to get reliable results (Ranjan & Foropon 2021).

DISCUSSION

Contribution and Limitations

This chapter contributes to both: theory and practice. For theory, it summarises the current literature on CI in healthcare and at the same time shows a research gap in this field. CI papers that are adaptable to the healthcare context are also considered. General AI and big data methods that can also be applied to this industry are also consulted. The literature was divided into the three dimensions of the CI cycle: data collection, analysis, and dissemination. For practice, CI tools and requirements to establish a good CI process in healthcare and many inspirations for every part of the CI process are shown. For the analysis phase, especially text mining and networks are taken into consideration.

Finding literature for the whole healthcare industry, in general, is also challenging because each field has different attributes. There are articles focused on hospitals, biotechnology, and pharmaceuticals. Two articles give an overview of the industry as a whole, but only for the US. Different countries apply different laws, in particular, product approvals function differently, e.g. in the US, the Food and Drug Administration (FDA) and in Europe the European Medicine Agency (EMA) is responsible for pharmacy and medical devices. There are few papers about different countries.

Future Research

Future research should focus on simulation methods to bring often mentioned "scenario planning" into practice. Already Canongia (2007) stated that there is a lack of research in simulation and modelling. As the industry is often represented as a semantic network for analysis purposes, e. g. agent-based models (ABM) can serve as simulation methods to plan and prescribe future scenarios. Often data is only visualised and there is no real "intelligence" built (Lòpez-Robles et al. 2020). Future research should focus more on prediction and prescription from a foresight point of view, as there are already many papers about analysis and description from the insight perspective. In the area of open-source intelligence (OSINT) there is also an enormous research potential as well as in the field of "trademark" as a data source for CI. Experiments and surveys about the reason, why more sophisticated methods and tools are seldom used should be conducted. Another interesting research area is the observation of managers believing in intuition-based subjective judgements rather than in analytical studies (Sauter & Free 2005). Having a look at the healthcare sectors, medical technology and CI is not found in a single paper which opens opportunities for future research in this field.

CONCLUSION

It is conspicuous, that with variation in time and country, approaches of CI in healthcare strongly differ as regulations and insurance systems vary from country to country. Over time, processes are automised and novel data gathering as well as data analysis and dissemination tools are developed. From manual, intuition-based subjective work CI changes to broader access, more objective, more diverse, more sophisticated methods which are invented in theory already, but are seldom practically used in companies (Ranjan & Foropon 2021). One reason could be that decision-makers often prefer intuition-based judgements of domain experts to analytical studies which could lead to biases (Sauter & Free 2005). Another reason is the missing expertise in this area. More forecasting and less ex-post analysis are important. In the analysis phase, there was no scenario planning using a simulation found.

REFERENCES

Adil, B., Abdelhadi, F., Mohamed, B. and Haytam, H. 2019. "A spark based big data analytics framework for competitive intelligence," in Proceedings of the 1st International Conference on Smart Systems and Data Science (ICSSD), Rabat, Morocco, pp. 1–6.

Acharya, A., Singh, S. K., Pereira, V., and Singh, P. 2018. "Big data, knowledge co-creation and decision making in the fashion industry," *International Journal of Information Management* (42), pp. 90–101.

Ahmad, A. 2015. "Business intelligence for sustainable competitive advantage", in *Sustaining Competitive Advantage Via Business Intelligence, Knowledge Management, and System Dynamics (Advances in Business Marketing and Purchasing, Vol. 22A)*, Quaddus, M. and Woodside, A. G. (eds.), Emerald Group Publishing Limited, Bingley, pp. 3–220.

Amiri, N. S., Shirkavand S., Chalak M., and Rezaeei, N. 2017. "Competitive intelligence and developing sustainable competitive advantage," *AD-minister* (30), pp. 173–194.

Blohm, I., Antretter, T., Sirén, C., Grichnik, D., & Wincent, J. 2022. "It's a Peoples Game, Isn't It?! A comparison between the investment returns of business angels and machine learning algorithms," *Entrepreneurship Theory and Practice* 46(4), pp. 1054–1091.

Buck-Luce, C. 2011. "Pharma 3.0 and the new healthcare eco-system," Keynote address delivered at Pharma CI Conference, New Jersey, US.

Boncella, R. J. 2003. "Competitive intelligence and the web", *Communications of Association of Information Systems* (12), pp. 327–340.

Botta, M. and Cutler, D. 2014. "Meaningful use: Floor or ceiling?", *Healthcare* (2), pp. 48–52.

Caya, O. and Bourdon, A. 2016. "A framework of value creation from business intelligence and analytics in competitive sports," in Proceedings of the 2016 49th Hawaii International Conference on System Sciences (HICSS), Koloa, US, pp. 1061–1071.

Canongia, C. 2007. "Synergy between Competitive Intelligence (CI), Knowledge Management (KM) and Technological Foresight (TF) as a strategic model of prospecting - the use of biotechnology in the development of drugs against breast cancer," *Biotechnology Advances* (25), pp. 57–74.

Černý, J., Potančok, M. and Molnár, Z. 2019. "Using open data and Google search data for competitive intelligence analysis," *Journal of Intelligence Studies in Business* (9), pp. 72–81.

Dishman, P. and Calof, J. 2008. "Competitive intelligence: A multiphasic precedent to marketing strategy," *European Journal of Marketing* (42), pp. 766–778.

Evans, M. 2005. "Global CI – best practice methods," in Conference proceedings of the Competitive Intelligence conference, Somerset West, ZAF.

Farley H. F. and Freyn S. 2022. "Competitive intelligence: A precursor to a learning health system," *Health Services Management Research* (36), pp. 82–88.

Fatti, A. C. and Du Toit, A. S. A. 2012. "Competitive intelligence in the South African pharmaceutical industry," *ProQuest Dissertations & Theses Global* (2572695767).

Festervand, J. and Lumpkin, T. 1990. "Building an effective competitive intelligence system for healthcare service providers", *Health Marketing Quarterly* (7), pp. 51–63.

Freyn, S.L. and Farley, F. 2020. "Competitive intelligence: A prescription for US health care?", *Foresight* (22), pp. 617–632.

Ghannay, J and Mamlouk, Z. 2012. "Synergy between competitive intelligence and knowledge management—a key for competitive advantage," *Journal Intelligence Study Business* (2), pp. 23–34.

He, W., Shen, J., Tian, X., Li, Y., Akula, V., Yan, G., and Tao, R. 2015. "Gaining competitive intelligence from social media data: Evidence from two largest retail chains in the world," *Industrial Management & Data Systems* (115), pp. 1622–1636.

Isabelle, D., Horak, K., McKinnon, S., and Palumbo, C. 2020. "Is porter's five forces framework still relevant? A study of the capital/labour intensity continuum via mining and IT industries," *Technology Innovation Management* (10), pp. 28–41.

Itani, O.S. 2017. "Social media use in B2b sales and its impact on competitive intelligence collection and adaptive selling: Examining the role of learning orientation as an enabler," *Industrial Marketing Management* (66), pp. 64–79.

Jeong, B., Ko, N., Son, C., and Yoon, J. 2021. "Trademark-based framework to uncover business diversification opportunities: Application of deep link prediction and competitive intelligence analysis," *Computers in Industry* (124), pp. 1–13.

Kahlon, R. S. and Tse, M.-C. 2013. "Finding new competitive intelligence: Using structured and unstructured data," in Proceedings of the 8th European Conference on Innovation and Entrepreneurship, Brussels, BEL, pp. 842–846.

Khurram, A., Hassan, S., and Khurram, S. 2020. "Revisiting porter five forces model: Influence of non-governmental organizations on competitive rivalry in various economic sectors," *Pakistan Social Sciences Review* (4), pp. 1–15.

Köseoglu, M. A., Ross, G., and Okumus, F. 2016. "Competitive intelligence practices in hotels," *International Journal of Hospitality Management* (53), pp. 161–172.

Kordon, A. 2020. "Applied artificial intelligence-based systems as competitive advantage," in Proceedings of the IEEE 10th International Conference on Intelligent Systems (IS), Varna, BGR, pp. 6–18.

Krakowski, S., Luger, J., and Raisch, S. 2022. "Artificial intelligence and the changing sources of competitive advantage," *Strategic Management Journal*, pp. 1- 28.

Lee, M. and Lee, S. 2017. "Identifying new business opportunities from competitor intelligence: An integrated use of patent and trademark databases," *Technological Forecasting and Social Change* (119), pp. 170–183.

Lewis, D. 2006. "Marketing masterclass: Harnessing intelligence for competitive advantage," *Journal of Medical Marketing* (6), pp. 276–281.

López-Robles, J. R., Otegi-Olaso, J. R., Porto-Gomez, I., Gamboa-Rosales, H., and Gamboa-Rosales, N. K. 2020. "Understanding the intellectual structure and evolution of Competitive Intelligence: A bibliometric analysis from 1984 to 2017," *Technology Analysis & Strategic Management* (32), pp. 604–619.

Luu, T. 2014. "Knowledge sharing and competitive intelligence", *Marketing Intelligence & Planning* (32), pp. 269–292.

Maguire, S., Suluo, H., and Ojiako, U. 2010. "Competitor intelligence: The real value from E.R.P. II?" in Proceedings of the UK Academy for Information Systems Conference. 36

Marks, M. A., Mathieu, J. E., and Zaccaro, S. J. 2001. "A temporally based framework and taxonomy of team processes", *Academy of Management Review* (26), pp. 356–376.

Miller A and Tucker C. 2014. "Health information exchange, system size and information silos," *Journal of Health Economics* (33), pp. 28–42.

Mori, J., Kajikawa, Y., Kashima, H., and Sakata, I. 2012. "Machine learning approach for finding business partners and building reciprocal relationships," *Expert Systems with Applications* (39), pp. 10402–10407.

Park, H. and Yoon, J. 2014. "Assessing coreness and intermediarity of technology sectors using patent co-classification analysis: The case of Korean national R&D," *Scientometrics* (98), pp. 853–890.

Park, I. and Yoon, B. 2018. "Technological opportunity discovery for technological convergence based on the prediction of technology knowledge flow in a citation network," *Journal of Informetrics* (12), pp. 1199–1222.

Park, H., Yoon, J., and Kim, K. 2013. "Identification and evaluation of corporations for merger and acquisition strategies using patent information and text mining," *Scientometrics* (97), pp. 883–909.

Porter, M. E. 1979. "How competitive forces shape strategy," *Harvard Business Review*, pp. 137–145.

Ranjan, J. and Foropon, C. 2021. "Big data analytics in building the competitive intelligence of organizations," *International Journal of Information Management* (56).

Reyes, D. D. L., Trajano, D., Manssour, I. H., Vieira, R., and Bordini, R. H. 2021. "Entity Relation Extraction from News Articles in Portuguese for Competitive Intelligence Based on BERT," in *Intelligent Systems. BRACIS 2021. Lecture Notes in Computer Science (13074)*, Britto, A. and Valdivia Delgado, K. (eds.), Springer, Cham.

Rodriguez-Salvador, M. and Castillo-Valdez, P. F. 2021. "Integrating science and technology metrics into a competitive technology intelligence methodology," *Journal of Intelligence Studies in Business* (11), pp. 69–77.

Sauter, V. L. 2005. "Competitive intelligence systems: Qualitative DSS for strategic decision making," *SIGMIS Database* (36), pp. 43–57.

Schwarz, J. O., Ram, C., and Rohrbeck, R. 2019. "Combining scenario planning and business wargaming to better anticipate future competitive dynamics," *Futures* (105), pp. 133–142.

Sheng, M. L., Chang, S., Teo, T., and Lin, Y. 2013. "Knowledge barriers, knowledge transfer, and innovation competitive advantage in healthcare settings," *Management Decision* (51), pp. 461–478.

Shi, Z. (M.), Lee, G. M., and Whinston, A. B. 2016. "Toward a better measure of business proximity: Topic modeling for industry intelligence," *MIS Quarterly* (40), pp. 1035–1056.

Silva, J., del Carmen Vidal Pacheco, L., Parra Negrete, K., Cómbita Niño, J., Lezama, O. B. P. and Varela, N. 2019. "Design and development of a custom system of technology surveillance and competitive intelligence in SMEs" *Procedia Computer Science* (151), pp. 1231–1236.

Spetz, J., Burgess, J., and Phibbs, C. 2014. "The effect of health information technology implementation in veterans health administration hospitals on patient outcomes," *Healthcare Journal of Delivery Science and Innovation* (2), pp. 40–47.

Staudt, J., Yu, H., Light, R. P., Marschke, G., Börner, K., and Weinberg, B. A. 2018. "High-impact and transformative science (HITS) metrics: Definition, exemplification, and comparison," *PLoS ONE* (13): e0200597, pp. 1–23.

Trong Tuan, L. 2013. "Corporate social responsibility, upward influence behavior, team processes and competitive intelligence", *Team Performance Management* (19), pp. 6–33.

Vaughn, T., Koepke, M., Levey, S., Kroch, E., Davis, L., Hatcher, C. Tompkins, C. and Baloh, J. 2014. "Governing board, C-suite, and clinical management perceptions of quality and safety structures, processes, and priorities in US hospitals," *Journal of Healthcare Management* (59), pp. 111–128.

Webster, J. and Watson, R. T. 2002. "Analyzing the past to prepare for the future: Writing a literature review," *MIS Quarterly* (26), pp. 13–23.

Wisnowski, J., Castillo, F., Karl, A., and Rushing, H. 2015. "Harness the power of JMP®: Big data and social media for competitor analytics," JMP Discovery Conference.

Wu, S., Sun, J., and Tang, J. 2013. "Patent partner recommendation in enterprise social networks," in Proceedings of the 6th ACM international conference on Web search and data mining (WSDM '13), New York, USA, pp. 43–52.

Zheng, Z. (E.), Fader, P., and Padmanabhan, B. 2012. "From business intelligence to competitive intelligence: Inferring competitive measures using augmented site-centric data," *Information Systems Research* (23), pp. 698–720.

III

Clinical Applications

Nilmini Wickramasinghe, Freimut Bodendorf, and Mathias Kraus

Ultimately, to impact healthcare delivery a critical success factor is concerned with clinical applications. Such applications directly sit at the patient-clinician coal face and naturally have a direct bearing on the quality and value of the care received.

Possible clinical applications and their implications for delivering better patient-centred high-value clinical outcomes, or not, is thus the focus of this section. The chapters that make up this section address key aspects as follows:

Chapter 10: Machine Learning for Healthcare Applications: Possibilities and Barriers, by Nalika Ulapane et al., unpacks several machine learning applications and in doing so presents key barriers and facilitators.

Chapter 11: A Systematic Review of Prediction Models for Chronic Opioid Use Following Surgery, by Tong Lei Liu et al., presents evidence from the literature which serves to highlight the impact of analytics, machine learning, and/or artificial intelligence for identifying overuse and possible addiction with opioids.

Chapter 12: Addressing Challenges in the Emergency Department with Analytics and AI, by Josh Ting et al., identifies opportunities for analytics and artificial intelligence to support and facilitate effective and efficient deployment of essential care in one of the critical areas in hospitals, the emergency department.

DOI: 10.1201/9781032699745-12

Chapter 13: Using Simulators to Assist with Mental Health Issues: The Impact of a Sailing Simulator on People with ADHD, by Gurdeep Sarai et al., discusses the growing use of simulators, their advantages, and the benefits of physical activity for people with attention deficit hyperactivity disorder (ADHD) offered by the VSail Sailing Simulator.

Chapter 14: A Possible Blockchain Architecture for Healthcare: Insights from Catena-X, by Nalika Ulapane et al., addresses vital privacy and security concerns with sensitive healthcare data and presents a private blockchain architecture model that is developed from outside of healthcare.

Given the breadth and depth of clinical care today, no section can even try to capture all the major issues; rather, the focus of this section is to highlight and illustrate a few important areas including privacy and security, risk mitigation, supporting and guiding superior decision making, as well as providing more effective and efficient care. In the aforementioned chapters, these issues are illustrated by specific use case examples, but the themes are generally applicable to all areas of clinical applications and should always be considered when designing and developing responsible clinical decision-support solutions. Rapid advances in machine learning, analytics, and artificial intelligence have opened the door to numerous possibilities that are both exciting and have tremendous potential for supporting better care delivery and better clinical outcomes. However, it is also important to proceed with caution, employing best practices including incorporating user-centred design and design science principles to ensure heterogeneous user needs are addressed. In addition, it is vital to be responsible and have appropriate security and privacy measures in place and ensure the highest levels of accuracy in all results that are generated so that the ensuing decisions do indeed serve to realize better clinical outcomes, high-quality care, and high-value care.

CHAPTER 10

Machine Learning for Healthcare Applications

Possibilities and Barriers

Nalika Ulapane, Amir Eslami Andargoli, and Nilmini Wickramasingh

INTRODUCTION

Healthcare for a long time has been a domain for human experts. However, with recent advancements in electronic data acquisition and record keeping, computer infrastructure, algorithms and techniques, and Artificial Intelligence (AI) applications, the environment is shaping up for AI to be used to improve medical practice [1]. Research into areas such as the use of the concept of digital twins in healthcare [2–5] is a prime example. The use of AI for healthcare has the potential to improve clinical practice by reducing the cognitive burden on clinicians, increasing precision and personalisation of care through enhanced use of data, and improving patient outcomes and cost implications [2–5].

AI applications are developed on machine learning principles. Numerous algorithms have been developed over time based on these machine learning principles, to make sense of data by making data-driven inferences. These machine learning algorithms are recently being used to make sense of health data as well. It has been well observed that different machine learning algorithms serve different purposes, and each algorithm tends to have unique strengths and weaknesses. As such, it is

DOI: 10.1201/9781032699745-13

important for practitioners who develop AI applications to have a summary understanding of these algorithms, including their merits and demerits. Having that understanding will help practitioners to choose the right algorithms for the right purposes. To help practitioners along those lines, we attempt in this chapter to present a summary classification and a list of strengths and weaknesses of different machine learning algorithms that were found through a scoping review. Our scoping review covers the application of artificial intelligence in a healthcare context. In the healthcare context, dementia is considered as a case study provided the current rising prevalence of dementia worldwide [6]. Thereby we attempt to answer the following research question through this chapter: What are the commonly used machine learning algorithms in AI applications related to dementia care, what are their strengths and weaknesses, and how may some of their persisting limitations be addressed?

METHOD

A scoping review of empirical studies that used AI-powered clinical decision support systems to support the implementation of the Global Action Plan for Dementia (GAPD) [6] was conducted using MEDLINE, EMBASE, PubMed, SCOPUS and Cumulative Index to Nursing and Allied Health Literature (CINAHL) databases. A search strategy was developed using keywords around three main concepts: Artificial intelligence, Dementia and Decision Support Systems, as shown in Table 10.1. Literature was

TABLE 10.1 Keywords for Scoping Review

Concept	Key Phrase
Artificial intelligence	("Artificial intelligence" OR "Analytics")
Dementia	("Dementia" OR "Alzheimer" OR "cognitive dysfunction" OR "cognitive impairment" OR "intellectual impairment" OR "mental impairment" OR "mental deficiency")
Decision support system	("Decision support system" OR "decision support tool" OR "reminder system" OR "reminding system" OR "alert system" OR "alerting system" OR "computer-assisted decision making" OR "computer-assisted diagnosis" OR "computer-assisted therapy" OR "expert system" OR "CDS" OR "order entry system" OR "computerized order entry" OR "computerized prescriber order entry" OR "computerized provider order entry" OR "computerized physician order entry" OR "electronic order entry" OR "automated order entry" OR "CPOE" OR "electronic prescribing" OR "electronic prescription" OR "computer-assisted drug therapy" OR "DSS")

TABLE 10.2 Inclusion and Exclusion Criteria

Inclusion Criteria:	Only articles that focussed on the application of AI in the development of decision support systems in dementia care were included. Therefore, papers should cover these three dimensions of AI, decision support systems and dementia care to be eligible for inclusion in this study. In this study, we included only primary research studies with both qualitative and quantitative methodologies that were published in peer-reviewed journals. Only articles that were published in English were included. No restrictions were placed on the date in order to be able to conduct a trend analysis later. Articles that were published until August 2021 using relevant keywords to AI, Dementia and decision support systems were included. Furthermore, no restrictions were placed on the type of participants and the location of the study. Any contextual setting would be eligible for inclusion.
Exclusion Criteria:	Articles that were published in a language other than English were excluded. Non-empirical studies, abstract-only publications, editorials, letters, books, book chapters, comments, dissertations, conference proceedings, and reviews were excluded. Further, studies that do not focus on the application of intelligent decision support systems for dementia care were excluded. The focus of the studies should be on all three topics of dementia, DSS and AI.

searched by combining the three key phrases in Table 10.1 through AND Boolean logic. Search results were imported into Endnote to remove duplicates and then uploaded into the Covidence software. Each article's title and abstract were screened against the inclusion and exclusion criteria in Table 10.2. Then, full texts of the articles included from the title and abstract screening were reviewed. The machine learning algorithms found in those articles reviewed are discussed in this chapter.

SUMMARY OF RESULTS

The summary of the characteristics of the included articles in this study is provided in Table 10.3. The filtering of the articles that occurred at each stage of reviewing is summarised in Figure 10.1. The first publication in this area that was included in this study was published in 2000. However, the majority of the publications included in these articles (approximately 80%) were published in the last decade indicating an increasing trend towards the application of AI in dementia as the field and the technology mature. Further, the articles often revealed that most of the publications deal with the application of AI-powered decision

TABLE 10.3 Overview of the Included Studies

Characteristics	Number of Studies (n = 28)
Year of Publication	
2000–2005	4
2006–2010	2
2011–2015	13
2016–2021	9
Dementia Types	
Alzheimer disease	8
MCI	1
Not specific (AD/MCI/SCI)	19
Dementia Area	
Diagnosis	22
Early detection	2
Treatment	2
Carer support & education	3

support systems not specific to any dementia types, and the focus was on the mix of types including Alzheimer's disease (AD), Mild Cognitive Impairment (MCI) and Subjective Cognitive Impairment (SCI). Most of the studies focused on diagnosis. The focus of discussion for this chapter is specifically the different types of machine learning algorithms that have been used in the included articles.

Then, the algorithms that were found are listed in Table 10.4 alongside their respective studies. Support Vector Machines (SVM) was the most common technique used in these studies.

The algorithms are grouped and presented in Figure 10.2. The grouping of machine learning algorithms in Figure 10.2 is twofold, that goes as supervised learning and unsupervised learning algorithms. Then, another observation was that most of the works had focused on classification problems. A classification problem usually involves two tasks. They are: (1) Determination of descriptive features from raw data to be fed as the inputs to a classifier; and (2) The classification task. Therefore, in Figure 10.2, the algorithms are further grouped according to whether they help in feature determination, or whether they help in classification. Rarely though, regression has also been attempted to compute different numerical values to help in prediction. The work by Bucholc 2019 (i.e., [7]) is an example. To include such attempts, a third section has also been added to Figure 10.2. The third section lists algorithms used for regression. Also, the older works (i.e., the works prior to 2010) have been

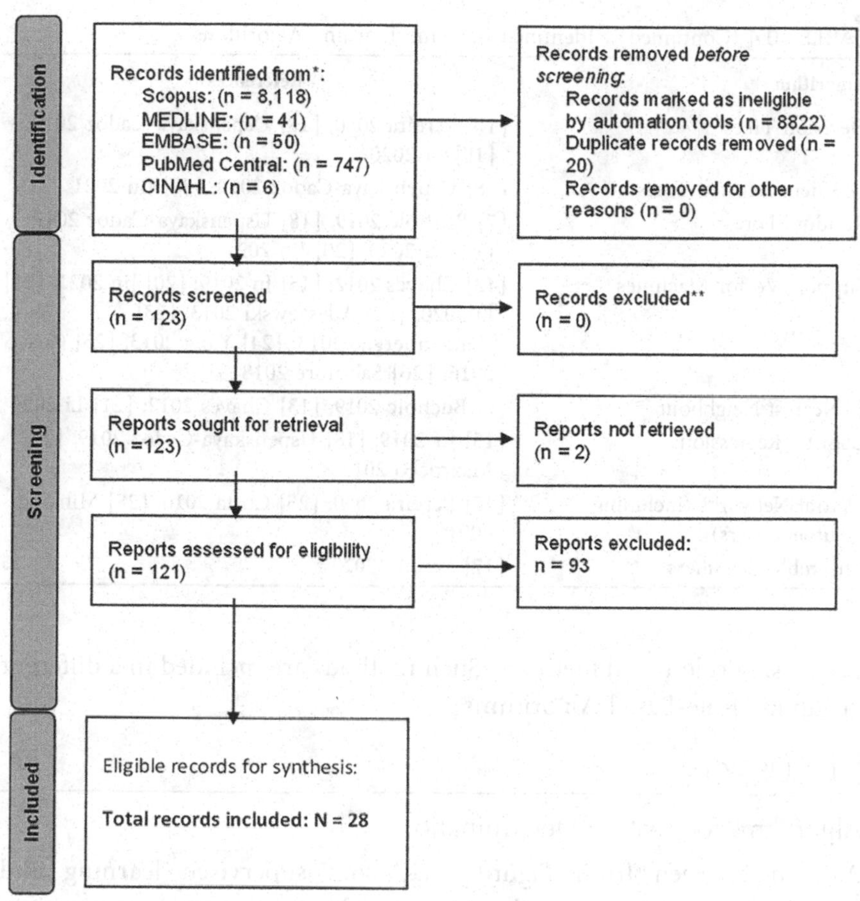

FIGURE 10.1 Scoping review flow diagram.

TABLE 10.4 Identified Machine Learning Algorithms

Algorithm	References
Rule-Based Algorithms	[8] Coulson 2000; [9] Man 2002; [10] Jimison 2004; [11] Colliot 2008
Kernel Ridge Regression	[7] Bucholc 2019
Support Vector Regression	[7] Bucholc 2019
k-Nearest Neighbor for Regression	[7] Bucholc 2019
Sparse Representation	[12] Xu 2015
Principal Component Analysis	[13] Chaves 2012
Linear Discriminant Analysis	[14] McEvoy 2009; [15] Ju 2019
Bayesian Networks	[16] Seixas 2014
Naïve Bayes	[17] Pereira 2020

(Continued)

TABLE 10.4 (Continued) Identified Machine Learning Algorithms

Algorithm	References
Decision Trees	[17] Pereira 2020; [18] Uspenskaya-Cadoz 2019; [19] Bi 2020
Gradient-Boosted Trees	[18] Uspenskaya-Cadoz 2019; [20] Jin 2021
Random Forest	[7] Bucholc 2019; [18] Uspenskaya-Cadoz 2019; [19] Bi 2020; [20] Jin 2021
Support Vector Machines	[13] Chaves 2012; [15] Ju 2019; [20] Jin 2021; [21] Li 2020; [22] Adaszewski 2013; [23] Vandenberghe 2013; [24] Yang 2013; [25] Costa 2016; [26] Salvatore 2018
K-Nearest Neighbour	[7] Bucholc 2019; [13] Chaves 2012; [21] Li 2020
Logistic Regression	[15] Ju 2019; [18] Uspenskaya-Cadoz 2019; [27] Mazzocco 2012
Neural Networks (including Autoencoders)	[17] Pereira 2020; [25] Costa 2016; [28] Mihailidis 2001
Ensemble Classifiers	[17] Pereira 2020

done using rule-based methods. Such methods are included in a different group as "Rule-Based Algorithms".

DISCUSSION

Algorithms for Feature Determination

As can be seen from Figure 10.2, both supervised learning and unsupervised learning algorithms are available for feature determination. The unsupervised learning algorithms Principal Component Analysis (PCA), Sparse Representation and Autoencoders have been used for feature determination. PCA and Sparse Representation are classically used techniques in statistics and machine learning applications for reducing the dimensionality of raw data. These techniques are often used to derive linearly independent features. These techniques are especially useful in image processing, specifically in image compression. They can be useful in medical applications when dealing with imaging, such as MRI image analysis. The main advantage of these techniques comes from reducing the volume of data while preserving a sufficient degree of informativeness. These techniques enable a degree of noise suppression as well. Working with features derived from such techniques makes the computational burden lighter than feeding raw data for classification. Autoencoders on the other hand are well-known intermediate layers

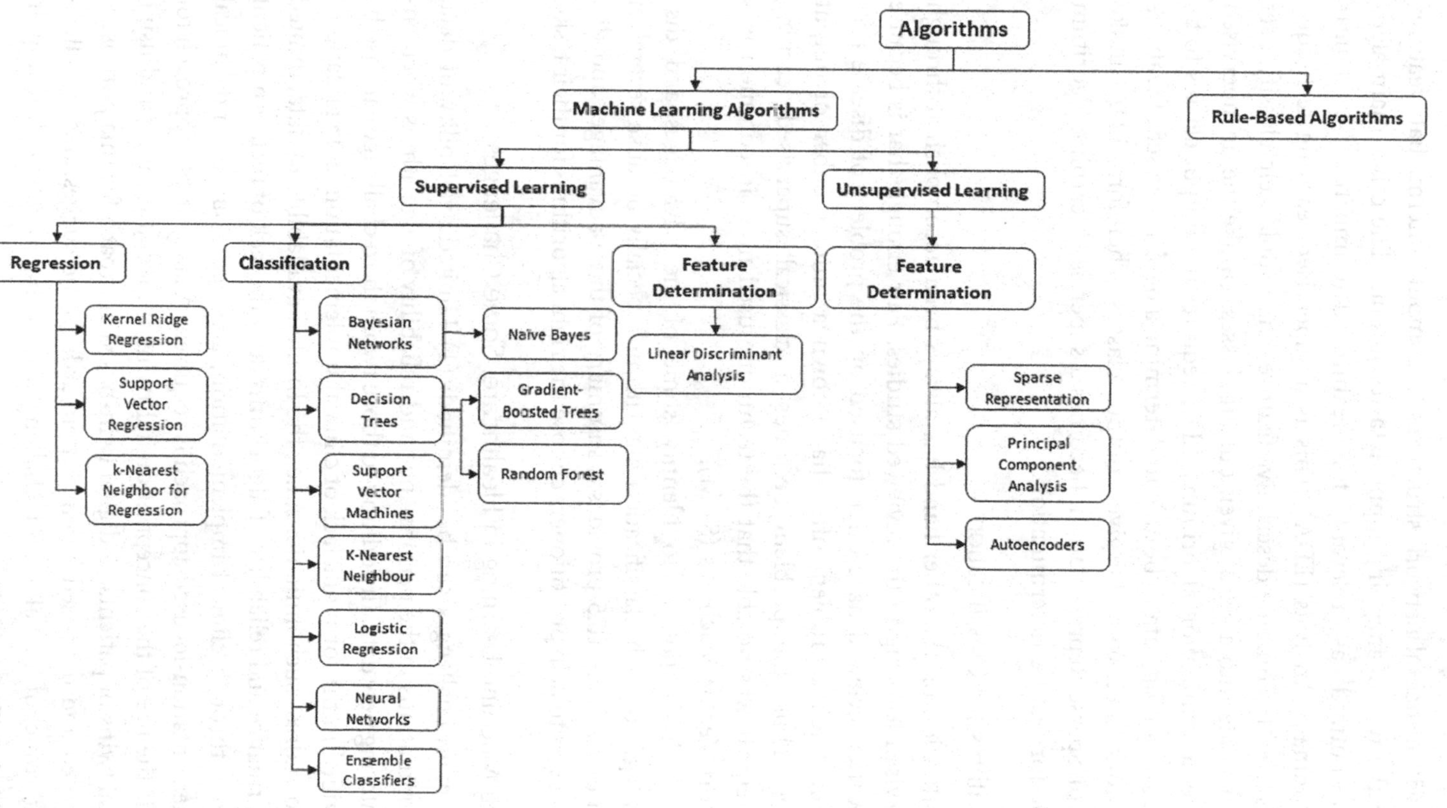

FIGURE 10.2 Grouping of algorithms.

used within neural network structures to compute intermediate features along the way of mapping input data to outputs. The other main algorithm noticed as relevant for feature determination is Linear Discriminant Analysis (LDA). This is a supervised learning technique and is used to compute descriptive features that would help classify a set of input data into a set of given output classes. Unlike the unsupervised feature determination algorithms, LDA requires the output classes to be given as training data to be able to determine a descriptive set of features that works well with the given output classes. Therefore, LDA unlike PCA or Sparse Representation, becomes a supervised learning algorithm usable for feature determination.

Algorithms for Classification

Classification on the other hand has always been accomplished through supervised learning in the reviewed studies. Fair enough that is because the works reviewed have often focused on the problem of disease prediction. Such a problem often has known a finite number of output classes. Thus, the problem becomes a classical supervised learning problem. It was notable that the technique used most in common was Support Vector Machines (SVM).

It is also important to identify some of the advantages and disadvantages of each classification algorithm, especially because several of them exist. Table 10.5 provides a summary of these advantages and disadvantages to help practitioners choose the right algorithms for their tasks.

Using Machine Learning in Healthcare: Some Challenges

Two main challenges can be identified: (1) Limited availability of data; (2) Limitations in the performance and reliability of algorithms when encountering new data. In addition to those two, a third challenge can also be identified in the form of a lack of clinical implementation and validation.

To address such limitations, i.e., the limited availability of data, limited performance and reliability of algorithms, and the lack of focus on patient journey through clinical implementation, a patient journey and clinical implementation-focused approach is required. A suggestable approach for this is the use of the concept of digital twins, aimed at creating and using digital twins of patients. A digital twin-based approach for this purpose is proposed and discussed herein. Afterwards, some suggestions for alleviating some of the aforesaid challenges of using machine learning in healthcare are discussed.

TABLE 10.5 Comparison of the Classification Algorithms

Classification Algorithm	Advantages	Disadvantages
Bayesian Networks – [29] Aghaie & Saeedi, 2009	• The output is a probability • Can presenting a problem as a graphical model • Easy to interpret	• Relies heavily on prior beliefs in inference processing • Inaccuracy of prior beliefs will propagate to distort the subsequent stages of the network • Relies on assumptions about data that may not hold true in reality • There is no universally accepted method to construct a network
Decision Trees – [30] Ptak-Chmielewska, 2016, [31] Mohamed, 2017	• Easy to interpret and visualise • Robust and automatic selection of features • Can be converted to a rule-based classifier • Minimal assumptions made about the data; nonparametric method • Can model highly nonlinear relationships • Can handle outliers and missing values	• Models can be unstable • Often suffers in accuracy • Likely to overfit • Often requires large training sets to achieve stable and reliable models
Support Vector Machines – [31] Mohamed, 2017	• Training is relatively easy • Scales relatively well to the high dimensional data • Easy to control the trade-off between model complexity and accuracy • Can deal with both continuous and categorical data • Can capture nonlinear relationships in the data • No assumptions are required regarding the data as SVM is a non-parametric method • Prediction accuracy is usually high • Can usually generalise well	• Difficulty to interpret unless the features are interpretable • Needs a good kernel function • Lacks transparency in results because SVM is a non-parametric method

(Continued)

TABLE 10.5 (Continued) Comparison of the Classification Algorithms

Classification Algorithm	Advantages	Disadvantages
	• An SVM model becomes a unique solution because it solves a convex optimisation problem • Robust and able to deal with data that contains errors	
K-Nearest Neighbours – [31] Mohamed, 2017	• Little to no training is required • Simple and easy to interpret and implement • Can deal with noisy data	• No model is learned so to speak; makes use of training data every time when running • Can be sensitive to irrelevant features • A lazy algorithm; takes time to run • Needs large memory to store training examples
Logistic Regression – [32] Westreich, *et al.*, 2010	• Simple and easy to interpret • Efficient training and usage	• Can overfit with high dimensional data • Difficult to solve nonlinear problems • Requires minimal multicollinearity between input features • Sensitive to outliers • Assumes a log-linear relationship, parametric method
Neural Networks – [31] Mohamed, 2017	• Can be used to solve linear and nonlinear programming problems • No prior knowledge about the data or the process is required; no assumptions about data are made • Usually successful in solving challenging classification, clustering, and regression problems	• The success of a model usually depends on the quantity of the data • Difficult to interpret (black box) • Difficult to choose an optimal neural network structure

Using Machine Learning in Healthcare: Some Possibilities

The proposed use of digital twins of patients along patient journeys is illustrated in Figures 10.3 and 10.4. In Figure 10.3, a patient journey is illustrated over time, across multiple clinical encounters where the patient meets a clinician. As mentioned before, the digital twin in this patient journey is a digital representation of the patient. In Figure 10.4, the patient journey within a single clinical encounter is illustrated. The complete patient journey involving the digital twin is described across Ten distinct steps. These steps are marked and labelled in the illustration.

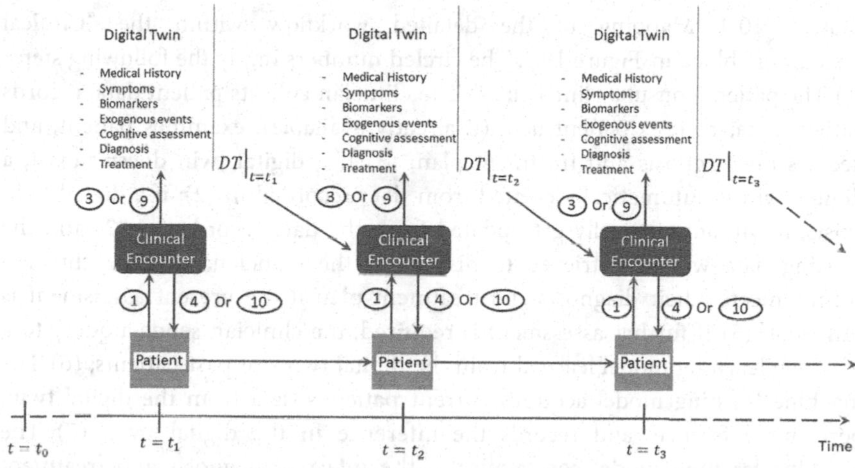

FIGURE 10.3 Mapping of a digital twin incorporated proposed clinical workflow along time. The circled numbers imply the following steps: (1) The patient consults clinician; (2) The clinician collects patient data, records patient data, reviews patient data (if already available), examines patient, and decides on diagnosis and treatment plan; (3) If a digital twin doesn't exist, a digital twin is automatically created from data recorded in (2); if a digital twin exists, it will automatically get updated from the data recorded in (2) and the existing data will be retrieved to display to the clinician; (4) The clinician communicates their diagnosis and treatment plan if the present assessment is sufficient; (5) If further assessment is required, the clinician sends a query to a machine learning model learned from the digital twins of past patients; (6) The machine learning model acquires current patient's data from the digital twin, performs inference, and records the inference in the digital twin; (7) The machine learning model communicates the inferred diagnosis and treatment plan to the clinician; (8) The clinician makes an augmented decision on diagnosis and treatment plan and records it; (9) The digital twin is automatically updated according to data recorded in (8); (10) The clinician communicates their augmented diagnosis and treatment plan.

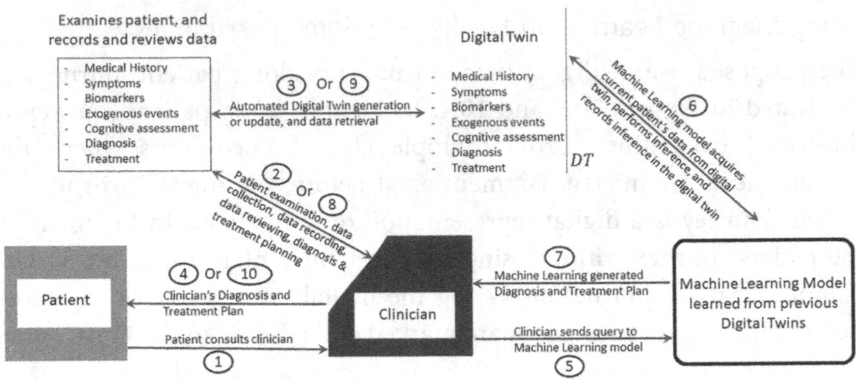

FIGURE 10.4 Mapping of the detailed workflow within the "Clinical Encounter" block in Figure 10.3. The circled numbers imply the following steps: (1) The patient consults clinician; (2) The clinician collects patient data, records patient data, reviews patient data (if already available), examines patient, and decides on diagnosis and treatment plan; (3) If a digital twin doesn't exist, a digital twin is automatically created from data recorded in (2); if a digital twin exists, it will automatically get updated from the data recorded in (2) and the existing data will be retrieved to display to the clinician; (4) The clinician communicates their diagnosis and treatment plan if the present assessment is sufficient; (5) If further assessment is required, the clinician sends a query to a machine learning model learned from the digital twins of past patients; (6) The machine learning model acquires current patient's data from the digital twin, performs inference, and records the inference in the digital twin; (7) The machine learning model communicates the inferred diagnosis and treatment plan to the clinician; (8) The clinician makes an augmented decision on diagnosis and treatment plan and records it; (9) The digital twin is automatically updated according to data recorded in (8); (10) The clinician communicates their augmented diagnosis and treatment plan.

How Might the Limited Availability of Data Be Addressed through the Suggested Digital Twin Approach?

The trivial solution for the limited data constraint lies in collecting more data. The collection of more data is facilitated by the proposed patient journey in several steps. The conjoined steps (2) and (8) serve to electronically record details about patients, as well as decisions made by clinicians alongside time stamps. One can argue that recording data as such is essentially the same as Electronic Health Records (EHR) or Electronic Medical Records (EMR), and thus, the question of "what's different?" obviously arises. The difference can be understood as such. The HER/EMR system is typically a passive storage of information that requires significant manual intervention to make sense of. In contrast, the digital twin architecture has provision for machine learning frameworks to be incorporated at the backend. These facilitate automated and tailored training of machine learning algorithms. This also allows the production of machine learning inferences to support clinicians in their decision-making. As such, the digital twin architecture becomes a decision support system that can provide automated inferences of decisions regarding a patient based on data-driven deterministic or probabilistic inference. Such use of machine learning algorithms at the backend is what is involved with steps (6) and (7). Note that in step (7), the inference made by a respective machine learning model also gets recorded in the digital twin along with the respective time stamp in addition to the inference getting displayed to the clinician as well. As such, the use of digital twins facilitates the recording of data, and thereby enables addressing the issue with "limited data". Three modalities can be identified in the data recorded according to the proposed patient journey. The three modalities are: (1) Patient history and progress (i.e., details about the patient) with time stamps; (2) Decisions made by clinicians alongside timestamps; (3) Inferences made by machine learning algorithms alongside time stamps. Those three modalities of data, when collected over time, can facilitate systematically captured clinical evidence. Such evidence can be useful for further generation of knowledge while improving the capability of machine learning algorithms. They can also enable quality control and help improve clinical practice and patient outcomes in the long run. Such provisions and opportunities can be foreseen regarding addressing the issue of limited data through using digital twins.

Another aspect together with limited data, is the issue with incomplete data in healthcare. Although deep learning techniques at present have been successful in many complex classification tasks, the prerequisite for that success is access to good-quality data. This prerequisite often becomes unrealistic especially in the healthcare sphere, at least at the present since medical data comes at a cost. Each data feature in the medical setting usually requires a medical test. This results in costs and time, and at times, side effects to patients. This also results quite often in incomplete datasets with missing data features, inhibiting the training of machine learning models. As a solution for this challenge, doing more tests to complete the datasets is not practical. But a possible solution in terms of machine learning lies in training different models that match the available data features, rather than training one model to match the rich data points and removing the incomplete data points. However, to enable this approach, the collection of data (which may be incomplete) over a longer period of time becomes necessary. This is again a place where the digital twin setup brings value as it helps with recording data over time.

How Might the Limitations in Performance and Reliability of Algorithms Be Addressed?

As discussed earlier, three modalities of data can be recorded in the suggested digital twin approach. They are: (1) Patient history and progress (i.e., details about the patient) with their time stamps; (2) Decisions made by clinicians alongside timestamps; (3) Inferences made by machine learning algorithms alongside time stamps. The ultimate validation of a machine learning model in the medical context comes through comparing the machine learning predictions against implications caused by patient outcomes. To perform that validation, two sources of information collected over time are required. They are: (1) The machine learning predictions made over time; (2) Patient progress. Now, as per the three modalities of data collected from the digital twin architecture, the two required elements for validating machine learning models over time will automatically be collected. In addition to the two required elements, the clinician's decisions too will be recorded as a third mode of data. Sustained collection of all these modalities of data can yield a rich bank of data for sustained learning and relearning of machine learning models over time. This will facilitate an environment where machine learning models can be incorporated into clinical practice along the patient journey. This incorporation of machine learning models in the clinical workflow will over time give substantial data for validation. As such, the proposed digital twin architecture with patient journey has the potential to address the present limitations with algorithms as well through sustained learning, relearning, and assessment over time.

CONCLUSION

The use of artificial intelligence for healthcare applications is an emerging area. At the core of this emergence lies machine learning algorithms. Different machine learning algorithms serve different purposes and have unique strengths and weaknesses. In that backdrop, we attempted the answer through this chapter the research question: What are the commonly used machine learning algorithms in AI applications related to dementia care, what are their strengths and weaknesses, and how may some of their persisting limitations be addressed? In an attempt to answer that question, we presented a summary of machine learning algorithms found through a scoping review about the use of artificial intelligence applications in a healthcare context. The healthcare context focused on dementia diagnosis and care. We presented in this chapter a grouping and a list of strengths and weaknesses of different machine learning algorithms. Our grouping and the list of strengths and weaknesses will be useful for practitioners in choosing the right algorithm for the right purpose. We also discussed how some of the challenges persisting at present for the use of machine learning in healthcare can be addressed using concepts like digital twins.

REFERENCES

1. Yu, K. H., Beam, A. L. and Kohane, I. S., 2018. Artificial Intelligence in Healthcare. *Nature Biomedical Engineering* 2(10), pp.719–731.
2. Björnsson, B., Borrebaeck, C., Elander, N., Gasslander, T., Gawel, D. R., Gustafsson, M., Jörnsten, R., Lee, E. J., Li, X., Lilja, S. & Martínez-Enguita, D., 2020. Digital Twins to Personalize Medicine. *Genome medicine* 12, pp.1–4.
3. Wickramasinghe, N., Jayaraman, P. P., Forkan, A. R. M., Ulapane, N., Kaul, R., Vaughan, S. and Zelcer, J., 2021. A Vision for Leveraging the Concept of Digital Twins to Support the Provision of Personalized Cancer Care. *IEEE Internet Computing* 26(5), pp.17–24.
4. Wickramasinghe, N., Ulapane, N., Andargoli, A., Ossai, C., Shuakat, N., Nguyen, T. and Zelcer, J., 2022. Digital twins to enable better precision and personalized dementia care. *JAMIA open* 5(3), p.ooac072.
5. Wickramasinghe, N., Ulapane, N., Nguyen, T. A., Andargoli, A., Ossai, C., Shuakat, N. and Zelcer, J., 2022. Towards Discovering Digital Twins of Dementia Patients: Matching the Phases of Cognitive Decline. *Alzheimer's & Dementia* 18, p.e066336.
6. World Health Organization. 2017. "Global Action Plan on the Public Health Response to Dementia 2017–2025."
7. Bucholc, M., Ding, X., Wang, H., Glass, D. H., Wang, H., Prasad, G., Maguire, L. P., Bjourson, A. J., McClean, P. L., Todd, S., Finn, D. P., and Wong-Lin, K. 2019. "A Practical Computerized Decision Support System for Predicting the Severity of Alzheimer's Disease of an Individual," *Expert Systems with Applications* (130), pp. 157–171.
8. Coulson, J. S. 2000. "Shhhh: An Expert System for the Management of Clients with Vocally Disruptive Behaviors in Dementia," *Educational Gerontology*.

9. Man, D. W. K., Tam, S. F., and Hui-Chan, C. W. Y. 2002. "Learning to Live Independently with Expert Systems in Memory Rehabilitation," *NeuroRehabilitation* 18(1), pp. 21–29.
10. Jimison, H., Pavel, M., McKanna, J., and Pavel, J. 2004. "Unobtrusive Monitoring of Computer Interactions to Detect Cognitive Status in Elders," *IEEE Transactions on Information Technology in Biomedicine.*
11. Colliot, O., Chételat, G., Chupin, M., Desgranges, B., Magnin, B., Benali, H., Dubois, B., Garnero, L., Eustache, F., and Lehéricy, S. 2008. "Discrimination between Alzheimer Disease, Mild Cognitive Impairment, and Normal Aging by Using Automated Segmentation of the Hippocampus," *Radiology* 248(1), pp. 194–201.
12. Xu, L., Wu, X., Chen, K., and Yao, L. 2015. "Multi-Modality Sparse Representation-Based Classification for Alzheimer's Disease and Mild Cognitive Impairment," *Computer Methods and Programs in Biomedicine.*
13. Chaves, R., Ramírez, J., Górriz, J. M., Illán, I. A., Gámez-Río, M., and Carnero, C. 2012. "Effective Diagnosis of Alzheimer's Disease by Means of Large Margin-Based Methodology," *BMC Medical Informatics and Decision Making.*
14. McEvoy, L. K., Fennema-Notestine, C., Roddey, J. C., Hagler Jr, D. J., Holland, D., Karow, D. S., Pung, C. J., Brewer, J. B., and Dale, A. M. 2009. "Alzheimer Disease: Quantitative Structural Neuroimaging for Detection and Prediction of Clinical and Structural Changes in Mild Cognitive Impairment," *Radiology.*
15. Ju, R., Hu, C., Zhou, P., and Li, Q. 2019. "Early Diagnosis of Alzheimer's Disease Based on Resting-State Brain Networks and Deep Learning," *IEEE/ACM Transactions on Computational Biology and Bioinformatics.*
16. Seixas, F. L., Zadrozny, B., Laks, J., Conci, A., and Muchaluat Saade, D. C. 2014. "A Bayesian Network Decision Model for Supporting the Diagnosis of Dementia, Alzheimer[U+05f3]S Disease and Mild Cognitive Impairment," *Computers in Biology and Medicine.*
17. Pereira, T., Cardoso, S., Guerreiro, M., Mendonça, A. d., Madeira, S. C., and for the Alzheimer's Disease Neuroimaging, I. 2020. "Targeting the Uncertainty of Predictions at Patient-Level Using an Ensemble of Classifiers Coupled with Calibration Methods, Venn-Abers, and Conformal Predictors: A Case Study in Ad," *Journal of Biomedical Informatics.*
18. Uspenskaya-Cadoz, O., Alamuri, C., Wang, L., Yang, M., Khinda, S., Nigmatullina, Y., Cao, T., Kayal, N., O'Keefe, M., and Rubel, C. 2019. "Machine Learning Algorithm Helps Identify Non-Diagnosed Prodromal Alzheimer's Disease Patients in the General Population," *The Journal of Prevention of Alzheimer's Disease.*
19. Bi, X. A., Hu, X., Wu, H., and Wang, Y. 2020. "Multimodal Data Analysis of Alzheimer's Disease Based on Clustering Evolutionary Random Forest," *IEEE Journal of Biomedical and Health Informatics.*

20. Jin, H., Chien, S., Meijer, E., Khobragade, P., and Lee, J. 2021a. "Learning from Clinical Consensus Diagnosis in India to Facilitate Automatic Classification of Dementia: Machine Learning Study," *JMIR Mental Health.*
21. Li, Z., Dong, A., and Zhou, J. 2020. "Research of Low-Rank Representation and Discriminant Correlation Analysis for Alzheimer's Disease Diagnosis," *Computational and Mathematical Methods in Medicine.*
22. Adaszewski, S., Dukart, J., Kherif, F., Frackowiak, R., and Draganski, B. 2013. "How Early Can We Predict Alzheimer's Disease Using Computational Anatomy?," *Neurobiology of Aging.*
23. Vandenberghe, R., Nelissen, N., Salmon, E., Ivanoiu, A., Hasselbalch, S., Andersen, A., Korner, A., Minthon, L., Brooks, D. J., Van Laere, K., and Dupont, P. 2013. "Binary Classification of 18f-Flutemetamol Pet Using Machine Learning: Comparison with Visual Reads and Structural Mri," *NeuroImage.*
24. Yang, S. T., Lee, J. D., Chang, T. C., Huang, C. H., Wang, J. J., Hsu, W. C., Chan, H. L., Wai, Y. Y., and Li, K. Y. 2013. "Discrimination between Alzheimer's Disease and Mild Cognitive Impairment Using Som and Pso-Svm," *Computational and Mathematical Methods in Medicine.*
25. Costa, L., Gago, M. F., Yelshyna, D., Ferreira, J., Silva, H. D., Rocha, L., Sousa, N., and Bicho, E. 2016. "Application of Machine Learning in Postural Control Kinematics for the Diagnosis of Alzheimer's Disease," *Computational Intelligence and Neuroscience.*
26. Salvatore, C., and Castiglioni, I. 2018. "A Wrapped Multi-Label Classifier for the Automatic Diagnosis and Prognosis of Alzheimer's Disease," *Journal of Neuroscience Methods.*
27. Mazzocco, T., and Hussain, A. 2012. "Novel Logistic Regression Models to Aid the Diagnosis of Dementia," *Expert Systems with Applications.*
28. Mihailidis, A., Fernie, G. R., Mihailidis, A., and Barbenel, J. C. 2001. "The Use of Artificial Intelligence in the Design of an Intelligent Cognitive Orthosis for People with Dementia," *Assistive Technology.*
29. Aghaie, A., and Saeedi, A. 2009. "Using Bayesian Networks for Bankruptcy Prediction: Empirical Evidence from Iranian Companies," 2009 International Conference on Information Management and Engineering: IEEE, pp. 450–455.
30. Ptak-Chmielewska, A. 2016. "Statistical Models for Corporate Credit Risk Assessment-Rating Models," *Acta Universitatis Lodziensis. Folia Oeconomica* 3(322), pp.87–8111.
31. Mohamed, A. E. 2017. "Comparative Study of Four Supervised Machine Learning Techniques for Classification," *International Journal of Applied* 7(2), pp. 1–15.
32. Westreich, D., Lessler, J., and Funk, M. J. 2010. "Propensity Score Estimation: Neural Networks, Support Vector Machines, Decision Trees (Cart), and Meta-Classifiers as Alternatives to Logistic Regression," *Journal of Clinical Epidemiology* 63(8), pp. 826–833.

CHAPTER 11

A Systematic Review of Prediction Models for Chronic Opioid Use Following Surgery

Tong Lei Liu, Stephen Vaughan, and Nilmini Wickramasinghe

INTRODUCTION

Post-operative pain is a common clinical dilemma affecting 80% of patients following surgery and is the most common concern among postoperative patients (1). Despite the increasing prevalence of opioid dependence and toxicity, opioid analgesia remains the mainstay of postoperative pain management (2,3). It is now well-established that adverse effects of medium to long-term opioid use including constipation, mood dysregulation, and sleep-disordered breathing contribute significantly to morbidity and mortality (4). Such risks are further amplified in populations with existing chronic diseases such as diabetes and cardiovascular disease (5,6).

In the United States of America, the economic cost of opioid analgesia misuse is estimated to be $8.5 billion annually (7). Similarly in Australia, the cost of extra-medical opioid use between July 2015 to June 2016 is estimated to be $5.6 billion (8). Predicting and identifying patients at risk of chronic opioid use presents an opportunity to implement alternative analgesic regimens and strategies to mitigate risks associated with opioid use (9). A previous systematic review has explored predictors of chronic

DOI: 10.1201/9781032699745-14

opioid use in the medical and surgical population and identified various characteristics associated with chronic opioid use, including age, sex, previous opioid use, and known diagnosis of chronic pain syndrome or anxiety disorders (10).

With the increase in the availability of data from electronic medical records and accessibility to computational power, there has been an expansion in the development and validation of prediction models in medical research (11). Despite this, there is a research gap in the integration and synthesis of these widely available studies. To date, our research question has not been explored by systematic reviews inclusive of studies utilising predictive modelling techniques. The aim of this study is to conduct a systematic review to identify, describe and compare currently available predictive modelling studies of chronic opioid use following surgery.

METHODS

We followed the Preferred Reporting Items for Systematic Reviews and Meta-analyses (PRISMA) guidelines to ensure systematic and transparent reporting (12). The research question was developed following guidance from CHecklist for critical Appraisal and data extraction for systematic Reviews of prediction Model Studies (CHARMS) (13). Study details and prespecified search strategy were registered through PROSPERO (ID: CRD42022354944). Our research question was first identified following the PICO strategy (population - patients with postoperative pain, intervention - prediction model for chronic opioid use, comparison - no specific comparator, outcome - persistent opioid use >3 months after surgery). Our aim was to systematically search, compare and synthesise studies presenting prognostic predictive models for chronic opioid use following surgery.

Search Strategy

A search of OVID MEDLINE, OVID Embase, Pubmed and Scopus from inception to July 2022 was conducted using a specified search strategy. We also conducted a manual search through Google Scholar and the British Journal of Anesthesia. All resulting articles were imported to Endnote X9 for review. Titles and abstracts were screened after the removal of duplicates. The full text of articles potentially meeting the selection criteria were evaluated for inclusion in the systematic review.

Selection Criteria

We included original studies developing and validating prediction models for chronic opioid use following surgery. Studies evaluating chronic pain, but not opioid use, did not meet our research objective and were thus excluded. Studies specifically investigating cancer-related pain or paediatric patients were excluded due to differences in usual standard practice and underlying pathophysiology. References identified by the search strategy were independently reviewed by 2 reviewers (TL, SV) using Rayyan (14). Disagreements were resolved by a third reviewer (NW).

Data Extraction

A standardised data extraction form was developed following recommendations from the CHecklist for critical Appraisal and data extraction for systematic Reviews of prediction Model Studies (CHARMS) (13). Data extraction was extracted by two independent reviewers (TL, SV). Data relating to the source of data, participants and sample size, outcomes, predictors and selection, model development and validation, and model performance were extracted.

Risk of Bias

Two reviewers (TL, SV) assessed the quality of studies following the Prediction model Risk of Bias Assessment Tool (PROBAST) (15). Several domains, including participants, predictors, outcome and analysis were assessed through questioning and answered by "high", "low" or "unclear" risk of bias. Disagreements were resolved by a third reviewer (NW).

RESULTS

After database searches from inception to July 2022, 410 abstracts were reviewed and we identified 20 articles for full-text screening, of which 10 articles met the predefined inclusion criteria for inclusion in the systematic review (Figure 11.1).

Source of Data and Participants

All 10 studies obtained data from cohort studies which is considered an optimal source of data for predictive model development. Nine studies obtained data from retrospective cohort designs and one study obtained data from prospective cohort design. Data was sourced from

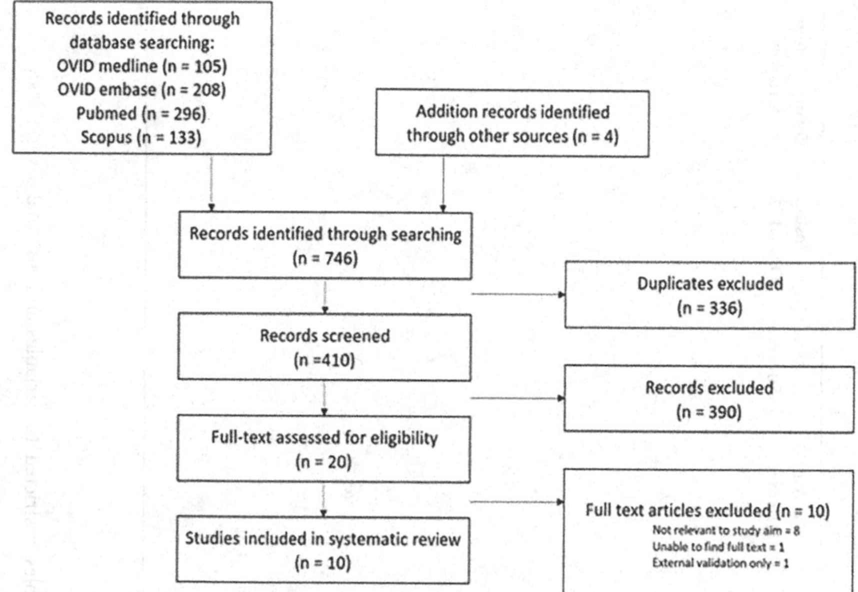

FIGURE 11.1 Consort diagram for included studies.

multiple sites in five studies. Six studies featured populations undergoing orthopaedic surgery, two studies were of populations undergoing neurosurgery, one study was of a population undergoing gynaecological surgery, and one study was non-specific and included participants undergoing any surgery. All 10 studies were from the United States of America. One study excluded patients with preoperative opioid use. The risk of bias for participants was high for two studies (Gabriel et al., Kunze et al.) due to unexplained exclusion criteria.

Candidate Predictors

The number of candidate predictors considered for inclusion in the final model varied between 10 to 216 variables. This commonly included demographic, social, premorbid, preoperative, intraoperative, and postoperative variables. The method of predictor selection was overall handled well with most studies incorporating a backwards variable selection process such as recursive feature selection. Only one study selected all candidate predictors without a variable selection method. The number of variables selected for model development ranged from four to 216 variables (Table 11.1). The overall risk of bias for predictors was low.

TABLE 11.1 Predictor Variables Included for Final Model Development

	Age	Gender	Race	BMI	Pre-op Opioid Use	Pre-op Pain Level	Psychiatric History	Smoking History	Duration of Surgery	Postop Opioid Dose	Postop Opioid Duration
Anderson et al. 2021 (16)	X		X		X						
Gabriel et al. 2022 (17)	X	X		X	X		X	X		X	
Grazal et al. 2022 (18)	X				X		X			*	
Karhade et al. 2020 (19)	X				/			X			
Karhade et al. 2019 (20)		X			/		X	X			
Karhade et al. 2019 (21)	X				/						X
Rodriguez et al. 2022 (22)	X				/			X	X		
Singh et al. 2023 (23)[1]	X				X		X				
Kunze et al. 2021 (24)	X		X	X	#	X					
Lu et al. 2020 (25)	X				X	X					

Notes

/ = non-opioid analgesics.

* = any postoperative opioid use.

1 = 3 models were developed but only the restricted model is shown (full - 216 variables, restricted 10 variables and minimal 5 variables).

= excluded from study.

Model Outcomes

Outcome definitions were inconsistent across studies. Nine studies dichotomised the outcome as a binary variable. Of these, seven studies defined chronic opioid use as persistent opioid use after 90 days following index procedure or surgery, one study defined chronic opioid use as persistent opioid use after 30 days of follow-up, and one study considered any additional opioid use following index procedure as chronic opioid use. Only one study defined chronic opioid use as a continuous outcome (number of pills used postoperatively). The risk of bias was high for reporting bias as only five studies evaluated opioid use through an objective measurement such as prescription filling, rather than self-reported measurements. The risk of bias for outcome variables was also high for studies that used non-standardised outcome definitions (Tables 11.2 and 11.3).

Model Development and Evaluation

Regularised logistic regression was the best-performing model in six studies, with elastic-net regularisation being the most common method of regularisation. Tree-based ensemble methods such as random forest and gradient-boosted machines also presented good performance. Only one study developed a high-performing neural network. AUROC or c-statistic was reported in all 10 studies and ranged between 0.75–0.95 for the best performing model. Calibration was reported through intercept and slope or graphically in seven studies.

Internal validation was overall handled poorly, with eight studies adopting a hold-out set through random or non-random splits for internal validation. Only two studies utilised bootstrapping for internal validation. Cross-validation was not explored as a method for internal validation. External validation was not explored in any studies. The risk of bias was overall high for analysis due to inappropriate methods for internal validation (random splits).

Presentation of Model

5 studies presented a web-based application where end-users can freely access and manually input predictor variables to obtain a predicted risk for chronic opioid use. Risk scores and nomograms were not utilised in any study.

TABLE 11.2 Risk of Bias

Study	ROB				Applicability			Overall	
	Participants	Predictors	Outcome	Analysis	Participants	Predictors	Outcome	ROB	Applicability
Anderson et al. 2021 (16)	+	+	+	-	-	+	+	-	-
Gabriel et al. 2022 (17)	-	+	-	-	+	+	+	-	+
Grazal et al. 2022 (18)	+	+	+	-	-	+	+	-	-
Karhade et al. 2020 (19)	+	+	+	-	+	+	+	-	+
Karhade et al. 2019 (20)[1]	+	+	+	-	+	+	+	-	+
Karhade et al. 2019 (21)[2]	+	+	+	-	+	+	+	-	+
Rodriguez et al. 2022 (22)	+	+	-	-	+	+	-	-	-
Singh et al. 2023 (23)	+	+	+	-	+	+	+	-	+
Kunze et al. 2021 (24)	-	+	-	-	+	+	-	-	-
Lu et al. 2020 (25)	+	?	-	-	+	-	+	-	-

Notes

1 Development of machine learning algorithms for prediction of prolonged opioid prescription after surgery for lumbar disc herniation.

2 Development of Machine Learning Algorithms for Prediction of Sustained Postoperative Opioid Prescriptions After Total Hip Arthroplasty.

TABLE 11.3 Overview of Study Methodology and Model Performance for Included Studies

Author	Data Source	Outcome	Predictor Selection	Types of Predictors Included	Missing Data	Same Size (n)	Internal Validation	Best Performing Model	Discrimination	Calibration
Anderson et al. 2021 (16)	Cohort study (R), USA	Opioid use >90 days after index procedure Prescription filling	Multimodal	7 variables	Multiple imputation	10,919	Random split [N]	Gradient boosting machine	AUC = 0.77 (0.74–0.80)	Brier = 0.10
Gabriel et al. 2022 (17)	Cohort study (R), USA	Opioid use >90 days after index procedure Self-reported	Included all predictors	37 variables	Nil missing data	1,042	Random split [N]	Balanced bagging classifier	AUC = 0.95	N/A
Grazal et al. 2022 (18)	Cohort study (R), USA	Opioid use > 90 days after index procedure Prescription filling	Feature selection using Boruta Algorithm	5 variables	Multiple imputation	6, 760	Random split [N]	Artificial neural network	AUC = 0.71 (0.68–0.74)	Brier = 0.21
Karhade et al. 2020 (19)	Cohort study (R), USA	Opioid use >90 days after index procedure Prescription filling	Recursive feature selection with random forest algorithms	6 variables	Multiple imputation	8,435	Random split [N]	Elastic-net penalised logistic regression	AUC = 0.70	Intercept = 0.06, slope = 1.02, Brier = 0.039
Karhade et al. 2019 (20)	Cohort study (R), USA	Opioid use >90 days after index procedure Prescription filling	Recursive feature selection with random forest algorithms	8 variables	Multiple imputations	5,413	Random split [N]	Elastic-net penalised logistic regression	AUC = 0.81	Intercept = 0.06, slope = 1.02, Brier = 0.039
Karhade et al. 2019 (21)	Cohort study (R), USA	Opioid use > 90 days after index procedure Prescription filling	Recursive feature selection with random forest algorithms	4 variables	Multiple imputations	5,507	Random split [N]	Elastic-net penalised logistic regression	AUC = 0.77	Intercept = 0.01, slope = 0.97, Brier = 0.052

(Continued)

TABLE 11.3 (Continued) Overview of Study Methodology and Model Performance for Included Studies

Author	Data Source	Outcome	Predictor Selection	Types of Predictors Included	Missing Data	Same Size (n)	Internal Validation	Best Performing Model	Discrimination	Calibration
Rodriguez et al. 2022 (22)	Cohort study (P), USA	Number of pills used postoperatively	Backward elimination with bootstrapping or CV	7 variables	Multiple imputations	382	Bootstrap [Y]	Penalised regression	AUC = 0.69 (0.57–0.79)	Intercept = −0.27, slope = 0.94, Brier = 0.12
Singh et al. 2023 (23)	Cohort study (R), USA	Filling opioid prescription in post-discharge days 4 to 90 AND days 91 to 180.	Multimodal	3 models - 216, 10, 5 variables	Mean imputation or bootstrap	24,040	Non-random split [N]	Elastic-net logistic regression	AUC = 0.87 (0.85–0.88)	Calibration curve only: slight overprediction for all models
Kunze et al. 2021 (24)	Cohort study (R), USA	Any additional opioid prescription filling following the index procedure	Recursive feature selection with random forest	7 variables	Multiple imputations	775	Random split [N]	Elastic-net penalised logistic regression.	AUC = 0.75 (0.65–0.83)	Intercept = −0.07, slope = 1.06, Brier = 0.13
Lu et al. 2020 (25)	Cohort study (R), USA	Opioid consumption within 30 days of 6-month follow-up	Recursive feature selection with random forest	11 variables	Multiple imputations	381	Bootstrap [Y]	Random forest	AUC = 0.81 (0.79–0.84)	Intercept = 0.01, slope = 0.95, Brier = 0.13

DISCUSSION

The preceding served to present a systematic review identifying 10 clinical prediction models to support perioperative care by predicting chronic opioid use following surgery. The most prominent predictors for chronic opioid use were demographics (age, gender), preoperative opioid use, psychiatric history, and smoking history. Patients with preoperative opioid use were excluded in one study despite being a known predictor for chronic opioid use (Kunze et al.). It is difficult to ascertain whether surgery has impacted chronic opioid use in patients already taking chronic opioid analgesics. Such differences in exclusion criteria introduce heterogeneity and present a barrier to direct comparison between studies included in this systematic review. The risk of bias was deemed to be high in all studies and thus cannot be recommended for implementation in routine clinical practice.

Among the included studies, the sample size varied between 381 to 24,040 participants. Convenience sampling was adopted for all studies without attempting more rigorous sampling methods. Power calculation for studies with smaller sizes was not performed and the rationale for this was not explored by the authors. In future studies, there is room for improvement in attempting sample size calculations a priori as per recommendations from Riley et al (26). Missing data was handled appropriately across the studies, with eight studies adopting methods of multiple imputation. Exclusion of cases with missing data through listwise deletion was not inappropriately performed in any study.

The authors developed and validated various predictive models including regularised logistic regression, random forest, gradient-boosted machines, and neural networks. Performance of models as evaluated in internal validation ranged from fair to excellent with all studies reporting AUROC between 0.69–0.95 for their best performing model. Elastic-net logistic regression being the most frequent best-performing model may suggest underlying data that is highly complex and multi-dimensional. Indeed, the number of included predictors varied greatly between four to 216 variables. With the inclusion of large numbers of candidate predictor variables and without a method for valid predictor selection, the final models are often overly complex and vulnerable to overfitting. Regularisation or penalisation has likely reduced the effect of overfitting when the performance of models was evaluated through internal validation (27).

Sample hold-out through random or non-random split was adopted as the method for internal validation in eight studies. The major disadvantage of this method is the reduction in performance of developed models due to inefficiencies in sample size utilisation (28). This inefficiency may be overcome through resampling techniques such as bootstrapping or cross-validation where each sample may be utilised in both the development and validation group (28). Despite this, only two studies maximised sample size efficiencies through resampling techniques (Rodriguez et al., Lu et al.). Reporting of calibration is inconsistent across studies, with only six studies comprehensively reporting calibration intercept, slope, and curve. One study did not report on calibration (Gabriel et al.).

External validation is a process that allows us to examine model performance and degree of overfitting through out-of-sample evaluation. External validation closely mirrors real-world performance but was not explored for any of the included studies. This presents a significant barrier to clinical translation as the models were not evaluated on a diverse range of patients more representative of those encountered in clinical practice. Furthermore, models with large numbers of predictor variables present challenges with clinical interpretation. This poses further challenges in translation to clinical practice when the underlying modelling mechanisms are "black box" and poorly interpretable to clinicians. Simpler algorithms, such as logistic regression, offer easier interpretability and familiarity to clinicians less experienced with machine learning (29).

In order to facilitate clinical utility, five studies presented the model via a freely accessible online web application, thereby improving real-world accessibility and utility (30). To practically predict patients for chronic opioid use following surgery and identify opportunities for intervention, the web applications should only include variables readily available in the preoperative period. However, the inclusion of postoperative predictors for the web application was evident in one study (Lu et al.).

Applicability to a broader population is poor. Half of the included studies were conducted at single sites and all studies were from the United States of America. Furthermore, two of the studies included populations strictly of military personnel and six studies were of patients undergoing orthopaedic procedures and surgeries only. Due to the lack of diversity in patient populations, the findings of this systematic review may not be generalisable to a broader surgical population. This is highly relevant due to the differences in clinical practice across countries with different standards of care and healthcare systems (31).

This systematic review has identified 10 models with the aim of predicting chronic opioid use following surgery. In the preoperative period, these models propose an opportunity to identify patients susceptible to persistent opioid use and its associated adverse effects, allowing for the timely implementation of harm mitigation strategies. Whilst we acknowledge the pivotal role of opioid analgesia in postoperative pain and that complete avoidance of opioid therapy is unfeasible, the potential for significant harm warrants personised preventative strategies. Previous studies have identified evidence-based prescribing guidelines, the use of multimodal and opioid-sparing analgesia, and prescription monitoring systems to be effective methods of preventing opioid dependence following surgery (32). If integrated into routine clinical practice, the prediction of patients likely to experience chronic opioid use following surgery can facilitate earlier engagements of the above interventions. Despite these advantages, care must be given when applying these prediction models to clinical practice due to the inherent risks of bias and poor generalisability of included studies.

This systematic review highlights the paucity of evidence available to predict chronic opioid use following surgery that sufficiently addresses a diverse surgical population. Further attempts at model development and validation should be encouraged to utilise standardised outcome definitions and follow guidelines for clinical prediction models to reduce bias and improve applicability.

Despite these shortcomings, the increasing availability of data and advancements in machine learning techniques, as demonstrated in the included studies, reveal opportunities for artificial intelligence augmentation in all aspects of healthcare. Such intervention has the potential to transform the healthcare landscape by identifying patients prior to clinical diagnosis or onset of symptoms and signs of disease. Further research into novel prediction models and synthesis of such models are necessary to encourage integration into routine clinical practice.

CONCLUSION

The presented systematic review compared and summarised 10 models for the prediction of chronic opioid use following surgery. These studies further confirmed our understanding of predictor variables that are instrumental in the development of chronic opioid use. Despite the inherent risk of bias, these studies provide utility in predicting patients who may benefit from early risk reduction strategies. However, generalisability to non-orthopaedic populations outside the United States of America may be limited due to a lack of diversity in data. Future studies should aim to address the limitations identified in this review to facilitate safe and evidence-based translation of artificial intelligence in clinical practice.

REFERENCES

1. Apfelbaum JL, Chen C, Mehta SS, Gan TJ Postoperative Pain Experience: Results from a National Survey Suggest Postoperative Pain Continues to Be Undermanaged. *Anesthesia & Analgesia.* 2003;97(2):534–540. Available at https://anesthesia.bidmc.harvard.edu/ADEL/Pain/Documents/APS/Anesth%20Analg-2003-Apfelbaum-534-40.pdf
2. AIHW. Opioid Harm in Australia: And Comparisons between Australia and Canada Canberra: Australian Government; 2018 [Available from: https://www.aihw.gov.au/reports/illicit-use-of-drugs/opioid-harm-in-australia/summary.
3. Donovan PJ, Arroyo D, Pattullo C, Bell A Trends in Opioid Prescribing in Australia: A Systematic Review*.. *Australian Health Review.* 2020;44(2): 277–287.
4. Els C, Jackson TD, Kunyk D, Lappi VG, Sonnenberg B, Hagtvedt R, et al. Adverse Events Associated with Medium- and Long-term Use of Opioids for Chronic Non-cancer Pain: An Overview of Cochrane Reviews. *Cochrane Database of Systematic Reviews.* 2017;10(10):Cd012509.
5. Nalini M, Khoshnia M, Kamangar F, Sharafkhah M, Poustchi H, Pourshams A, et al. Joint Effect of Diabetes and Opiate Use on All-cause and Cause-specific Mortality: the Golestan Cohort Study. *International Journal of Epidemiology.* 2021;50(1):314–324.
6. Khodneva Y, Muntner P, Kertesz S, Kissela B, Safford MM Prescription Opioid Use and Risk of Coronary Heart Disease, Stroke, and Cardiovascular Death among Adults from a Prospective Cohort (REGARDS Study). *Pain Medicine.* 2016;17(3):444–455.
7. Schuchat A, Houry D, Guy GP, Jr. New Data on Opioid Use and Prescribing in the United States. *JAMA.* 2017;318(5):425–426.
8. Makate M, Whetton S, Tait R, Chrzanowska A, Donnelly N, McEntee A, et al. Quantifying the Social Costs of Pharmaceutical Opioid Misuse and Illicit Opioid Use to Australia in 2015/16. *Health SoP*; 2020.
9. Lawal OD, Gold J, Murthy A, Ruchi R, Bavry E, Hume AL, et al. Rate and Risk Factors Associated with Prolonged Opioid Use after Surgery: A Systematic Review and Meta-analysis. *JAMA Network Open.* 2020;3(6): e207367-e.
10. Karmali RN, Bush C, Raman SR, Campbell CI, Skinner AC, Roberts AW Long-term Opioid Therapy Definitions and Predictors: A Systematic Review. *Pharmacoepidemiology and Drug Safety.* 2020;29(3):252–269.

11. Yang C, Kors JA, Ioannou S, John LH, Markus AF, Rekkas A, et al. Trends in the Conduct and Reporting of Clinical Prediction Model Development and Validation: A Systematic Review. *Journal of the American Medical Informatics Association*. 2022;29(5):983–989.
12. Page MJ, McKenzie JE, Bossuyt PM, Boutron I, Hoffmann TC, Mulrow CD, et al. The PRISMA 2020 Statement: An Updated Guideline for Reporting Systematic Reviews. *Systematic Reviews*. 2021;10(1):89.
13. Moons KGM, de Groot JAH, Bouwmeester W, Vergouwe Y, Mallett S, Altman DG, et al. Critical Appraisal and Data Extraction for Systematic Reviews of Prediction Modelling Studies: The CHARMS checklist. *PLoS Med*. 2014;11(10):e1001744-e.
14. Ouzzani M, Hammady H, Fedorowicz Z, Elmagarmid A Rayyan—A Web and Mobile App for Systematic Reviews. *Systematic Reviews*. 2016;5(1):210.
15. Wolff RF, Moons KGM, Riley RD, Whiting PF, Westwood M, Collins GS, et al. PROBAST: A Tool to Assess the Risk of Bias and Applicability of Prediction Model Studies. *Annals of Internal Medicine*. 2019;170(1):51–58.
16. Anderson M, Hallway A, Brummett C, Waljee J, Englesbe M, Howard R Patient-Reported Outcomes After Opioid-Sparing Surgery Compared With Standard of Care. *JAMA Surgery*. 2021;156(3):286–287.
17. Gabriel RA, Harjai B, Prasad RS, Simpson S, Chu I, Fisch KM, Said ET Machine learning approach to predicting persistent opioid use following lower extremity joint arthroplasty. *Reg Anesth Pain Med*. 2022;47(5): 313–319.
18. Grazal CF, Anderson AB, Booth GJ, Geiger PG, Forsberg JA, Balazs GC A Machine-Learning Algorithm to Predict the Likelihood of Prolonged Opioid Use Following Arthroscopic Hip Surgery. *Arthroscopy*. 2022;38(3): 839–847.
19. Karhade AV, Cha TD, Fogel HA, Hershman SH, Tobert DG, Schoenfeld AJ, Bono CM, Schwab JH Predicting prolonged opioid prescriptions in opioid-naïve lumbar spine surgery patients. *Spine J*. 2020;20(6):888–895.
20. Karhade AV, Chaudhary MA, Bono CM, Kang JD, Schwab JH, Schoenfeld AJ Validating the Stopping Opioids after Surgery (SOS) score for sustained postoperative prescription opioid use in spine surgical patients. *The Spine Journal*. 2019;19(10):1666–1671.
21. Karhade AV, Schwab JH, Bedair HS Development of Machine Learning Algorithms for Prediction of Sustained Postoperative Opioid Prescriptions After Total Hip Arthroplasty. *J Arthroplasty*. 2019;34(10):2272–2277.
22. Rodriguez IV, Cisa PM, Monuszko K, Salinaro J, Habib AS, Jelovsek JE, Havrilesky LJ, Davidson B Development and Validation of a Model for Opioid Prescribing Following Gynecological Surgery. *JAMA Netw Open*. 2022;5(7):e2222973–e2222973.
23. Singh V, Fiedler B, Sicat CS, Bi AS, Slover JD, Long WJ, Schwarzkopf R Impact of preoperative opioid use on patient-reported outcomes following primary total knee arthroplasty. *European Journal of Orthopaedic Surgery & Traumatology*. 2023;33(4):1283–1290.

24. Kunze KN, Polce EM, Alter TD, Nho SJ Machine Learning Algorithms Predict Prolonged Opioid Use in Opioid-Naïve Primary Hip Arthroscopy Patients. *JAAOS Global Research & Reviews*, 2021;5(5).
25. Lu Y, Beletsky A, Cohn MR, Patel BH, Cancienne J, Nemsick M, Skallerud WK, Yanke AB, Verma NN, Cole BJ, Forsythe B Perioperative Opioid Use Predicts Postoperative Opioid Use and Inferior Outcomes After Shoulder Arthroscopy. *Arthroscopy*. 2020;36(10):2645–2654.
26. Riley RD, Ensor J, Snell KIE, Harrell FE, Martin GP, Reitsma JB, et al. Calculating the Sample Size Required for Developing a Clinical Prediction Model. *BMJ*. 2020;368:m441.
27. Ying X An Overview of Overfitting and Its Solutions. *Journal of Physics: Conference Series*. 2019;1168(2):022022.
28. Steyerberg EW, Harrell FE, Jr. Prediction Models Need Appropriate Internal, Internal-external, and External Validation. *Journal of Clinical Epidemiology*. 2016;69:245–247.
29. Petch J, Di S, Nelson W Opening the Black Box: The Promise and Limitations of Explainable Machine Learning in Cardiology. *Canadian Journal of Cardiology*. 2022;38(2):204–213.
30. Kappen TH, van Klei WA, van Wolfswinkel L, Kalkman CJ, Vergouwe Y, Moons KGM Evaluating the Impact of Prediction Models: Lessons Learned, Challenges, and Recommendations. *Diagnostic and Prognostic Research*. 2018;2(1):11.
31. Kaafarani HMA, Han K, El Moheb M, Kongkaewpaisan N, Jia Z, El Hechi MW, et al. Opioids after Surgery in the United States versus the Rest of the World: The International Patterns of Opioid Prescribing (iPOP) Multicenter Study. *Annals of Surgery*. 2020;272(6): 879–886. Doi: 10. 1097/SLA.0000000000004225. PMID: 32657939. Available at https:// pubmed.ncbi.nlm.nih.gov/32657939/
32. Burns S, Urman R, Pian R, Coppes OJM Reducing New Persistent Opioid Use after Surgery: A Review of Interventions. *Current Pain and Headache Reports*. 2021;25(5):27.

CHAPTER 12

Addressing Challenges in the Emergency Department with Analytics and AI

Josh Ting, Belal Alsinglawi, Muhammad Nadeem Shuakat, and Nilmini Wickramsinghe

INTRODUCTION

Post COVID19, we have seen a surge in emergency department (ED) attendance within Epworth Richmond Emergency Department which is based in Melbourne, Australia. This has contributed to overcrowding which has also been reported by various emergency departments around the world (Bouillon-Minois et al., 2021; Kamis et al., 2021; Morley et al., 2018; O'Dowd, 2020). The effects of overcrowding on patient outcomes are pronounced, increasing wait time, prolonging pain and suffering, decreasing patient satisfaction, increasing rate of ambulance diversions, and putting public safety at risk. Moreover, on the provider side, it leads to increased staff burnout, decreased productivity, and increased costs for the hospital (Derlet and Richards, 2000).

Crowding can be seen as a lack of patient flow. El-Bouri et al. (2021) have defined it as the way in which patients are moved through a healthcare facility. High Patient flow can be achieved by the effective balance of supply and demand through various points in the system. Subsequently, we can then break down each different point in the system

DOI: 10.1201/9781032699745-15

conceptually using the Input-throughput-output Model (ITO Model) (Asplin et al., 2003; Weintraub et al., 2010).

The ten major causes of ED overcrowding at each different point of the system as well as their associated solutions have been reviewed extensively by Morley et al. (2018). Yet, studies like Mumma et al. (2014) in the past which showed a paradoxical increase in demand for emergency services with increasing capacity have illustrated that the patient flow problem is multivariate, and not a simple demand-capacity problem to be solved.

With this in mind, we think that one of the most important processes impacted is the cognitive capacity of ED staff. Cognitive capacity drives clinical decision making and its effects ripple down from an executive level of resource allocation to the intimate patient care of diagnosis and management. When cognitive capacity is overloaded, error rates increase, patient care is compromised, and further resources are diverted to rectify the errors (Croskerry, 2014). Moreover, we have seen advances in recent years in artificial intelligence acting as a decision support tool in optimising patient flow in hospitals with potential applications in forecasting, bed management, and seasonal flow predicting (Ellahham and Ellahham, 2019). As a result, we would like to conduct this scoping review to survey the evidence for AI-based interventions in improving patient flow in the ED.

METHODS

Study Design

We conducted a scoping review of the literature on applications of artificial intelligence in the emergency department in improving patient flow. PRISMA guidelines were used to guide the construction of the scoping review, however they were not strictly adhered to.

Inclusion Criteria

Articles which met the following criteria were included in the study (1) Scopus Journal Cite Score > 3 (2) Use of AI/ML Algorithms and techniques (3) study concerns Emergency service delivery (4) Not a review.

Search Strategy

To identify eligible studies, we developed a comprehensive search strategy using MeSH terms, and keywords for the general concepts of artificial intelligence, emergency department, and decision support. We noted that patient flow was not used as a keyword in the literature widely and thus decision support was used to narrow down the range of records. Medline and Embase on Ovid were searched on 27th May 2022. A most recent 5-year limit was used. Only English publications and human studies were considered. A title word restriction was applied. The full search strategy for all databases is shown in Appendix A.

Study Selection

Study selection was entered into Zotero Citation management software, and duplicates were removed. For each study, the title, abstract and full text were independently screened by pairs of reviewers for inclusion criteria. Disagreements were resolved via discussion.

Data Processing and Analysisis

Narrative Synthesis was performed including textural commentaries and tabular representations.

RESULTS

Search Yield

Results for the search are available in Figure 12.1 below. Of the 136 records identified through the database, 38 duplicates were removed, leaving 107 unique records. After a title and abstract screen of the remaining 107 studies, 42 studies were left to undergo a full-text eligibility screen which left 29 studies to be included in the final analysis.

Article Characteristics

Details of the design of the study are available in Table 12.1, and the types of comparators used are available in Table 12.2.

The majority of study designs were retrospective studies (n = 14) or secondary analyses (n = 10). Only 1 case-control study, clinical trial study, cross-sectional study, and prospective study were included.

We found that 8 studies (28%) did not have a comparator. The majority of studies (n = 13) compared their performance with other AI algorithms. Some studies (n = 4) compared against non-AI clinical decision-making tools (i.e., ESI in triage). (Table 12.3)

Intervention Characteristics

Of the 4 interventions (14%) which acted on the input of patient flow into the emergency department, we found some applications in clinical

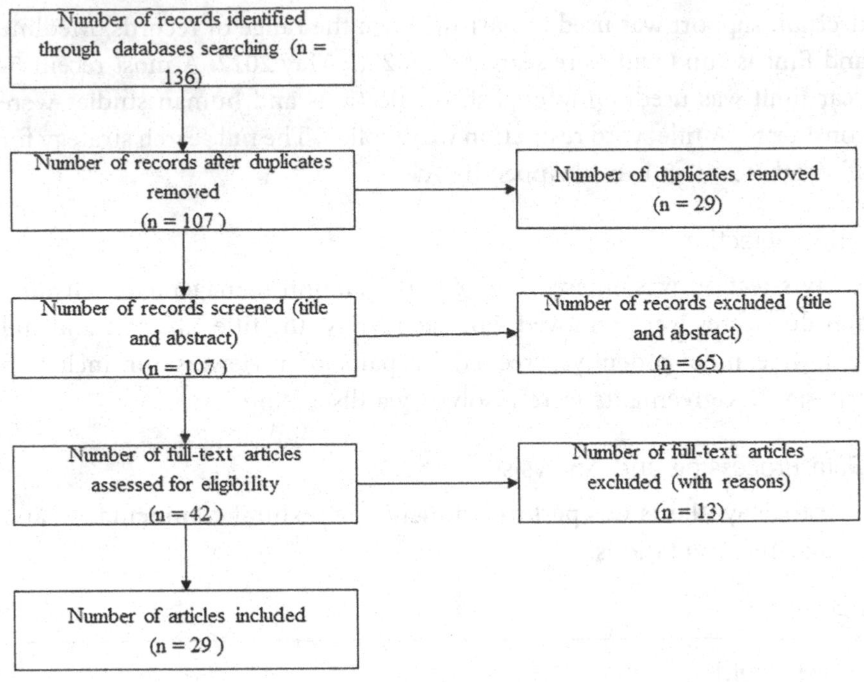

FIGURE 12.1 PRISMA study for study selection.

TABLE 12.1 Study Design of Included Studies

Study Design	COUNTA of Titles
Case-control study Total	1
Clinical Trial Total	1
Cross-Sectional Study Total	1
Not Stated Total	1
Prospective Observational Study Total	1
Retrospective Cohort Study Total	14
Secondary analysis Total	10
Grand Total	**29**

TABLE 12.2 Comparators of Included Studies

Comparator Category	COUNTA of Titles
AI-Algorithms Total	13
Human Total	3
Non-AI Clinical Decision-Making Tool Total	4
None Total	8
Other Total	1
Grand Total	**29**

TABLE 12.3 Intervention Type Relative to Patient Flow

ED Flow – Input-throughput-output Model	*ED Flow – Subcategory*	*AI Application – SubCategory*	COUNTA of Titles
Input – ED Admissions	From Community	Clinical State Detection/ Diagnosis Total	3
	Referral	Prediction of Patient Flow Total	1
Input – ED Admissions Total			4
Output – Patient Disposition	ED to Hospital	Clinical State Detection/ Diagnosis Total	10
		Prediction of Patient Flow Total	2
	Patient Readmission	Prediction of Patient Flow Total	1
Output – Patient Disposition Total			13
Throughput – LOS	LOS	Prediction of Patient Flow Total	1
	Operations	Operations Streamlining Total	1
	Phase 1 – Triage & Initial Evaluation	Clinical State Detection/ Diagnosis Total	10
		Risk Stratifying Total	3
	Phase 2 – diagnostic testing and treatment	Clinical State Detection/ Diagnosis Total	3
		Risk Stratifying Total	3
		Test Results Prediction Total	1
Throughput – LOS Total			22
Grand Total			**39**

*The grand total does not add up to n=29 as some papers were included in multiple categories

state detection/diagnosis (n = 3) and a paper (n = 1) on directly predicting patient flow.

On the output side of the equation, the majority of papers (n = 10) acted on clinical state detection/diagnosis, and directly predicted patient flow (n = 2) to facilitate hospital admissions from the emergency department. There were 2 papers which directly predicted patient readmission back into the emergency department.

Taking a closer look at throughput, we followed the Input-throughput-output model and conceptualized the process into two different phases – phase 1 of Triage and Initial Evaluation, then phase 2 of

TABLE 12.4 Categories of AI's Intended Purpose

AI Application – Category	*AI Application – SubCategory*	COUNTA of Titles
Classification	Clinical State Detection/Diagnosis Total	6
	Risk Stratifying Total	6
Classification Total		12
Prediction	Clinical State Detection/Diagnosis Total	10
	Operations Streamlining Total	1
	Prediction of Patient Flow Total	5
	Test Results Prediction Total	1
Prediction Total		17
Grand Total		**29**

diagnostic testing and treatment. The majority of papers (n = 20) acted along those 2 phases to increase the efficiency in the ED. We also found 1 paper on streamlining operations more generally across the entire process, and 1 paper on predicting patient flow length of stay. (Table 12.4)

Of the 12 papers where AI performed classification tasks, 6 studies (50%) were around clinical state detection/diagnosis. The remaining 6 papers (50%) were on risk stratifying. Of the 17 papers where AI performed predictive tasks, 10 papers were on clinical state detection diagnosis (59%), 5 papers on prediction of patient flow (29.5%), 1 paper (6%) on streamlining operations, and 1 paper (6%) on test results prediction.

Of the 29 papers, there were multiple techniques used in various papers resulting in a count of 59 in Table 12.5. The majority of techniques (n = 26) were medium in explainability. Gradient-boosted Algorithms (n = 12) and Random Forest (n = 12) were the most commonly used techniques.

DISCUSSION

Summary of Current State

The field of AI and patient flow in the ED is a vast and complex one, with a wide range of applications and techniques used. From predicting patient outcomes, length of stay (Chen C.-H. et al., 2020), and readmission rates to streamlining workflow and providing clinical decision support, the potential for AI to improve patient flow in the ED is undeniable. However, as our study has shown, this is still a relatively new and disjointed field of research, with a low number of studies available for analysis.

TABLE 12.5 AI Algorithm Techniques

Explainability (low/mid/high)	*AI Technique (Single)*	COUNTA of Titles
High	Neural network (NN)	7
High Total		7
Low	k-nearest neighbor (kNN)	1
	Support Vector Machines (SVM)	5
Low Total		6
Low to Medium	Gradient Boosted Algorithms	12
	Natural Language Processing (NLP)	2
Low to Medium Total		14
Medium	Classification and regression tree (CART)	2
	Logistical Regression (LR)	9
	Optimal Classification Tree (OCT)	1
	Partial least squares classification	1
	Random Forest (RF)	12
	Regularised Regression	1
Medium Total		26
Medium to High	Gradient Boosted Algorithms	1
Medium to High Total		1
N/A	Not Mentioned	5
N/A Total		5
Grand Total		**59**

*does not add up to 30 as some papers contain more than 1 technique

This lack of research can be attributed to a number of factors. Firstly, the complexities of the emergency setting and the high knowledge barrier of both computer science and clinical medicine required for successful research in the field can be significant barriers to advancing this field of research. Additionally, access to electronic health records (EHRs) and the tools and data they provide are crucial for training and testing AI models.

We have also noted that not all studies in this field are intended to provide solutions to the entire problem, some were undertaken to provide insights into improvements in clinical processes rather than improving patient flow. Regardless, they provide insights into specific components of the problem and contribute to a larger body of work. Additionally, the field of AI and patient flow in the ED encompasses a wide range of AI applications, from clinical to nonclinical, which can further complicate the research landscape.

Despite these challenges, the potential for AI to improve patient flow in the ED is undeniable and further research in this field is crucial in order to fully realise its potential. Collaboration between computer science and clinical experts will remain crucial in future research endeavours.

Gaps and Potential for Future Research

In our analysis, we identified significant gaps in the current research on the application of AI in improving patient flow in emergency department settings. These include a lack of a unified model and problem deconstruction approach, a lack of unified performance measures for patient flow, a lack of emphasis on patient flow outcomes in addition to clinical outcomes, a lack of exploration of non-clinical applications of AI, and a need for improvement and evolution of research design. Additionally, there is a need for elevated standards in ML model construction and greater attention to ethical and legal considerations in this field of research.

Unified Model and Problem Deconstruction

With the current state of research, there is a general lack of evidence to fully solve the complex issue of patient flow. Research endeavours tend to occur in isolation, with various limitations specific to the researcher's situation, such as limited access to data, financial constraints, a shortage of skilled personnel, or unexplored perspectives. To address this, we suggest adopting a unified approach to understanding the patient flow issue, by reaching a collective understanding and approach to breaking down the problem into smaller components.

For example, in our scoping review, we have adopted the input-throughput-output model (Asplin et al., 2003; Elamir, 2018) to contextualise our analysis. However, we observed that the majority of studies within our study did not utilise this model, which would have been advantageous in connecting their work to the broader goal of enhancing patient flow. The model allowed us to break down patient flow through the ED into 3 parts, input with ED admission, throughput through the emergency department, and output as discharge. Further, as an initial attempt, we have abstracted AI's intended application into 6 categories: Clinical state detection/diagnosis, Risk stratification, Operations Streamlining, Prediction of Patient Flow, and Test Results Prediction. Overall, this allows us to deconstruct the patient flow problem by parts of the ED flow & AI application. Within this structure, future studies can identify the highest-yielding subsystem to optimise to have the largest improvements in patient flow.

Another key area in need of unification identified in our research was the focus of numerous studies on specific subsets of patients, such as those with stroke, intra-abdominal sepsis, or cardiopulmonary arrest. (Fernandes et al., 2020; Kijpaisalratana et al., 2022; Levartovsky A. et al., 2021; Sung et al., 2021). While these studies were useful in improving outcomes for those specific patient groups, they made it challenging to standardise results from a patient flow research perspective. This highlights the need for more advanced algorithms that can account for multiple comorbidities.

Unified Performance Measures

In our results, we found a lack of measurement surrounding the successful implementation of AI interventions in enhancing patient flow. Measuring emergency department performance is a complex process, as outlined by Austin et al. (2020), who categorised performance measures into five categories, cost, clinical (adverse events, readmission), process (patient and provider satisfaction), proportion (admission rate, treatment followup rate) and time (length of stay, waiting time).

As the field of research shifts towards implementation and adoption, there are a few key considerations to keep in mind. Firstly, Blomberg S.N. et al. (2021) have shown that even if AI does demonstrate superior performance to their counterparts, a lack of education on the technology can lead to non-compliance in the human workforce. Therefore, measures related to patient and provider experience will become increasingly important. Furthermore, as noted by Austin et al. (2020), decisions around implementation are often made based on budget and funding considerations. Thus, cost-based performance measures will play an increasing role in light of the challenges in aligning financial incentives between technology vendors and health systems (Taylor and Haimovich, 2021).

Inclusion of Patient Flow Outcomes

Our review found that the majority of studies applied AI to clinical state detection and diagnosis, and patient flow was not among their primary outcomes. This is likely due to the fact that the utilisation of AI in enhancing patient outcomes is more advanced than its use in improving flow, whether in the classification task of diagnosis, risk stratification, or predictive tasks. AI clinical decision support has been used for some decades in medicine (Patel et al., 2018), and applications have mainly focused on improving clinical outcomes as they are more directly measurable, such as stroke detection and diagnosis, and treatment outcome prediction (Jiang et al., 2017).

On the other hand, patient flow is a complex process affected by a range of factors such as patient characteristics, healthcare resource availability, and organisational policies (Cooke et al., 2010; Elamir, 2018). No study that we reviewed directly predicted ED admission (input) or discharge (output) using AI. Although the primary authors of these studies did not connect clinical outcomes with patient flow, we made our own implicit link by using predictions of clinical state as a proxy for hospital admission, an approach also noted by El-bouri (2021).

We recommend future studies on improving patient outcomes to also include patient flow as a secondary outcome, to future improve patient outcomes from a systemic approach.

Exploration of Non-Clinical Application

Another observation from our review was the limited number of studies on non-clinical applications, such as documentation (Greenbaum et al., 2019). We believe this represents an area of untapped opportunity for future research as non-clinical processes such as documentation, scheduling, and registration are less complex than clinical processes such as diagnosis and treatment, yet they can greatly contribute to streamlining work processes and enhancing patient flow.

Improved Quality of Overall Research Design

The current state of research on improving patient flow in the emergency department (ED) is in need of improvement. Our review found that many studies are retrospective in nature, which limits their applicability in the clinical setting. Furthermore, the authors of the studies we reviewed (Bertsimas D. et al., 2019; Irvin et al., 2022; Kijpaisalratana et al., 2022) have also recognised this as a limitation. Therefore, it is crucial for future studies to include clinical trials and prospective cohort studies, such as the eRADAR trial (Faqar-Uz-Zaman et al., 2021) to better measure efficacy. Additionally, our review found that many studies have limitations and biases such as class imbalance problems, self-reported bias, small sample size, interobserver variability, and selection bias (Goto et al., 2019; Hong et al., 2018; Konikoff T. et al., 2020; Levartovsky A. et al., 2021;

Sung et al., 2021). Accurate identification and resolution of these limitations and biases are crucial for ensuring the success of machine learning in this field.

Moreover, many studies have demonstrated superiority in the performance of their AI algorithm relative to their comparators (Blomberg S.N. et al., 2021; Costantino et al., 2017; Irvin et al., 2022; Obeid et al., 2019; Pearce C. et al., 2019; Raita et al., 2019) but drawing true conclusions of superior performance is still difficult overall due to the lack of comparators to clinician judgment. Most comparators in our studies were AI algorithms, which is expected as this field of research is very new and most are in the development phase selecting the best algorithm to move forward with. There is a need for later-stage implementation research due to the novelty of such a field of research.

In addition, we found that there is a lack of standardisation across studies in their study designs, methods, and evaluations. A universal dataset with EHR data from multiple hospitals, a strict definition of patient types, predefined machine learning types, and a standardised definition of comorbidities in patients will help researchers benchmark and compare models, and allow more research efforts to build on each other (El-Bouri et al., 2021). Moreover, many studies have limitations in terms of generalisability as the models were developed and tested at one specific clinical site, and external validation and generalisability remain a challenge (Bertsimas D. et al., 2019; Goto et al., 2019; Greenbaum et al., 2019; Kijpaisalratana et al., 2022; Li et al., 2020). Hunter-Zinck et al. (2019) did realise that retraining the models on new datasets at new clinical sites can happen in an automated and efficient fashion. However, there is a secondary issue at play – can different studies build upon the work of each other? El-Bouri et al. (2021) have noted that authors access data and build models around those access from hospitals that are affiliated with the authors. This presents a challenge in building upon previous work and creating models that can be universally applied. A universally accessible dataset could serve as a benchmark for patient flow research.

Elevated Standards in ML Model Construction

AI Algorithm Used

The inclusion protocol revealed nine machine-learning techniques utilised in the literature to improve patient flow in EDs. There are references to neural networks and natural language processing studies that utilised their potential in clinical decision support systems and improved patient flow in the emergency department. The application of machine learning models in relation to intervention type and patient flow has revealed a dynamic landscape of approaches. With 12 and 12 studies, respectively, Gradient-Boosted Algorithm (GB) and Random Forest (RF) are the most commonly utilised models. These models have been extensively investigated and shown to be effective in numerous ED machine learning task applications; nonetheless, their implementation in the context of patient flow may necessitate consideration of certain details. In addition, the data indicate that there are only two studies on Natural Language Processing (NLP), a promising area of research in healthcare, especially in the context of patient flow. In addition, the results indicate that five publications were not mentioned in terms of the models used, indicating a lack of reporting of the nature of machine learning applied and investigated in these studies. This emphasises the need for additional study to understand the strengths and drawbacks of different models in ED setting, as well as the significance of transparent reporting of the exact models employed in studies to promote replication and comparison. In addition, it requires increased efforts to investigate novel techniques and approaches, such as natural language processing (NLP) and deep neural networks in order to gain insights and optimise the patient flow.

Explainability

Explainable machine learning (xML) aims to produce machine learning models that are transparent and human-understandable. In contrast to traditional "black box" models, which are difficult to understand and interpret. ML models often use approaches like feature importance, partial dependence plots, and locally interpretable model-independent explanations (such as SHAP and LIME) to make the model's decision-making process more clear. Also, xML models often use simpler models, such as decision trees, linear regression, and logistic regression, which are easier for people to interpret. xML's purpose is to develop models that are not only accurate but also transparent and human-comprehensible. This can be especially crucial in fields such as healthcare and emergency departments, where decisions made by the model might have a huge impact on the lives of patients.

In recent years, the application of explainable machine learning models in the context of intervention type relative to patient flow in the emergency department has been a subject of intense study. Several studies have explored and analysed xAI; nonetheless, the majority of the machine learning models employed are difficult to comprehend. This can be a significant challenge in healthcare, especially in emergency departments where time is of the essence and transparency is essential.

12 and 12 research, respectively, indicated Gradient-Boosted algorithms (GB) and Random Forest (RF) as the most often employed models according to Table 12.5. These models are renowned for their precision and performance, although they are not always obvious to interpret. This can make it difficult to comprehend the reasoning behind the model's predictions and their inner workings, which can be detrimental in the healthcare sector, where trust and transparency are essential.

On the other hand, models such as logistical regression (LR) have been utilised often in the literature, with nine identified investigations. Logistic regression is a simplistic and interpretable model whose predictions are easy to comprehend, making it suited for healthcare applications. However, it may not always be the optimal solution for more complex problems in dynamic environments requiring crucial decision-making, such as the ED.

In addition, Classification and Regression Tree (CART) and Optimal Classification Tree (OCT) models were only identified in two and one investigations, respectively. These models are based on basic decision criteria and are clearly interpretable, making them suited for healthcare applications where explainability is crucial, especially in emergency departments. Moreover, there were two studies using natural language processing (NLP), which is a relatively new topic of research in xML in healthcare, especially in terms of patient flow in emergency rooms. However, it is recognised that NLP models are complex and difficult to read, which may be a drawback in this subject. The data also indicate that five studies of the employed models were not reported, indicating a lack of transparency in these investigations. This emphasises the need for additional study to understand the strengths and drawbacks of different models in this setting, as well as the significance of transparent reporting of the exact models employed in studies to promote replication and comparison. In addition, it urges more efforts to investigate explainable machine learning algorithms that might provide transparency and confidence in emergency department projections.

The general interpretability of a machine learning model is another essential technical aspect of xAI. Additionally, it is essential to distinguish between local and global interpretability. Local interpretability refers to the ability to comprehend the logic underlying a particular prediction made by the model, whereas global interpretability refers to the capacity to comprehend the model's entire operation. Local interpretability is critical in the context of intervention type in relation to patient flow in emergency rooms since it enables healthcare practitioners to comprehend the reasons behind specific predictions produced by the model. In emergency departments, where time is of the essence and swift choices must be made, this might be especially crucial. A model that employs logistic regression, for instance, would be more locally interpretable given that it is based on simple decision principles and is easily understood by healthcare professionals.

Alternatively, global interpretability is also essential since it enables healthcare practitioners to perceive the model's entire operation, which can help ensure that the model makes accurate predictions. For instance, gradient-boosted algorithms and Random Forest, which are examples of globally complex models, may not be as readily interpretable, but they are still capable of delivering excellent accuracy and performance. When designing a machine learning model for intervention type in relation to patient flow in emergency rooms, it is crucial for researchers in this field to examine both local and global interpretability. By selecting models that can be interpreted both locally and internationally, it is possible to ensure that the model's predictions are accurate and that healthcare practitioners can realise the reasons behind them. Also, approaches such as feature importance and partial dependence plots can be utilised to improve the interpretability of the models.

The application of Artificial Intelligence (AI) in healthcare has the potential to revolutionise patient flow and clinical decision-making. However, the quality of research in this field is often limited by the quality of datasets used to train AI models. Studies that utilise datasets from electronic health records (EHRs) often suffer from data issues, entry errors, and inconsistent coding practices. This can lead to inconclusive datasets that do not accurately represent the population being studied. On the other hand, some studies have found that using datasets with errors can be beneficial for the model's learning process as it allows the model to learn from these errors, rather than spending time normalising the data (Horng et al., 2017). The context in which the AI is being applied determines the quality of datasets that are required.

Another issue that arises in AI research is the limited number of inputs used in the construction of machine learning algorithms. Many studies have noted that their algorithms only take into account a limited set of inputs, such as ECG data, potentially missing other important confounders and data inputs that could lead to better models (Chen C.-H. et al., 2020; Goto et al., 2019; Irvin et al., 2022; Raita et al., 2019; Sung et al., 2021) However, Bertsimas et al. (2019) have highlighted the potential of AI to integrate a multitude of inputs and outperform human biases or non-AI clinical decision rules (i.e., PECARN rules) which only take into account isolated findings. However, the lack of access to comprehensive data, such as EHRs, will still serve as the bottleneck in limiting the number of inputs used in these studies (Sung et al., 2021).

An issue which was significant in algorithm performance was the issue of false positives. In various studies (Horng et al., 2017; Obeid et al., 2019; Sung et al., 2021) false positives were viewed as a barrier for clinical adoption as it can lead to false positive alert fatigue and staff burnout. However, Nguyen et al. (2021) have noted the insight that thresholds for alerts can be adjusted to clinical sites based on their risk tolerance to avoid alarm fatigue. This further stresses the importance of having safeguards and human oversights to ensure adaptability to dynamic situations.

AI models present an exciting opportunity in that updating the accuracy of the prediction models themselves can happen in an automated and scalable fashion from healthcare records, which does not require any extra human effort (Raita et al., 2019; Tollinton et al., 2020). However, there may be challenges in obtaining new training datasets from different clinical sites due to a lack of incentive between healthcare systems for data exchange (Jiang et al., 2017). Additionally, the narrow scope of machine learning tasks, such as only reporting certain radiographic features, can lead to significant costs and challenges in integration into clinical workflows (Irvin et al., 2022; Obeid et al., 2019). To improve the quality of research in this field, it is important to focus on obtaining high-quality datasets, using a wide range of inputs, and having safeguards in place to ensure adaptability to dynamic situations.

Ethical and Legal Considerations

It is important to note that ethical and legal considerations are often overlooked in the literature surrounding the implementation of AI in healthcare. Given the prevalence of AI in healthcare today, these considerations are becoming more and more important and have far-reaching consequences. This is a crucial field to consider, especially as we move towards the implementation phase of research for various stakeholders. In the papers reviewed, we found a lack of discussion on ethical and legal implications. To address this, we will be using frameworks primarily from Gerke (2020) to examine the ethical and legal implications for 1) Vendors 2) Algorithms 3) Patients 4) Clinicians 5) Hospitals.

Vendors

IP law and the commercial protection of technology for vendors are critical issues when it comes to data sharing in the healthcare industry. The need for large-scale data sharing is evident, but there are many obstacles that companies and healthcare providers must navigate. Tensions between entities, such as a lack of trust, can make it difficult to share data effectively. As Gerke (2020) has noted, legal frameworks can help resolve these tensions and promote more data sharing. Future papers can review the various causal factors that contribute to the lack of data sharing and collaboration, particularly in the context of EHR data in the ED department. Furthermore, researching legal frameworks that can be set up to address these causal factors can help to facilitate more effective data sharing.

Algorithm

The lack of transparency and the "black box" nature of some technology systems is a significant concern for many healthcare providers and patients. Physicians may not fully understand how these systems work, which can make it difficult to troubleshoot problems or explain the system's decisions to patients. Additionally, there are important legal questions about who bears responsibility if something goes wrong. To address these issues, vendors should ensure that they provide clear instructions on how their systems make decisions, and make it easy for users to understand the system's logic. Bias is also a major concern in this context (Gerke et al., 2020). If the dataset used to train these systems is not representative of the population it will be used with, it can lead to discrimination and unfair outcomes. Future research can delve into explainable model construction, and training dataset requirements required for the emergency setting.

Patient

Informed consent is a crucial issue when it comes to the use of AI in healthcare. Clinicians must consider how much education to provide to patients about the complexities of AI and the potential for bias, especially in the case of black box algorithms. The level of transparency needed to explain these issues to patients can be especially challenging in emergency settings.

Data privacy and protection is another important consideration. Patients have the right to have their personal information protected, and hospitals and vendors must take steps to ensure that patient data is kept secure and used only for the purposes for which it was collected. This raises questions about obtaining consent from patients when using data from EHRs for research purposes, especially in a time-poor and stressful setting in the emergency department.

Ensuring the safety and effectiveness of AI systems is also of paramount importance. Good training data is crucial, but data sharing can be an issue. Transparency is also critical, ideally, the systems should be open for public examination (Gerke et al., 2020). Hospitals must also have a system in place to monitor the performance of these systems and take action if any issues arise, including remedies in the patient flow system.

Clinician

The use of AI in healthcare raises important legal questions about liability and responsibility in the event of patient harm (Gerke et al., 2020). If a clinician harms a patient based on the suggestion of an AI algorithm, even if the clinician acted in good faith, it would still be considered medical malpractice. The fear of litigation may discourage clinicians from using AI, but it is important to remember that they are the final decision maker and the AI is there to help augment their decision-making and quality assurance. Gerke (2020) has noted product liability and compensation funds as potential solutions. It is important to consider whether patients and clinicians will be willing to accept these changes and what legal frameworks will need to be put in place to avoid litigation and clearly define responsibility and remedies for malpractice. This is especially important in emergency departments where there is a great temptation to use algorithms as a tool to rely on in a resource-intensive, time-poor, high-stress setting.

Hospital

As we move towards an IoT era, the infrastructure is becoming increasingly vulnerable to cyber security attacks. In the emergency department, which is a very dynamic and fragile system, this is especially important given the time-poor and high-stress setting. Malfunctions in underlying technology can be very stressful for clinicians and life-threatening for patients. To mitigate these risks, it is important to implement robust firewalls and encryption measures. Legal frameworks to increase the standards of cybersecurity will be crucial to ensure the safety and security of patients and healthcare providers.

Limitations

Our systematic review of multiple studies on the use of artificial intelligence (AI) in patient flow within the emergency department (ED) represents a novel contribution to the field. Despite this, the heterogeneity in study designs, AI applications, comparators, and the focus of different parts of the ED department make it challenging to draw specific conclusions. Furthermore, some studies lack transparency in the construction of their models, making it difficult to comment on their results.

It is important to note that the limitations of the review may include limitations in the search strategy, as the keywords generated may not have been exhaustive enough to capture the list of specific AI techniques used. Additionally, certain exclusion criteria, such as papers that were not in English, did not self-classify as AI/ML, or had a journal citation score less than 3, may have also limited the scope of the review.

Furthermore, we acknowledge that patient flow was not the primary outcome of some papers included in the review. Therefore, some inferences were made in repurposing the potential use cases of the AI applications. Despite these limitations, our review provides valuable insights into the current state of the literature on AI in patient flow within the ED.

Finally, this study was set out to investigate how AI is employed to address patient flow in the emergency department in the literature. What we note from our investigation – whilst there is some use of AI/ML, there exists the opportunity to leverage advances in this regard to provide better emergency operations which will in turn result in better clinical outcomes and higher patient satisfaction. We urge further research in this area.

REFERENCES

Asplin, B.R., Magid, D.J., Rhodes, K.V., Solberg, L.I., Lurie, N., Camargo, C.A., 2003. A conceptual model of emergency department crowding. *Annals of Emergency Medicine* 42, 173–180. 10.1067/mem.2003.302

Austin, E.E., Blakely, B., Tufanaru, C., Selwood, A., Braithwaite, J., Clay-Williams, R., 2020. Strategies to measure and improve emergency department performance: a scoping review. *Scandinavian Journal of Trauma, Resuscitation and Emergency Medicine* 28, 55. 10.1186/s13049-020-00749-2

Bertsimas D., Dunn J., Steele D.W., Trikalinos T.A., Wang Y., 2019. Comparison of Machine Learning Optimal Classification Trees with the Pediatric Emergency Care Applied Research Network Head Trauma Decision Rules. *JAMA Pediatrics* 173, 648–656. 10.1001/jamapediatrics.2019.1068

Blomberg S.N., Christensen H.C., Lippert F., Ersboll A.K., Torp-Petersen C., Sayre M.R., Kudenchuk P.J., Folke F., 2021. Effect of Machine Learning on Dispatcher Recognition of Out-of-Hospital Cardiac Arrest during Calls to Emergency Medical Services: A Randomized Clinical Trial. *JAMA Network Open* 4, e2032320. 10.1001/jamanetworkopen.2020.32320

Bouillon-Minois, J.-B., Raconnat, J., Clinchamps, M., Schmidt, J., Dutheil, F., 2021. Emergency Department and Overcrowding During COVID-19 Outbreak; a Letter to Editor. *Academic Emergency Medicine* 9, e28. 10.22037/aaem.v9i1.1167

Chen C.-H., Hsieh J.-G., Cheng S.-L., Lin Y.-L., Lin P.-H., Jeng J.-H., 2020. Early short-term prediction of emergency department length of stay using natural language processing for low-acuity outpatients. *American Journal of Emergency Medicine*. 38, 2368–2373. 10.1016/j.ajem.2020.03.019

Cooke, D., Rohleder, T., Rogers, P., 2010. A dynamic model of the systemic causes for patient treatment delays in emergency departments. *Journal of Modelling in Management* 5, 287–301. 10.1108/17465661011092650

Costantino, G., Falavigna, G., Solbiati, M., Casagranda, I., Sun, B.C., Grossman, S.A., Quinn, J.V., Reed, M.J., Ungar, A., Montano, N., Furlan, R., Ippoliti, R., 2017. Neural networks as a tool to predict syncope risk in the Emergency Department. *Europace* 19, 1891–1895. 10.1093/europace/euw336

Croskerry, P., 2014. ED cognition: any decision by anyone at any time. *CJEM* 16, 13–19. 10.2310/8000.2013.131053

Derlet, R.W., Richards, J.R., 2000. Overcrowding in the nation's emergency departments: Complex causes and disturbing effects. *Annals of Emergency Medicine* 35, 63–68. 10.1016/S0196-0644(00)70105-3

Elamir, H., 2018. Improving patient flow through applying lean concepts to the emergency department. *Leadership in health services (Bradford, England)* 31, 293–309. 10.1108/LHS-02-2018-0014

El-Bouri, R., Taylor, T., Youssef, A., Zhu, T., Clifton, D.A., 2021. Machine learning in patient flow: a review. *Progress in Biomedical Engineering* 3, 022002. 10.1088/2516-1091/abddc5

Ellahham, S., Ellahham, N., 2019. Use of artificial intelligence for improving patient flow and healthcare delivery. *Journal of Computer Science & Systems Biology* 12, 2.

Faqar-Uz-Zaman, S.F., Filmann, N., Mahkovic, D., von Wagner, M., Detemble, C., Kippke, U., Marschall, U., Anantharajah, L., Baumartz, P., Sobotta, P., Bechstein, W.O., Schnitzbauer, A.A., 2021. Study protocol for a prospective, double-blinded, observational study investigating the diagnostic accuracy of an app-based diagnostic health care application in an emergency room setting: the eRadaR trial. *BMJ Open* 11, e041396. 10.1136/bmjopen-2020-041396

Fernandes, M., Vieira, S.M., Leite, F., Palos, C., Finkelstein, S., Sousa, J.M., 2020. Clinical decision support systems for triage in the emergency department using intelligent systems: a review. *Artificial Intelligence in Medicine* 102, 101762.

Gerke, S., Minssen, T., Cohen, G., 2020. Ethical and legal challenges of artificial intelligence-driven healthcare. *Artificial Intelligence in Healthcare*, 295–336. 10.1016/B978-0-12-818438-7.00012-5

Goto, T., Camargo, C.A.J., Faridi, M.K., Freishtat, R.J., Hasegawa, K., 2019. Machine Learning-Based Prediction of Clinical Outcomes for Children During Emergency Department Triage. *JAMA network open, Comment in: JAMA Network Open.* 2019 Jan 4;2(1), e186926 PMID: 30646201 [https://www.ncbi.nlm.nih.gov/pubmed/30646201] 2, e186937. 10.1001/jamanetworkopen.2018.6937

Greenbaum, N.R., Jernite, Y., Halpern, Y., Calder, S., Nathanson, L.A., Sontag, D.A., Horng, S., 2019. Improving documentation of presenting problems in the emergency department using a domain-specific ontology and machine learning-driven user interfaces. *International Journal of Medical Informatics* 132, 103981. 10.1016/j.ijmedinf.2019.103981

Hong, W.S., Haimovich, A.D., Taylor, R.A., 2018. Predicting hospital admission at emergency department triage using machine learning. *PloS ONE* 13, e0201016.

Horng, S., Sontag, D.A., Halpern, Y., Jernite, Y., Shapiro, N.I., Nathanson, L.A., 2017. Creating an automated trigger for sepsis clinical decision support at emergency department triage using machine learning. *PLoS ONE* 12, e0174708. 10.1371/journal.pone.0174708

Hunter-Zinck, H.S., Peck, J.S., Strout, T.D., Gaehde, S.A., 2019. Predicting emergency department orders with multilabel machine learning techniques and simulating effects on length of stay. *Journal of the American Medical Informatics Association* 26, 1427–1436. 10.1093/jamia/ocz171

Irvin, J.A., Pareek, A., Long, J., Rajpurkar, P., Eng, D.K.-M., Khandwala, N., Haug, P.J., Jephson, A., Conner, K.E., Gordon, B.H., Rodriguez, F., Ng, A.Y., Lungren, M.P., Dean, N.C., 2022. CheXED: Comparison of a Deep Learning Model to a Clinical Decision Support System for Pneumonia in the Emergency Department. *Journal of Thoracic Imaging* 37, 162–167. 10.1097/RTI.0000000000000622

Jiang, F., Jiang, Y., Zhi, H., Dong, Y., Li, H., Ma, S., Wang, Y., Dong, Q., Shen, H., Wang, Y., 2017. Artificial intelligence in healthcare: past, present and future. *Stroke and Vascular Neurology* 2. 10.1136/svn-2017-000101

Kamis, C., Stolte, A., West, J.S., Fishman, S.H., Brown, T., Brown, T., Farmer, H.R., 2021. Overcrowding and COVID-19 mortality across U.S. counties: Are disparities growing over time? *SSM – Population Health* 15, 100845. 10.1016/j.ssmph.2021.100845

Kijpaisalratana, N., Sanglertsinlapachai, D., Techaratsami, S., Musikatavorn, K., Saoraya, J., 2022. Machine learning algorithms for early sepsis detection in the emergency department: A retrospective study. *International Journal of Medical Informatics* 160, 104689. 10.1016/j.ijmedinf.2022.104689

Konikoff T., Goren I., Yalon M., Yanai H., Dotan I., Ollech J., 2020. Machine learning as a decision-support tool for selecting patients with crohn's disease for abdominopelvic CT in the emergency department. United Eur. Gastroenterol. J., 28th United European Gastroenterology Week, UEG. *Virtual* 8, 380–381. 10.1177/2050640620927345

Levartovsky A., Barash Y., Ben-Horin S., Ungar B., Soffer S., Amitai M.M., Klang E., Kopylov U., 2021. Machine learning for prediction of intra-abdominal abscesses in patients with Crohn's disease visiting the emergency department. *Therapeutic Advances in Gastroenterology* 14. 10.1177/17562848211053114

Li, Y., Zeng, L., Li, Z., Mao, Q., Liu, D., Zhang, L., Zhang, H., Xie, Y., Liu, G., Gan, X., Yang, F., Zhou, S., Ai, S., Tang, H., Zhong, Q., Lu, H., Zhang, H., Talmy, T., Zhang, W., Chen, L., Bai, X., Jiang, J., Zhang, L., 2020. Emergency trauma care during the outbreak of corona virus disease 2019 (COVID-19) in China. *World Journal of Emergency Surgery* 15, 33. 10.1186/s13017-020-00312-5

Morley, C., Unwin, M., Peterson, G.M., Stankovich, J., Kinsman, L., 2018. Emergency department crowding: A systematic review of causes, consequences and solutions. *PLoS One* 13, e0203316. 10.1371/journal.pone.0203316

Mumma, B.E., McCue, J.Y., Li, C.-S., Holmes, J.F., 2014. Effects of Emergency Department Expansion on Emergency Department Patient Flow. *Academic Emergency Medicine* 21, 504–509. 10.1111/acem.12366

Nguyen, M., Corbin, C.K., Eulalio, T., Ostberg, N.P., Machiraju, G., Marafino, B.J., Baiocchi, M., Rose, C., Chen, J.H., 2021. Developing machine learning models to personalize care levels among emergency room patients for hospital admission. *Journal of the American Medical Informatics Association* 28, 2423–2432. 10.1093/jamia/ocab118

Obeid, J.S., Weeda, E.R., Matuskowitz, A.J., Gagnon, K., Crawford, T., Carr, C.M., Frey, L.J., 2019. Automated detection of altered mental status in emergency department clinical notes: a deep learning approach. *BMC Medical Informatics and Decision Making* 19, 164. 10.1186/s12911-019-0894-9

O'Dowd, A., 2020. Emergency departments must not return to pre-covid days of overcrowding and lack of safety, says college. *BMJ* 369, m1848. 10.1136/bmj.m1848

Patel, S.J., Chamberlain, D.B., Chamberlain, J.M., 2018. A Machine Learning Approach to Predicting Need for Hospitalization for Pediatric Asthma Exacerbation at the Time of Emergency Department Triage. *Academic Emergency Medicine* 25, 1463–1470. 10.1111/acem.13655

Pearce C., McLeod A., Rinehart N., Patrick J., Fragkoudi A., Ferrigi J., Deveny E., Whyte R., Shearer M., 2019. POLAR Diversion: Using General Practice Data to Calculate Risk of Emergency Department Presentation at the Time of Consultation. *Applied Clinical Informatics* 10, 151–157. 10.1055/s-0039-1678608

Raita, Y., Goto, T., Faridi, M.K., Brown, D.F.M., Camargo, C.A.J., Hasegawa, K., 2019. Emergency department triage prediction of clinical outcomes using machine learning models. *Crit Care* 23, 64. 10.1186/s13054-019-2351-7

Sung, S.-F., Hung, L.-C., Hu, Y.-H., 2021. Developing a stroke alert trigger for clinical decision support at emergency triage using machine learning. *International Journal of Medical Informatics* 152, 104505. 10.1016/j.ijmedinf.2021.104505

Taylor, R.A., Haimovich, A.D., 2021. Machine Learning in Emergency Medicine: Keys to Future Success. *Academic Emergency Medicine* 28, 263–267. 10.1111/acem.14189

Tollinton, L., Metcalf, A.M., Velupillai, S., 2020. Enhancing predictions of patient conveyance using emergency call handler-free text notes for unconscious and fainting incidents reported to the London Ambulance Service. *International Journal of Medical Informatics* 141, 104179. 10.1016/j.ijmedinf.2020.104179

Weintraub, B., Jensen, K., Colby, K., 2010. Improving hospital-wide patient flow at Northwest Community Hospital. *Managing Patient Flow in Hospitals: Strategies and Solution, 2nd ed. Oak Brook*, IL: Joint Commission Resources, 129–151.

APPENDIX A

TABLE 12.6 Synthesised SWOTs

Strength - Positive Findings So Far	Opportunity - What This Means
1. Superior Performance - Better sensitivity/performance than existing benchmark comparators. Adept at handling non-linear relationships 2. Integration - Directly improves clinical workflow, reduces cognitive load 3. Safety - Some algorithms have demonstrated safety with good power 4. Explainability - Some algorithms are highly interpretable, highly explainable, simple 5. Streamlined Iteration Process - Incorporate data which are already available in the patient's electronic health record. No additional data collection or computational burden on clinicians (since it is data in the ECG) 6. Interoperability - New algorithms can be incorporated into existing clinical software (i.e., ECG)	1. Improve efficiency (i.e., flow through ED) and allocation of finite resources (i.e., reduce unnecessary imaging, and tests) 2. Planning of flow (i.e., Disposition planning) can be more proactive instead of reactive 3. Predicting risks early in presentation to trigger intervention 4. Opportunity to be adopted and change practice guidelines 5. The software can be customised/ adapted to each clinical site (i.e., thresholds adjusted, new training data set) 6. Training of new datasets in an automated, efficient scalable way in real-time than existing guidelines (i.e., using software rather than fixed guidelines) which leads to the models becoming more and more accurate over time
Weakness/Gaps	**Threat - Consequence of the Weakness**
1. Low Explainability - some algorithms used have low explainability for clinicians 2. Retrospective Nature - Most studies currently use EHR to collect events retrospectively rather than prospectively 3. Limitations of studies - Limited set of predictors (input features), Small sample size. Biases from missing values 4. Incomprehensive assessment - Some applications (i.e., ECG software) fail to take into account useful features (i.e., demographic information, health behaviours) 5. False Positives - may cause unnecessary burden	1. False Positive Alert fatigue 2. False diagnosis due to not taking into account important information (i.e., demographic data) 3. Adoption by various hospitals could be an issue 4. Lack of trust in the algorithm from clinical staff resulting in a lack of compliance 5. Friction in adoption by various hospitals due to lack of generalisability, lack of assessment of resourcing, and costing needs. 6. A narrow scope of output may not be practical in a clinical environment. I.e., reporting a diagnosis without the background past medical history

(*Continued*)

TABLE 12.6 (Continued) Synthesised SWOTs

Strength – Positive Findings So Far	Opportunity – What This Means
6. Lack of Generalisability – most studies, and algorithm is specific to 1 clinical site, not generalised to other sides 7. Leap of Faith – Prediction without diagnosis and treatment may be too big of a leap of faith for clinicians 8. Practical Adoption Measures – Impact of healthcare costs and patient outcomes not assessed, results not out yet 9. Narrow scope – does not report on other features on the radiograph yet that a radiologist would report	

APPENDIX B FULL SEARCH STRATEGY

Database Medline on Ovid

1. exp artificial intelligence/ OR algorithms/ OR "Internet of Things"/ OR Neural Networks, Computer/ OR Natural Language Processing/ OR digital twin*.tw. OR virtual self.tw. OR machine learning.tw. OR deep learning.tw. OR artificial intelligence.tw. OR internet of things.tw. OR computational model*.tw. OR neural network*.tw. OR natural language processing.tw.
2. exp Emergency Medical Services/ OR Emergency Department*.tw. OR ED.tw. OR Emergency Service*.tw. OR Emergency Medicine.tw. OR Emergency care.tw.
3. Decision Making, Computer-Assisted/ or Decision Support Systems, Clinical/ or Decision Support Techniques/ or Decision Making/ or decision support.tw.
4. 1 and 2 and 3
5. 4 and 2017:2022.(sa_year).
6. Limit 5 to english language

7. Limit 5 to humans

8. "emergency*".ti.

9. 7 and 8

Database Embase

1. exp artificial intelligence/ OR algorithms/ OR "Internet of Things"/ OR Neural Networks, Computer/ OR Natural Language Processing/ OR digital twin*.tw. OR virtual self.tw. OR machine learning.tw. OR deep learning.tw. OR artificial intelligence.tw. OR internet of things.tw. OR computational model*.tw. OR neural network*.tw. OR natural language processing.tw.

2. exp Emergency Medical Services/ OR Emergency Department*.tw. OR ED.tw. OR Emergency Service*.tw. OR Emergency Medicine.tw. OR Emergency care.tw.

3. Decision Making, Computer-Assisted/ or Decision Support Systems, Clinical/ or Decision Support Techniques/ or Decision Making/ or decision support.tw.

4. 1 and 2 and 3

5. and 2017:2022.(sa_year).

6. Limit 5 to english language

7. Limit 5 to humans

8. "emergency*".ti.

9. 7 and 8

CHAPTER 13

Using Simulators to Assist with Mental Health Issues

The Impact of a Sailing Simulator on People with ADHD

Gurdeep Sarai, Oren Tirosh, Prem Prakash Jayaraman, and Nilmini Wickramasinghe

INTRODUCTION

The COVID-19 pandemic has caused a significant increase in mental health issues, leading to a surge in the number of adults being prescribed ADHD medication in Australia (Behrmann et al. 2022). According to the Australian Department of Health and Aged Care (DUSC, 2021, Economics, 2019), the number of patients receiving ADHD medication has grown at an annual rate of 12.43%, with a higher growth rate of 16% observed from 2018 to 2020. This growth rate is almost double that of the growth rate from 2014 to 2017 (9%). The number of prescriptions has also increased, with an average annual growth rate of 10.25% and the highest growth rate of 17.67% observed from 2018 to 2020. As a result, more adults are now receiving ADHD medication than children.

Attention-deficit hyperactivity disorder (ADHD) is a neurodevelopmental disorder that affects individuals across their lifespan (Martin et al. 2006). The global prevalence of ADHD in children is estimated to

DOI: 10.1201/9781032699745-16

be around 5%, while in adults, it is around 3–4% (Polanczyk and Rohde, 2007, Shaw et al. 2007, AADPA). In early childhood, symptoms of ADHD may include impulsiveness, hyperactive behaviour, and low frustration tolerance (Wilens et al. 2009). Longitudinal neuroimaging studies indicate that children with ADHD may be 2–3 years behind their peers in development. In adulthood, individuals with ADHD may experience memory problems, restlessness, and difficulty with mental focus. Notably, 4–11% of university students exhibit symptoms of ADHD (AADPA).

Separate from this, yet contemporaneous, have been the advances in technology and simulation solutions. In this paper, we outline research in progress work that aims to address the larger key research question of "What is the degree of fidelity with which a sailing simulator can reproduce the health benefits associated with real-life sailing?" This research-in-progress paper contribution is towards the feasibility of using inertial measuring units (IMU) to identify hand movement patterns and motor assessments that are beneficial in real-life sailing. The primary objectives of the research-in-progress paper are:

1. Objective 1: To measure the effect of sailing simulation on grip strength and postural balance in non-ADHD and ADHD participants
2. Objective 2: To measure the acceleration patterns of both hands in a sailing simulation between ADHD and non-ADHD students.
3. Objective 3: To understand the participants' perception of ADHD therapies and simulators as a part of their therapy.

The research design explores the use of a grounded theory mixed methods approach, with a quantitative method to look at the use of IMUs in measuring sailing simulation and motor assessments, along with a qualitative perspective that examines the perceptions of those with ADHD towards ADHD therapy and simulation. By combining both quantitative and qualitative data, we can understand how sailing simulation influences grip strength and postural balance, along with the perception and acceptance of sports simulators as a therapeutic intervention for individuals with ADHD. Preliminary testing has been conducted to consider all critical IMU aspects of the proposed research plan.

RELATED WORK

Physical Activity and ADHD

Regulating the course of neural development has the potential to improve ADHD symptoms (Shaw et al. 2011), suggesting that interventions targeting neural growth and development will be more effective than other treatments. Non-pharmacological treatments such as cognitive-based therapies or physical activity have demonstrated effectiveness. Engaging in physical exercise is one of the most advantageous strategies for treatment, providing numerous benefits and reducing symptoms (Xie et al. 2021). Physical therapy leads to enhanced coordination and motor function, while mental health improvements include processing speed, selective attention, and cognitive flexibility (Montalva-Valenzuela et al. 2022, Watemberg et al. 2007). However, challenges exist in introducing physical activity as a treatment for ADHD, with dropout rates of 17.5% (Vancampfort et al. 2016). This suggests a need for better engagement strategies and further studies to explore other forms of physical activity (Carta et al. 2014).

Physical Activity-Based Interventions

Physical exercise has a positive impact on health and well-being, including improving mood, quality of life, and mitigating stress. Research on physical activity and ADHD supports using exercise as an intervention strategy. Aquatics exercise programs and racquet sports have shown efficacy in improving cognitive, behavioural, and motor functions in children with ADHD (Chang et al. 2014, Pan et al. 2016). Sailing also offers numerous benefits for mental and physical health, including enhancing concentration, communication, mental wellness, endurance, and muscle strength (Cotterill and Brown, 2018). It has shown positive outcomes in improving quality of life, global functioning, social skills, outlook on life, and mental and physical health for individuals with disabilities and severe mental illnesses. Sailing may be a promising intervention for enhancing well-being, particularly for those with mental illnesses, and may be more engaging than standard rehabilitation methods.

Simulator-Based Interventions

Simulators are effective tools for adaptive training, which adjusts the task's complexity to the user's skill level (Guadagnoli and Lee, 2004). They can break down cognitive activities into components that are difficult to train individually (Lathan et al. 2002, Tenbrink and Dylla, 2017). For example, simulators can introduce factors involved in sailing gradually, preventing the operator from becoming overwhelmed. Studies using a horse-riding simulator have yielded positive results in various populations. A study by Borges et al. (2011) revealed that children with cerebral palsy spastic diplegia showed greater emotional happiness and overall satisfaction with the simulator than with conventional physical therapy. The simulator was also statistically superior in increasing postural control in a seated position compared to conventional therapy. Other studies have demonstrated the simulator's potential to enhance physiological functioning in elderly individuals, such as postural control, muscle activation, and dynamic stability (Kim and Lee, 2015, Mitani et al. 2008).

RESEARCH DESIGN

Participants

Study participants are divided into two groups: "non-ADHD" students and "ADHD" students aged 18–30. Both groups are screened for physical conditions and injuries. The ADHD group includes students with self-diagnosed ADHD and a higher BMI. Participants complete the APSS Screening Tool to determine those more vulnerable to adverse events caused by exercise. The ASRS-V1.1 Symptom Checklist is used for self-diagnosis of ADHD symptoms in the ADHD group.

Apparatus

Sailing Simulator: The simulator itself is a VSail-Trainer®, designed by the company Virtual Sailing Pty Ltd. It comprises one boat hull (size length: 230 cm, breadth: 150 cm). The simulator allows sailors to control the course and speed of the boat using a joystick and mainsheet, whilst being in a seated setup suitable for disabled individuals. The simulator has a range of tools and functionalities for researchers to design experiments around, such as the ability to adjust environmental conditions, boat characteristics, and sailor behaviours.

The Inertial Measuring Unit (IMU) is a form of accelerometer, composed of an electromechanical sensor that is designed to measure dynamic acceleration. In this case, two IMUs are placed on the back of each hand of the participant. This will look at the change in velocity for the rudder movement and mainsheet.

The Jamar hand dynamometer will be used to measure isometric grip force in the participants pre- and post-trial as part of their motor assessment.

Movement Assessment

Studies suggest that postural instability in adults with ADHD may contribute to difficulties with motor coordination and everyday activities related to balance and postural control. Grip strength differences in individuals with ADHD may be influenced by a combination of motor coordination deficits, attentional deficits, and medication use. The relevance of grip strength and postural balance in real-life sailing has been shown to improve both areas. Participants will undergo a pre and post-simulator training movement assessment. The first motor assessment test will be the strength component (Clarke et al. 2020, Hove et al. 2015, Jansen et al. 2019, Jeoung et al. 2014, Neely et al. 2017). The Jamar hand dynamometer will be used to assess grip strength before and after each scenario (Mathiowetz et al. 1984). Balance will be assessed through a force plate or through a Balance Error Scoring System to assess overall static balance before and after each scenario (Bell et al. 2011).

Interviews

Interviews can provide valuable insights into the perception and acceptance of sports simulators as a therapeutic intervention for individuals with ADHD. Including whether individuals with ADHD would be willing to use sports simulators regularly, and investigating potential benefits such as improved motor skills and ADHD symptoms, along with potential drawbacks. This can help with the development of more effective interventions for individuals with ADHD. The interviews are conducted as semi-structured in-depth interviews with a consistent set of questions, while the order of the questions may be adjusted based on responses.

DATA COLLECTION

Participant Setup

Before testing begins each participant is briefed on the simulator, equipment, and safety features. Participants sign a consent form and wear two IMUs on their hands and one on their chest. After being seated in the V-Sail simulator, participants are given an adaptation period to learn how to sail using the information provided in the HUD. Steering is introduced first, followed by the main sheet, which teaches participants how to adjust the main sail and coordinate the boat's speed based on wind direction. Participants also learn manoeuvres such as tacking and aligning the twin tails on the mainsail to use the wind to their advantage. The final step is to introduce the pneumatic rams, which allow participants to understand how the boat handles at certain angles relative to the wind.

Sailing Program

Participants will train on a Sydney 2000 Olympic Games Trapezoid course in the Sydney harbour. The course involves sailing upwind to the first buoy, then downwind past three buoys, and back upwind. The training program consists of 6 sprints per week for three weeks, with each sprint lasting 3–4 minutes on average. The sprints progressively increase in difficulty and challenge the participants' decision-making and technique accuracy. The wind speeds will be implemented through a blocked and serial schedule in the first and final weeks.

Data Analysis

Pre- and Post-Movement Assessment: The measurements obtained for both sets of pre- and post-scenarios are evaluated. To evaluate whether the mean difference between the two sets of data varies, a paired sample t-test is performed.

IMUS:

1. Average acceleration magnitude (AAM): The standard deviation of acceleration from the mean. More task stability is indicated by smaller values.
2. Root mean square (RMS): An evaluation of the fluctuating signal strength. Significant stability is indicated by smaller values.

Interviews: Thematic analysis

PRELIMINARY FINDINGS

The pilot study aimed to determine if IMU placement and hand movement are appropriate measures for testing and comparing real-life sailing. The study collected data from a healthy participant using two IMUs on the back of both hands in three different wind conditions (8, 12, and 16 knots). The approach was based on a previous study by Mackie and Legg (1999) that focused on how force output varies with wind speed, finding that force

TABLE 13.1 Differences between Both Hands and the Wind Speed, Expressed as an Average Acceleration Magnitude (AAM) and Root-Mean-Squared (RMS)

	Hand	8 Knots Wind Speed	12 Knots Wind Speed	16 Knots Wind Speed
Average acceleration magnitude (AAM) (m/s^2)	Left (Tiller)	9.52	9.53	9.56
	Right (Mainsheet)	9.76	9.76	9.8
Root mean square (RMS) (m/s^2)	Left (Tiller)	5.51	5.52	5.54
	Right (Mainsheet)	5.66	5.67	5.68

on the mainsheet increases with higher winds. Mackie and Legg (1999) also found a trend between force and wind through experience level in sailing. Specifically, the mainsheet force increased for club sailors with less experience, while the opposite trend was found for pro sailors. This is due to differences in sailing techniques found with experience as conditions get more difficult (Table 13.1).

The study aims to quantify the difference in acceleration for hand movement between ADHD and healthy students. The preliminary study showed variability in both AAM and RMS parameters with increasing wind speed. At 8 and 12 knots wind speed, there were similarities in the acceleration of both hands, while 16 knots showed less stability during the sprint. The results are consistent with Mackie and Legg's study, which found higher force in the mainsheet between wind speeds of 15 and 20 knots. The findings of the IMU showed an increase in acceleration for both hands as wind speed increased, similar to real-life sailing. The methodology allowed for finding variability in the set conditions in the simulator. The research gives an opportunity to see how the movement patterns of both ADHD and healthy students will progress with experience and differ when using the sailing simulator.

This study has a few parts worth considering and should help inform future research directions. With this research looking at the feasibility of IMUs, future research will focus on using the IMUs towards the comparison of movement in real-life sailing. In this current generation of human and computer interaction, simulator use will also provide insight into values, interests, and user experience giving a good basis for how simulators are taken as a form of therapy in managing ADHD.

CONCLUSION

This research-in-progress study has served to highlight a potential role for the use of simulators to address mental health/mental wellness issues.

Specifically, we have focused on the benefits of a sailing simulator to assist students with ADHD. To date, the application of simulators to assist with addressing mental health/mental wellness issues is embryonic at best; but we contend that the potential benefit of this approach justifies more research in this area. Our future work will apply more analytics techniques to capture longitudinal data so that we can further show the benefits of simulation to assist in this area. We believe our study will serve as one of the first to shed light on this major area.

ACKNOWLEDGEMENTS

This work was supported by Swinburne University of Technology and Research under the SUPRA program, in partnership with Northern Health and Virtual Sailing. This endeavour would not have been possible without the support of the Virtual Sailing team Norman Saunders, Mark Habgood and Jonathan Binns. Along with the added support by Northern Health from Peter Brooks.

REFERENCES

Behrmann, J. T., Blaabjerg, J., Jordansen, J. & Jensen De López, K. M. 2022. Systematic review: Investigating the impact of COVID-19 on mental health outcomes of individuals with ADHD. *Journal of Attention Disorders*, 26, 959–975.

Bell, D. R., Guskiewicz, K. M., Clark, M. A. & Padua, D. A. 2011. Systematic review of the balance error scoring system. *Sports Health*, 3, 287–295.

Borges, M. B. S., Werneck, M. J. D., Da Silva, M. D., Gandolfi, L. & Pratesi, R. 2011. Therapeutic effects of a horse riding simulator in children with cerebral palsy. *Arquivos De Neuro-Psiquiatria*, 69, 799–804.

Carta, M. G., Maggiani, F., Pilutzu, L., Moro, M. F., Mura, G., Cadoni, F., Sancassiani, F., Vellante, M., Machado, S. & Preti, A. 2014. Sailing for rehabilitation of patients with severe mental disorders: Results of a cross over randomized controlled trial. *Clinical Practice and Epidemiology in Mental Health*, 10, 73–79.

Chang, Y. K., Hung, C. L., Huang, C. J., Hatfield, B. D. & Hung, T. M. 2014. Effects of an aquatic exercise program on inhibitory control in children with ADHD: A preliminary study. *Archives of Clinical Neuropsychology*, 29, 217–223.

Clarke, M. L., Clapham, E. D. & Shim, M. 2020. Sailing as therapy: Adapted sailing on children with disabilities. *Palaestra*, 34, 37–43.

Cotterill, S. T. & Brown, H. 2018. An exploration of the perceived health, life skill and academic benefits of dinghy sailing for 9-13-year-old school children. *Journal of Adventure Education and Outdoor Learning*, 18, 227–241.

DUSC. 2021. Attention Deficit Hyperactivity Disorder: Utilisation Analysis. In: DHAC (ed.). Pharmaceutical Benefits Scheme (PBS), Drug Utilisation Sub-Committee (DUSC).

Economics, D. A. 2019. *The Social and Economic Costs of ADHD in Australia.* Australian ADHD Professionals Association (AADPA).

Guadagnoli, M. A. & Lee, T. D. 2004. Challenge point: A framework for conceptualizing the effects of various practice conditions in motor learning. *Journal of Motor Behavior*, 36, 212–224.

Hove, M. J., Zeffiro, T. A., Biederman, J., Li, Z., Schmahmann, J. & Valera, E. M. 2015. Postural sway and regional cerebellar volume in adults with attention-deficit/hyperactivity disorder. *Neuroimage-Clinical*, 8, 422–428.

Jansen, I., Philipsen, A., Dalin, D., Wiesmeier, I. K. & Maurer, C. 2019. Postural instability in adult ADHD – A pilot study. *Gait & Posture*, 67, 284–289.

Jeoung, B. J. 2014. The relationship between attention deficit hyperactivity disorder and health-related physical fitness in university students. *Journal of Exercise Rehabilitation*, 10, 367–371.

Kim, S. G. & Lee, J. H. 2015. The effects of horse riding simulation exercise on muscle activation and limits of stability in the elderly. *Archives of Gerontology and Geriatrics*, 60, 62–65.

Lathan, C. E., Tracey, M. R., Sebrechts, M. M., Clawson, D. M. & Higgins, G. A. 2002. Using virtual environments as training simulators: Measuring transfer. In Stanney, K. (Ed.) *Handbook of Virtual Environments: Design, Implementation, and Applications*, 403–414. New York: CRC.

Mackie, H. W. & Legg, S. J. 1999. Preliminary assessment of force demands in laser racing. *Journal of Science and Medicine in Sport*, 2, 78–85.

Martin, N. C., Piek, J. P. & Hay, D. 2006. DCD and ADHD: A genetic study of their shared aetiology. *Human Movement Science*, 25, 110–124.

Mathiowetz, V., Weber, K., Volland, G. & Kashman, N. 1984. Reliability and validity of grip and pinch strength evaluations. *Journal of Hand Surgery-American Volume*, 9a, 222–226.

Mitani, Y., Doi, K., Yano, T., Sakamaki, E., Mukai, K., Shinomiya, Y. & Kimura, T. 2008. Effect of exercise using a horse-riding simulator on physical ability of frail seniors. *Journal of Physical Therapy Science*, 20, 177–183.

Montalva-Valenzuela, F., Andrades-Ramirez, O. & Castillo-Paredes, A. 2022. Effects of physical activity, exercise and sport on executive function in young people with attention deficit hyperactivity disorder: A systematic review. *European Journal of Investigation in Health Psychology and Education*, 12, 61–76.

Neely, K. A., Wang, P., Chennavasin, A. P., Samimy, S., Tucker, J., Merida, A., Perez-Edgar, K. & Huang-Pollock, C. 2017. Deficits in inhibitory force control in young adults with ADHD. *Neuropsychologia*, 99, 172–178.

Pan, C. Y., Chu, C. H., Tsai, C. L., Lo, S. Y., Cheng, Y. W. & Liu, Y. J. 2016. A racket-sport intervention improves behavioral and cognitive performance in children with attention-deficit/hyperactivity disorder. *Research in Developmental Disabilities*, 57, 1–10.

Polanczyk, G. & Rohde, L. A. 2007. Epidemiology of attention-deficit/hyperactivity disorder across the lifespan. *Current Opinion in Psychiatry*, 20, 386–392.

Shaw, P., Eckstrand, K., Sharp, W., Blumenthal, J., Lerch, J. P., Greenstein, D., Clasen, L., Evans, A., Giedd, J. & Rapoport, J. L. 2007. Attention-deficit/hyperactivity disorder is characterized by a delay in cortical maturation. *Proceedings of the National Academy of Sciences of the United States of America*, 104, 19649–19654.

Shaw, P., Gilliam, M., Liverpool, M., Weddle, C., Malek, M., Sharp, W., Greenstein, D., Evans, A., Rapoport, J. & Giedd, J. 2011. Cortical development in typically developing children with symptoms of hyperactivity and impulsivity: Support for a dimensional view of attention deficit hyperactivity disorder. *American Journal of Psychiatry*, 168, 143–151.

Tenbrink, T. & Dylla, F. 2017. Sailing: Cognition, action, communication. *Journal of Spatial Information Science*, 3–33.

Vancampfort, D., Firth, J., Schuch, F. B., Rosenbaum, S., Probst, M., Ward, P. B., Van Damme, T., De Hert, M. & Stubbs, B. 2016. Dropout from physical activity interventions in children and adolescents with attention deficit hyperactivity disorder: A systematic review and meta-analysis. *Mental Health and Physical Activity*, 11, 46–52.

Watemberg, N., Waiserberg, N., Zuk, L. & Lerman-Sagie, T. 2007. Developmental coordination disorder in children with attention-deficit-hyperactivity disorder and physical therapy intervention. *Developmental Medicine and Child Neurology*, 49, 920–925.

Wilens, T. E., Biederman, J., Faraone, S. V., Martelon, M., Westerberg, D. & Spencer, T. J. 2009. Presenting ADHD symptoms, subtypes, and comorbid disorders in clinically referred adults with ADHD. *Journal of Clinical Psychiatry*, 70, 1557–1562.

Xie, Y. T., Gao, X. P., Song, Y. L., Zhu, X. T., Chen, M. G., Yang, L. & Ren, Y. C. 2021. Effectiveness of physical activity intervention on ADHD Symptoms: A systematic review and meta-analysis. *Frontiers in Psychiatry*, 12, 706625.

CHAPTER 14

A Possible Blockchain Architecture for Healthcare

Insights from Catena-X

Nalika Ulapane, Nilmini Wickramasinghe, Amir Eslami Andargoli, Belal Alsinglawi, Jan Miltner, Jule van de Logt, Pavlina Kröckel, Mathias Kraus, and Freimut Bodendorf

INTRODUCTION

Blockchain has emerged as the underlying technology of cryptocurrencies with the most prominent being Bitcoin [1]. Blockchain technology operates as a chain of blocks that digitally store information along with digital signatures [1]. This technology enabling peer-to-peer transfer of digital assets without intermediaries is identified as a key benefit in the cryptocurrency sector. However, the benefits of this technology are not limited to cryptocurrency alone. These benefits can be extended to other industries that require data and information sharing between peers. Hence the technology's applicability is currently being explored in different sectors. These include finance [2], healthcare [3], government [4], manufacturing and distribution [5], and more. The purposes of using this technology can be viewed as supply chain and workflow optimization [6,7]. A special emphasis goes towards increasing productivity and sustainability while protecting privacy and increasing trust between stakeholders.

DOI: 10.1201/9781032699745-17

Like any technology, blockchain has its implementation challenges [8]. In fact, some consider the implementation of blockchain technologies to be lagging and below par in contrast to the hype [8]. The pertinent issues vary depending on the industry. To understand some of these issues, we study Catena-X as a case study. Catena-X is a state-of-the-art collaborative and open data ecosystem being implemented at present. As of July 2022, there is little literature to be found claiming full and successful implementation. However, progress has been made and there is interest in onboarding partners and building platforms and relevant infrastructure, along with making the relevant policy and administrative changes [9–19]. Thus, Catena-X is an interesting example of a data ecosystem from which we can derive some insights about making use of blockchain features in industrial settings.

We first attempt to find some key considerations as identified by those who partner with Catena-X. We do this by way of a scoping review. We review the current literature available related to Catena-X. We also review some grey literature as well on this topic. We conducted a SWOT (Strengths, Weaknesses, Opportunities and Threats) analysis, taking into consideration the points reported in the literature. We contend that our analysis will help practitioners in different sectors to envisage the pros and cons as well as the enablers and barriers in implementing blockchain solutions in their sectors. We conclude by emphasizing the implications and potential benefits for the healthcare sector. We map out the insights derived from Catena-X, to be helpful, especially for the healthcare sector in exploring the use of private blockchain. We also present a suggested blockchain architecture for healthcare.

WHAT IS CATENA-X?

Catena-X is a Europe-based platform with a vision of continuous data exchange for all partners along the automotive value chain [20]. Offered by Catena-X are the network and the technology for data exchange, catering for one of the central challenges of the automotive industry. Enabling collaboration is a primary objective. With a powerful and holistic system, Catena-X ensures the economic viability of all network partners—from small and medium-sized enterprises (SME) to corporate groups [20]. The goal is to establish a globally operating network based on European values [20].

A SCOPING REVIEW ON CATENA-X

We started by searching the keyword "Catena-X" OR "Catena X" in academic databases such as Scopus and IEEE Xplore. However, a minimal number of results were found. Therefore, we repeated the same keyword search in Google Scholar—a more inclusive database. The search was carried out between 4th and 6th of May 2022. This search resulted in 175 results. These included a mix of peer-reviewed academic publications to grey literature such as industry reports and media articles. Since the search was done in Google Scholar, we had limitations in specifying where exactly the searched keywords would appear. For instance, in databases like Scopus, one can search for keywords specifically within the article Titles and Abstract. However, Google Scholar offered limited capability to allow such constrictions. This meant that our results could include the keyword Catena-X anywhere in the text, for example, even in the reference list or an acknowledgement. Therefore, we performed an Abstract review to find out which articles were relevant. This resulted in 16 articles being relevant, which had Catena-X mentioned within the text body of the article. These articles were taken forward for full-text review. From the full-text review, four more articles were found to be irrelevant, as some of the articles had the name Catena mentioned for things other than the Catena-X platform. Thus, our review ended up with the 12 Articles—[9] to [20]—which are considered for this chapter. Shown in Figure 14.1 is a flowchart depicting our search.

In the following step, we performed a SWOT analysis, i.e., find out the Strengths, Weaknesses, Opportunities, and Threats, related to Catena-X as reported in the available literature. The selected 12 articles were studied in search of specific issues regarding Catena-X. The related text segments were tabulated, and themes were assigned to the points raised. These themes eventually yielded a list of relevant issues. However, most

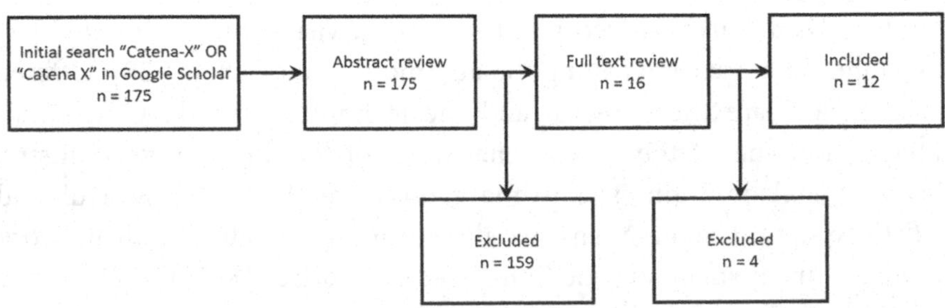

FIGURE 14.1 Flowchart depicting the literature search.

of the literature was either industry reports or media articles. Therefore, they were not very rigorous in the scientific or technical critique of Catena-X but rather pointed out the envisaged issues at a high level. This is understandable as it is still very early days for Catena-X; thus, there are minimal completed works reported yet. However, the importance of the results that can be found even at this stage, must not be undermined. This is how any major development starts, and identifying and envisaging issues at an early stage is extremely important. Therefore, we consider the points envisaged by these early articles as a great starting point for planning and brainstorming the viability of blockchain platforms for different sectors.

The issues found in the literature are tabulated and listed in the next section. Since the rigour of critique was lacking nevertheless as said before, most of the points we found in our search could be listed as "Opportunities". Only a few of the issues pointed at "Threats". However, the depth and richness of what we expected as "Strengths" and "Weaknesses" were not explicitly talked about in these articles at length. Therefore, for the sake of completeness, we went a step further and looked at some other material for what was missing. Since we set out to learn the challenges for "implementation," we referred to commercial and educational providers that offered Blockchain-related services rather than reading academic research. Thus, we selected IBM [21]—a renowned Blockchain service provider, and 101blockchains [22]—an education provider offering knowledge on Blockchain. We referred to the material published by IBM and 101blockcains and picked what they identified as Strengths and Weaknesses to fill the void in our analysis.

RESULTS FROM THE SCOPING REVIEW

In this section, we list out the identified Strengths, Weaknesses, Opportunities, and Threats. We list out the Strengths as identified in the IBM article in [23]. The weaknesses are listed as identified in the 101blockchains article in [24]. The Opportunities and Threats are listed from the findings of our literature review. Table 14.1 lists the findings. Appendices A, B, C and D, show our detailed analysis.

BLOCKCHAIN FOR HEALTHCARE

Most of the identified Strengths and Weaknesses of blockchain are general for many sectors. When speaking in the light of Catena-X, it turns out that the healthcare sector shows many similarities to the

TABLE 14.1 Summary of the SWOT Analysis

Strengths [23]	**Weaknesses** [9–19, 24]	**Opportunities** [9–19]	**Threats** [9–19]
Enhanced security	Node dependent	Increased efficiency	Lack of collaborative thinking
Greater transparency	Scalability challenges	Environmental friendliness	Lack of digital trust
Instant traceability	Interoperability Issues	Enhanced collaboration	Lack of financial resources
Increased efficiency and speed	Energy consumption	Smart factories	Lack of skills
Automation	Immutability of data	Team robotics	Lack of reliable technical foundations
	Not Completely Secure	Transparent value chain	Lack of reliable legal foundations
	Responsibility on the users	Optimized production	Lack of suitable business models
	Cost and Implementation Struggle	Increased average productivity	Requirement of new infrastructure
	Lack of maturity	Increased marginal productivity	Requirement of new rules and guidelines
	Require antitrust laws	Increased national product	Requirement of IP protection, trade secrets
	Require special corporate models	Increased trust	
		Digital twins	
		Increased transparency	
		Increased security	
		Increased autonomy	
		Enhanced interoperability	
		Enhanced sustainability	
		Improved infrastructure	
		Improved guidelines	
		Improved scalability	

automotive sector regarding the application of blockchain technology, highlighting the importance of considering the Strengths and Weaknesses prior to implementation. Most of the Opportunities and Threats are valid for the healthcare sector, although the interpretation should be slightly different. For instance, "environmental friendliness" refers to limiting the carbon footprint in the automotive value chain. While that point is certainly valid for the automotive sector, its validity to the healthcare sector is not that apparent unless one considers manufacturing pharmaceuticals and other necessities for healthcare. As such, while our findings are far from complete, the identified points from Catena-X and other providers at this stage can be used as a preliminary benchmark for the healthcare system to better explore the challenges unique to the healthcare sector.

To avoid some of the Weaknesses and Threats, it is almost certain that the Healthcare system should not use a public blockchain, but there appear to be benefits to designing and developing private blockchains. The following section and Table 14.2 summarize the key differences between public and private blockchains. Private blockchain becomes more suitable for the healthcare sector, especially because it deals with data sharing between specific stakeholders, such as payers, providers, patients, and healthcare organizations. Using private blockchain helps in managing the size of the blockchain and helps in increasing trust. Moreover, there is a significant value-based care perspective to be considered in data sharing in healthcare, as it enables more efficient and effective care through data checking, validation, recording, billing, and auditing. Finally, we point out that these findings are also not limited to the healthcare sector but are valid for other sectors as well.

TABLE 14.2 Summary of Key Differences between Public and Private Blockchains

	Public Blockchain	*Private Blockchain*
Access	Anyone	Single Organization
Authority	Decentralized	Partially Decentralized
Transaction Speed	Slow	Fast
Consensus	Permission less	Permissioned
Efficiency	Low	High
Data Handling	Read and write access to anyone	Read and write access to a single organization
Immutability	Full	Partial

PRIVATE VS PUBLIC BLOCKCHAIN

A public blockchain can be considered a blockchain network where anyone can join and participate [25]. There are minimal restrictions or vetting on who can or cannot join, or when someone wants to participate. Also, all participants can see the ledger and take part in the consensus process, thus ensuring greater decentralization, greater transparency, and equal rights to all participants, and thereby a greater potential for trust [25]. Ethereum is an example of a public blockchain platform [26].

However, the public blockchain architecture has its vulnerabilities too. For example, they can become slow with a growing number of participants and transactions. More so, since anybody can join and participate, public blockchains are vulnerable to the so-called 51% attack [27]. This describes a scenario where participants make communities offline and create a party consisting of a majority of the blockchain participants (i.e., ~51% or more). This majority can then deliberately act maliciously (if they wish to do so) within the blockchain, to corrupt the system and approve malicious or fraudulent transactions.

Therefore, in enterprise settings, there are reasons to not prefer the public blockchain architecture. The concerns are certainly valid for the healthcare setting too. This is where private blockchains come into play. Private blockchains are more like members-only clubs in which the members are vetted by a centralized authority, as opposed to being managed by an unmonitored public. Table 14.2 summarizes some of the main differences between public and private blockchains.

IMPLICATIONS FOR HEALTHCARE BILLING

Global healthcare systems must become more efficient and make better use of available resources due to issues including growing costs. Fraud and abuse are cited as one of the major causes of waste and inefficiency in healthcare systems, accounting for 10% of lost healthcare dollars [28]. To stop the rise in healthcare costs, healthcare systems are under pressure to identify and eliminate wasteful spending, including fraudulent billing [29]. However, every system is susceptible to fraud and corruption, regardless of whether it is predominantly public or private, well-funded or underfunded, or technically simple or complex [30]. For instance, the Australian healthcare system is similar to other fee-for-service healthcare systems in terms of features and fraud concerns [31]. It has proven challenging to accurately estimate non-compliant Medicare billing in Australia, although according to one observer, medical professionals' deliberate abuse costs the public $2–3 billion annually, or 10%–15% of the entire cost of the programs [32]. Most waste of money is not the result of premeditated fraud, but of poor practice and billing methods, and there is a narrow line between these practices and fraud [31]. Whether or not erroneous medical billing is intentional, the financial repercussions of inaccurate billing under Medicare have increased to the point that it is no longer viable to ignore the subject of how and why it is happening [31].

Traditional patient billing systems are seen to be too complex and prone to billing-related fraud [33]. Blockchain technology is expected to make invoicing easier and safer than traditional billing methods by facilitating payment processing and avoiding fraudulent transactions by employing decentralized record-keeping [34]. A function known as smart contracts is supported by blockchain technology. Organizations can improve the amount of funding they get depending on specific clinical results by using smart contract technologies. For instance, it may be possible to validate the quantity of a certain sort of intervention, along with the resources utilized and the results attained, and then link the entire dataset to a payment [33].

A PATHWAY THROUGH FEDERATED LEARNING

In traditional healthcare data-sharing systems, AI healthcare applications demand centralized data gathering and processing, which may be impractical in realistic healthcare applications due to the scale of contemporary healthcare networks and rising data privacy issues [35].

Access to large-scale data for model training and optimization is needed for reproducible and transferrable AI solutions. Access to big data in medical imaging presents considerable hurdles due to competition for scarce resources, despite the routine acquisition of massive volumes of medical and imaging data (e.g., healthcare and medical institutes). Cyber-attacks on AI medical infrastructure (e.g., adversarial attacks and data poisoning attacks) [36] can result in wrong predictions from AI applications and generate undesirable results (due to injecting false training data into AI models). Erroneous AI-generated results can in turn lead to life-threatening harm to patients.

To share medical data while retaining privacy poses a substantial challenge due to the transfer of the data over digitized medical systems. Such systems are vulnerable to hacking or malicious activities [36]. Google is credited with coining the term federated learning (FL), and researchers are now using FL to advance life-critical research. FL trains models of decentralized data on a massive corpus [37]. Simply stated, FL brings the code to the data rather than the data to the code; therefore, in principle, all data ownership and privacy issues are resolved [38]. Malicious attacks on FL infrastructure compromise users' privacy, especially in AI applications, which can lead to sophisticated attack tactics [39,40]. Thus, protecting sensitive health information, such as medical records, is challenging and paramount. The unprotected FL infrastructure itself faces privacy issues owing to "posing" by outside attackers, which is called a "local model attack." Hence, a multi-layer privacy-preserving FL architectural solution is needed. Recent improvements in Blockchain networks offer the promise of using this technology to address these infrastructure issues.

Researchers and developers have concentrated on developing methodologies, tools, platforms, and standards to assist in the process of quality medical data collection from medical institutions' sites for technology innovations while complying with data rules. Diverse data curation methods are available. However, the multi-dimensional evaluation between features in different resources is challenging. During optimization, each feature's importance should be considered. Therefore, a technical solution is needed. Multi-criteria decision-making optimization (MCDM) methods are useful for analyzing and qualifying the best options for medical dataset curation and annotation based on a predetermined set of features. Recently, MCDM methods have been used in medical applications [41], and they can handle the technological challenges associated with qualifying data curation and annotation AI applications. To this end, to the best of our knowledge, there is no study that has provided a complete solution for the FL infrastructure challenges based on Blockchain technology and formulated MCDM methods for technically challenging and privacy-preserving situations. This is considered a knowledge gap.

To bridge this gap, the following research proposed framework is proposed (Figure 14.2) and consists of two phases:

I. Formulation of a dynamic decision matrix that intersects between multi-dimensional datasets' attributes (features) (as a criterion) and curation methods (as alternatives) for each medically presented dataset (e.g., medical institute datasets). Then, developing MCDM methods to benchmark the best data curation methods to achieve and qualify annotated datasets for lung cancer data analytical and learning tasks, which are deemed to be essential

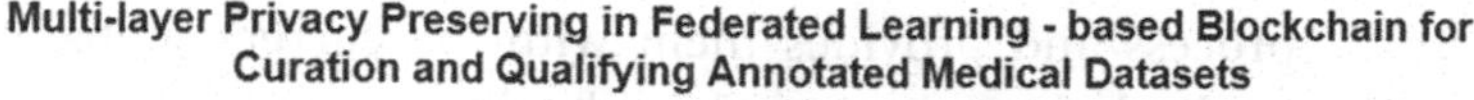

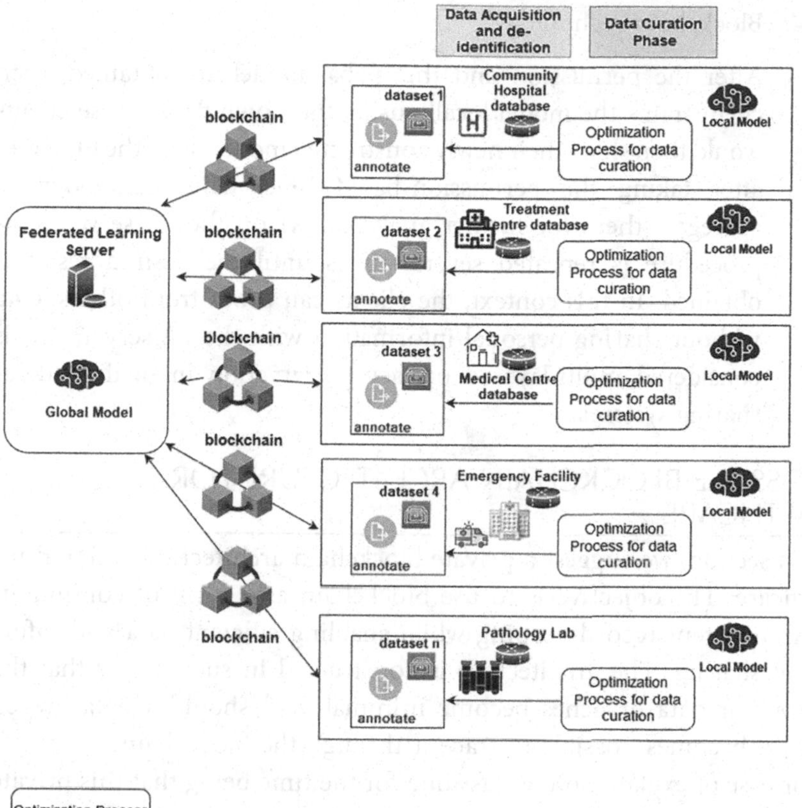

FIGURE 14.2 The proposed architecture for multilayer privacy preservation in Federated Learning-based Blockchain in medical data sharing systems.

research tasks to achieve AI application and output that are robust against uncertainty.

II. Application of FL-based Blockchain technology. The adoption of the necessary FL architecture to preserve data privacy in the second phase. This comprises two steps:

- Local learning and model transmission, designed to assure data privacy and cost reduction. In each round, the FL server selects a group of clients to engage in the learning process and provides them with the current global model. Each round in the FL server begins with choosing a group of clients to engage in the learning process and provides them with the current global model; the medical data sharing should take permission supported with Blockchain technology.

- After the permission and the global model are obtained, each client trains the model locally using their own data. These clients would then share their newly constructed models with the FL server after taking the permission-based Blockchain technology to aggregate them for further analytical AI on the FL server. This procedure is repeated several times until the desired result is obtained. In this context, the clients can profit from others' data without sharing personal information with the FL server; this is considered multi-layered privacy preservation in medical data-sharing systems.

A POSSIBLE BLOCKCHAIN ARCHITECTURE FOR HEALTHCARE

In this section, we suggest a private blockchain architecture, tailored for healthcare. The objective is to use blockchain as a form of continuous and transparent record-keeping while enabling efficient data and information sharing. The architecture is constructed in such a way that the chances for data breaches become minimal, and should a data breach occur, it becomes possible to trace it through the blockchain.

For ease of explanation, we assume for the time being that this private blockchain is implemented for a single hospital. Authorized stakeholders will have access to this system. A centralized administrative authority will govern who accesses this system. We emphasize that such an architecture can be expanded for broader usage across multiple hospitals and stakeholders. It can also be adapted for other industries.

Overview of the Blockchain Architecture

The architecture is composed of three components: (1) The data server; (2) The blockchain server; and (3) The stakeholder user interface. The overview of the architecture is illustrated in Figure 14.3 with communication links.

The Data Registers

The system functions on four data registers: (1) Register of authorized stakeholders; (2) Register of patients; (3) Register of patient data; and (4) Register of blockchain transactions (or the blockchain).

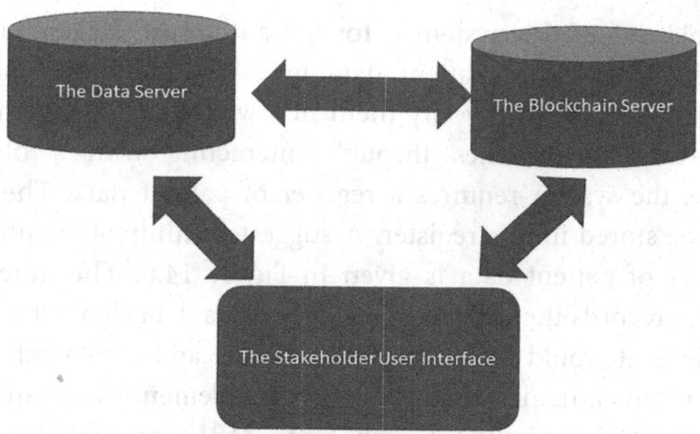

FIGURE 14.3 A suggested blockchain architecture for healthcare.

This private blockchain system functions on the premise that there is a register of authorized stakeholders already established. A suggested minimal architecture for the stakeholder register is given in Figure 14.4. As per the architecture in Figure 14.3, this register will be stored in the data server.

Similarly, it is assumed that at the point of admitting a patient, the patient's identification details are recorded. Therefore, this system functions on the premise that there is a register of patients already established. A suggested minimal architecture for the patient register is given in Figure 14.5. As per the architecture in Figure 14.3, this register will be stored in the data server.

Unique Stakeholder ID	Stakeholder's Name	Stakeholder's Date of Birth
---	---	---
---	---	---
---	---	---

FIGURE 14.4 A suggested minimal architecture for the register of authorized stakeholders.

Unique Patient ID	Patient's Name	Patient's Date of Birth
---	---	---
---	---	---
---	---	---

FIGURE 14.5 A suggested minimal architecture for the register of patients.

The objective of this system is for the authorized stakeholders to be able to efficiently store patient data in a database while having the capability to retrieve and verify them in a way that the system remains immune to data breaches through interacting with a blockchain. Therefore, the system requires a register of patient data. The patient's data will be stored in this register. A suggested minimal architecture for the register of patient data is given in Figure 14.6. The timestamp in Figure 14.6 records the date and time at which a data element was stored. A data element would include a data attribute and a data value. A data attribute means a name identifier for a data element; for example, for a cancer patient, the names CT scan or an MRI scan would be data attributes. A data value means the data entry corresponding to a data attribute. In our example of the cancer patient, this means actual CT scan report(s) or image(s), and MRI scan report(s) and image(s). As per the architecture in Figure 14.3, this register will be stored in the data server.

Lastly, a blockchain (or a register of blockchain transactions is required). A suggested minimal architecture for the blockchain is given in Figure 14.7. A row in the table in Figure 14.7 is one transaction. Three attributes are recorded in a blockchain element for each transaction as per the suggested minimal architecture. They are the timestamp, the transaction type, and the transaction hash. The timestamp will be stored in real value. The transaction type will also be stored in real value. There

Time Stamp	Transaction Type	Unique Stakeholder ID	Unique Patient ID	Data Attribute	Data Value
---	---	---	---	---	---
---	---	---	---	---	---
---	---	---	---	---	---

FIGURE 14.6 A suggested minimal architecture for the register of patient details.

Time Stamp	Transaction Type	Transaction Hash
---	---	---
---	---	---
---	---	---

FIGURE 14.7 A suggested minimal architecture for the blockchain.

are three transaction types allowed in this system. They are (1) Entry; (2) Retrieval; and (3) Verification. These transaction types are discussed in the next section. Each transaction will have a unique hash value and that is stored as a hash value under the transaction tab. Hash construction is discussed later. As per the architecture in Figure 14.3, this register will be stored in the blockchain server.

Types of Transactions

Three types of transactions are proposed for this system. They are (1) Data entry; (2) Data retrieval; and (3) Data verification.

A data entry transaction is an instance where an authorized stakeholder records some data about a patient. For example, consider a nurse saving an MRI scan of a cancer patient. The nurse would be the authorized stakeholder. The cancer patient would be the patient of interest. The stakeholder (i.e., the nurse) would interact with the system through the Stakeholder User Interface in Figure 14.3. The patient's data will be saved in the register of patient details (in Figure 14.6) that is stored in the data server (in Figure 14.3). These transactions begin at the stakeholder user interface (in Figure 14.3) and end at the stakeholder interface (in Figure 14.3) with an acknowledgement message after passing through the data server (in Figure 14.3). These data entry transactions get recorded in the blockchain with the keyword "Entry" under the transaction type (as in Figure 14.7).

A data retrieval transaction is an instance where an authorized stakeholder retrieves some data about a patient. For example, consider a doctor retrieving an MRI scan of a cancer patient. The doctor would be the authorized stakeholder. The cancer patient would be the patient of interest. The stakeholder (i.e., the doctor) would interact with the system through the Stakeholder User Interface in Figure 14.3. The patient's data would be available in the register of patient details (in Figure 14.6) that is stored in the data server (in Figure 14.3). These transactions begin at the stakeholder user interface (in Figure 14.3) and end back at the stakeholder user interface (in Figure 14.3) displaying the retrieved data, after passing through the data server to retrieve the respective data. These data retrieval transactions get recorded in the blockchain with the keyword "Retrieval" under the transaction type (as in Figure 14.7).

A data verification transaction is an instance where an authorized stakeholder verifies some data about a patient. For example, consider a pharmacist verifying a prescription for a cancer patient. The pharmacist would be the authorized stakeholder. The cancer patient would be the patient of interest. The stakeholder (i.e., the pharmacist) would interact with the system through the Stakeholder User Interface in Figure 14.3. The patient's data would be available in the register of patient details (in Figure 14.6) that is stored in the data server (in Figure 14.3). These transactions begin at the stakeholder user interface (in Figure 14.3) and end back at the stakeholder user interface (in Figure 14.3) displaying confirmation of verification, after passing through the data server to confirm the respective data. These data verification transactions get recorded in the blockchain with the keyword "Verification" under the transaction type (as in Figure 14.7).

The Stakeholder User Interface

The stakeholder user interface would have three interfaces according to the three transaction types discussed previously. Different components of the suggested minimal architectures for the user interfaces are provided in Figures 14.8 through 14.14.

Stakeholder and Patient Authentication

Once a transaction has been requested by a stakeholder, the data will be first transferred from the stakeholder user interface to the data server.

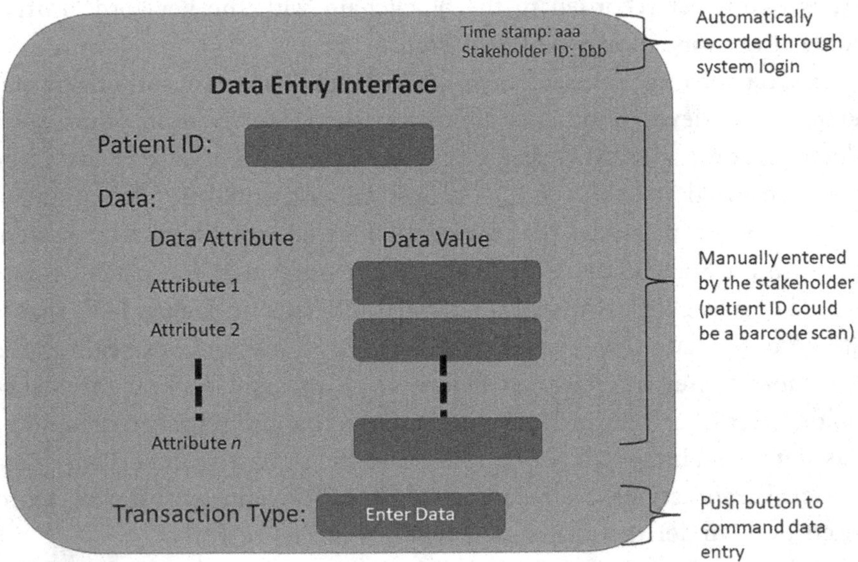

FIGURE 14.8 A suggested stakeholder interface architecture to begin data entry transactions.

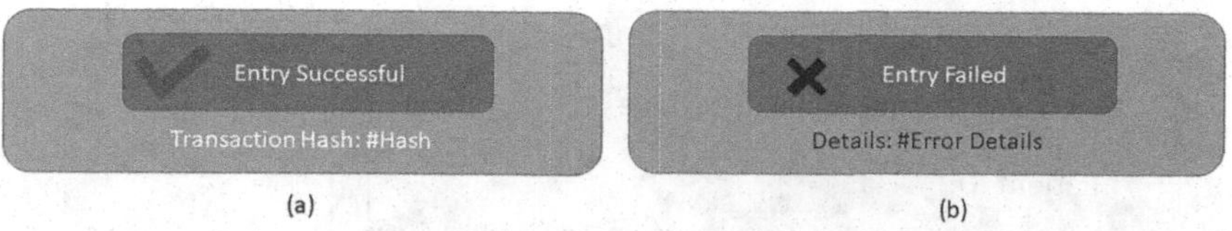

FIGURE 14.9 A suggested stakeholder interface architecture to indicate completion of data entry transactions: (a) Popup message to indicate success; (b) Popup message to indicate failure.

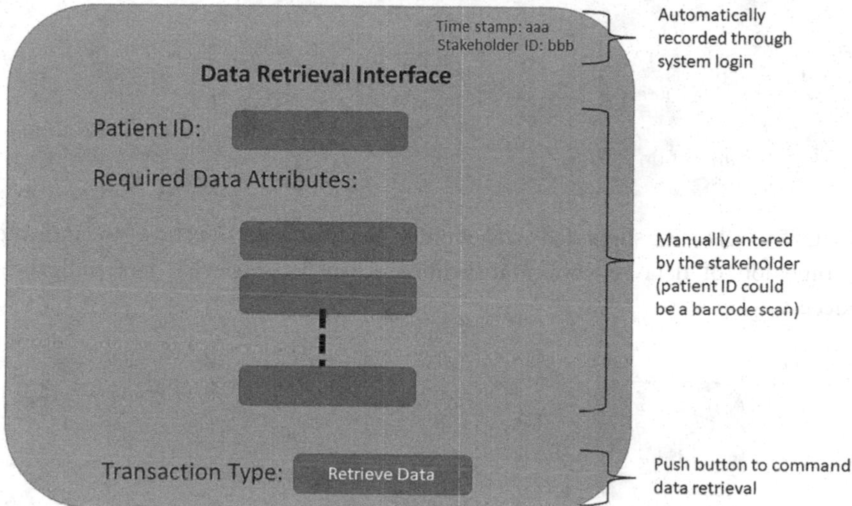

FIGURE 14.10 A suggested stakeholder interface architecture to begin data retrieval transactions.

Then, the first activity at the data server will be to authenticate the user and the patient. An algorithm is expected to run in the data server for this. This algorithm would extract the unique stakeholder and patient identifiers from the incoming data from the transaction. Then these unique identifiers will be compared with the information in the stakeholder and patient registers indicated in Figures 14.4 and 14.5. Only if the authentication is successful will the transaction proceed further. Success or error messages will bounce back to the user interface accordingly. Some example architectures for such success or error messages are given in Figures 14.9, 14.12 and 14.14.

Recording the Data in the Data Server

Once the authentication has been successful, the data of a particular transaction will be recorded in the data server.

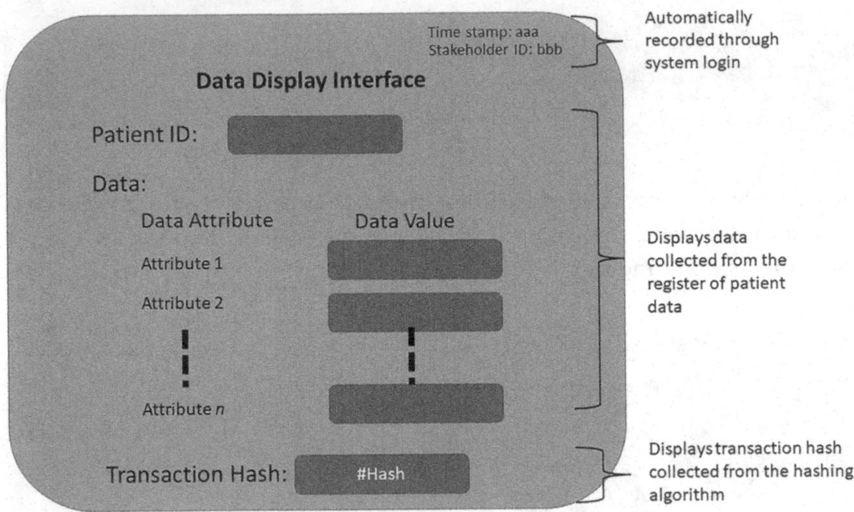

FIGURE 14.11 A suggested stakeholder interface architecture to indicate completion of data retrieval transactions: Displays retrieved data indicating success.

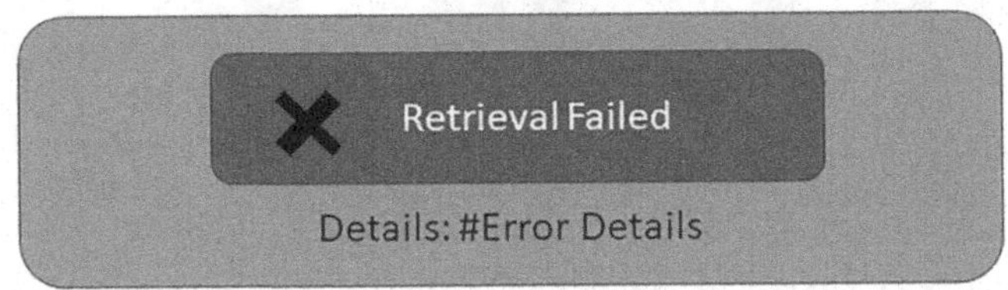

FIGURE 14.12 A suggested stakeholder interface architecture to indicate completion of data retrieval transactions: Popup message to indicate failure.

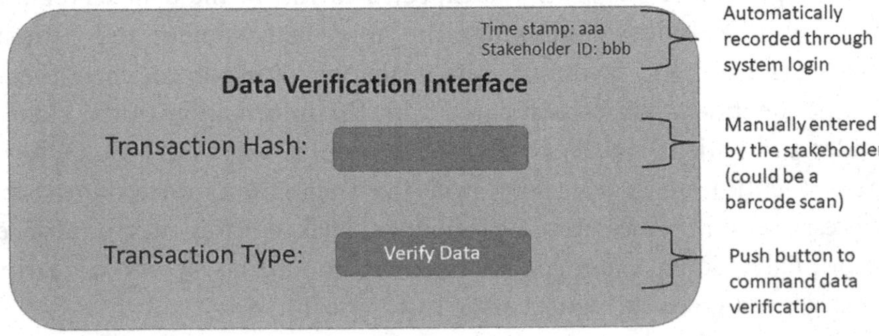

FIGURE 14.13 A suggested stakeholder interface architecture to begin data verification transactions.

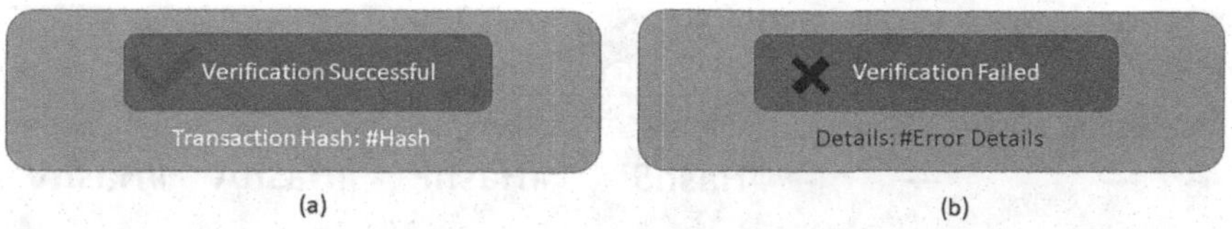

FIGURE 14.14 A suggested stakeholder interface architecture to indicate completion of data verification transactions: (a) Popup message to indicate success; (b) Popup message to indicate failure.

Time Stamp	Transaction Type	Unique Stakeholder ID	Unique Patient ID	Data Attribute	Data Value
---	---	---	---	---	---

Hashing

Time Stamp	Transaction Type	Unique Stakeholder ID	Unique Patient ID	Data Attribute	Data Value
---	---	#HashS	#HashP	#HashA	#HashV

FIGURE 14.15 A suggested architecture for hashing.

Hashing

The next action after verifying stakeholder and patient authentication and storing the data in the data server is to perform the hashing. Standard hashing algorithms have been designed and are readily available coming from the cryptocurrency sector. However, newer, more robust, and tailored hashing algorithms can also be designed. The hashing algorithm will also run in the data server. Every time a transaction request has been made it will transform the data of the transaction into hashes as shown in Figure 14.15.

Recording Transactions in the Blockchain

Once the hashing has been done, a transaction can be recorded in the blockchain. A suggested architecture for this recording is provided in Figure 14.16.

Time Stamp	Transaction Type	Unique Stakeholder ID	Unique Patient ID	Data Attribute	Data Value
---	---	#HashS	#HashP	#HashA	#HashV

Recording a Transaction in the Blockchain

Time Stamp	Transaction Type	Transaction Hash
---	---	#FullHash

#FullHash = #HashS&#HashP&#HashA&#HashV

FIGURE 14.16 A suggested architecture for recording a transaction in the Blockchain.

Using the Blockchain to Prevent Data Breach

A key benefit of this architecture lies in how it enables the use of the blockchain to prevent data breaches. Specifically, should any data alterations or deletions happen by directly accessing the data server from the backend, that can be caught. This can be caught through periodic crosschecking of the hashes between the blockchain and the data in the data server. A suggested architecture to perform this checking is shown in Figure 14.17.

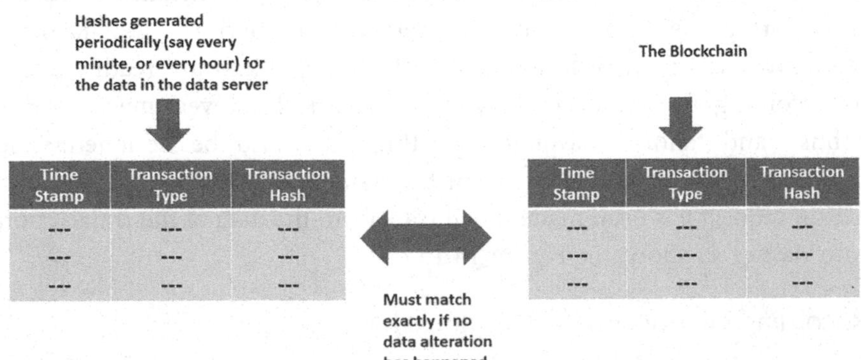

FIGURE 14.17 A suggested architecture for recording a transaction in the Blockchain.

DISCUSSION

The suggested private blockchain architecture for a healthcare setting has its advantages and limitations.

A key advantage is that such a system can be made immune to cyber-attacks by design. This can be done by keeping the system not connected to the internet, and making communication happen through intranets. If we are designing for just one hospital in one location, the hospital can have its servers located within the hospital premises and the system can be accessed via a local network from within the hospital. If it is to be expanded, say if we want to expand it to multiple hospitals, then too, we can have its unique server network including virtual private networks. However, when such expansions happen, there will be a possibility for third parties to monitor network activity and tap the transactions in numerous ways. This vulnerability can be addressed to a good extent through encryption, but there will be no way of guaranteeing 100% security.

Once we know that the system is by design quite immune to cyber-attacks, we can concede that threats would more likely come from the inside. Meaning, that we would know the vulnerability lies in a data breach happening from an authorized stakeholder who is using the network. In fact, a significant number of data breaches throughout the world have happened from the inside. Again, there is no 100% guarantee of preventing that. However, since we know that a threat lies from the inside, the blockchain architecture would provide some provision for tracing which user ID could have been responsible for any breach. This would at least enable some form of accountability, although any damage caused by any intentional data leaks, may not be accountable by any repercussion imposed on the party that has caused the leak.

On a positive note, there is also one challenge that can be addressed very well by such a blockchain architecture. That is, catching any data alterations or deletions that might happen deliberately, by mistake or by technical failure at the data server backend. Should such data alteration or deletion happen, that can be caught quickly through periodic checks with the blockchain as suggested in Figure 14.17.

Today, healthcare operations are generating volumes of data, moreover, these data are considerably sensitive, for example, genomic data. As such, it becomes vital for healthcare organizations and all healthcare stakeholders to consider responsible approaches to best manage these data and ensure appropriate levels of security and privacy to ensure the highest levels of trust between and within all parties and healthcare stakeholders. In this context, we see significant potential in private blockchains in increasing the data integrity in the healthcare sector. This chapter has served to provide a balanced perspective and highlight the key strengths and limitations as well as proffering a suitable architecture that could be adopted.

REFERENCES

1. Gayoso Martinez, V., Hernández-Álvarez, L. and Hernandez Encinas, L., 2020. Analysis of the cryptographic tools for blockchain and bitcoin. *Mathematics*, 8(1), p. 131.
2. Bozkus Kahyaoglu, S. and Aksoy, T., 2021. Survey on blockchain based accounting and finance algorithms using bibliometric approach. IntechOpen. Doi: 10.5772/intechopen.98207. Available at https://www.intechopen.com/chapters/76874
3. Epiphaniou, G., Daly, H. and Al-Khateeb, H., 2019. Blockchain and healthcare. In *Blockchain and Clinical Trial* (pp. 1–29). Springer, Cham.
4. Guarda, T., Augusto, M.F., Haz, L. and Díaz-Nafría, J.M., 2021, February. Blockchain and government transformation. In *International Conference on Information Technology & Systems* (pp. 88–95). Springer, Cham.
5. Kasten, J.E., 2020. Engineering and manufacturing on the blockchain: A systematic review. *IEEE Engineering Management Review*, 48(1), pp. 31–47.
6. Queiroz, M.M., Telles, R. and Bonilla, S.H., 2019. Blockchain and supply chain management integration: A systematic review of the literature. *Supply Chain Management*, 25(2), pp. 241–254. doi: https://doi.org/10.1108/SCM-03-2018-0143.
7. Evermann, J. and Kim, H., 2021. Workflow management on proof-of-work blockchains: Implications and recommendations. *SN Computer Science*, 2(1), pp. 1–22.
8. Luthra, S., Janssen, M., Rana, N.P., Yadav, G. and Dwivedi, Y.K., 2022. Categorizing and relating implementation challenges for realizing blockchain applications in government. *Information Technology & People*, (ahead-of-print).
9. Schulz, Wolfgang H., Franck, Oliver, Smolka, Stanley and Geilenberg, Vincent, 2022. Applicable knowledge for sustainability. The status of artificial intelligence in industrial production and the impact of future sustainability. In *Contemporary Studies in Economic and Financial Analysis, in: The New Digital Era: Digitalisation, Emerging Risks and Opportunities.* Volume 109, pp. 117–124, Emerald Group Publishing Limited.
10. Zhongming, Z., Linong, L., Xiaona, Y., Wangqiang, Z. and Wei, L., 2021. Automotive industry leaders partner to develop a shared approach to carbon

emissions data. Available at https://www.wbcsd.org/Programs/Cities-and-Mobility/Transforming-Urban-Mobility/Mobility-Decarbonization/News/Automotive-industry-leaders-partner-to-develop-a-shared-approach-to-carbon-emissions-data

11. Müller, T., Gaertner, N., Verzano, N. and Matthes, F., 2022. Barriers to the practical adoption of federated machine learning in cross-company collaborations. In *ICAART (3)* (pp. 581–588). Available at https://www.scitepress.org/Papers/2022/108675/108675.pdf
12. Langdon, C.S. and Schweichhart, K., 2020. Data Spaces: First Applications in Mobility and Industry (Part IV Solutions & Applications).
13. Johann, H., Klein, M. and Rieger, A., 2020. European Commission Horizon 2020 LC-MG-1-4-2018 Grant agreement ID: 814951.
14. Garrido, G.M., Sedlmeir, J., Uludağ, Ö., Alaoui, I.S., Luckow, A. and Matthes, F., 2022. Revealing the landscape of privacy-enhancing technologies in the context of data markets for the IoT: A systematic literature review. *Journal of Network and Computer Applications*, p. 103465. Available at https://arxiv.org/abs/2107.11905
15. Sautter, B., 2021. Shaping digital ecosystems for sustainable production: Assessing the policy impact of the 2030 vision for industry 4.0. *Sustainability*, 13(22), p. 12596.
16. Usländer, T., Schöppenthau, F., Schnebel, B., Heymann, S., Stojanovic, L., Watson, K., Nam, S. and Morinaga, S., 2021. Smart factory web—A blueprint architecture for open marketplaces for industrial production. *Applied Sciences*, 11(14), p. 6585.
17. Staab, P., Pietrón, D. and Hofmann, F., 2022. Sustainable digital market design: A data-based approach to the circular economy. Available at https://api-depositonce.tu-berlin.de/server/api/core/bitstreams/847a2922-a808-4185-b389-f13051bbd061/content
18. Ramesohl, S., Berg, H. and Wirtz, J., 2022. The circular economy and digitalisation-strategies for a digital-ecological industry transformation: A study commmissioned by Huawei Technologies Germany GmbH.
19. Berg, H., Bendix, P., Jansen, M., Le Blévennec, K., Bottermann, P., Magnus-Melgar, M., Pohjalainen, E. and Wahlström, M., 2021. *Unlocking the Potential of Industry 4.0 to Reduce the Environmental Impact of Production*. European Environment Agency, European Topic Centre on Waste and Materials in a Green Economy: Mol, Belgium.
20. Catena-X website. Link: https://catena-x.net/de/, date of last visit: July 28, 2022.
21. IBM Website. Link: https://www.ibm.com/au-en/, date of last visit: July 28, 2022.
22. 101blockchains Website. Link: https://101blockchains.com/, date of last visit: July 28, 2022.
23. Benefits of Blockchain, IBM Website. Link: https://www.ibm.com/au-en/topics/benefits-of-blockchain, date of last visit: July 28, 2022.

24. Disadvantages of Blockchain, 101blockchains Website. Link: https://101blockchains.com/disadvantages-of-blockchain/, date of last visit: July 28, 2022.
25. Public vs Private Blockchain, 101blockchains Website. Link: https://101blockchains.com/public-vs-private-blockchain/, date of last visit: October 9, 2022.
26. Wood, G., 2014. Ethereum: A secure decentralised generalised transaction ledger. Ethereum project yellow paper 151.2014, pp. 1–32.
27. Sayeed, S. and Marco-Gisbert, H., 2019. Assessing blockchain consensus and security mechanisms against the 51% attack. *Applied Sciences*, 9(9), p. 1788.
28. Joudaki, H., Rashidian, A., Minaei-Bidgoli, B., Mahmoodi, M., Geraili, B., Nasiri, M. and Arab, M., 2014. Using data mining to detect health care fraud and abuse: A review of literature. *Global Journal of Health Science*, 7(1), pp. 194–202.
29. Settipalli, L. and Gangadharan, G., 2021. Healthcare fraud detection using primitive sub peer group analysis. *Concurrency and Computation: Practice and Experience*, 33(23), p. e6275.
30. Dumitru, C.G., Batca, V. and Răileanu, Ş., 2011. The fraud in the health systems–A financial or ethic problem?. Revista de management comparat international/review of international comparative management, Faculty of Management, Academy of Economic Studies, Bucharest, Romania, vol. 12(6), pp. 319–325, December.
31. Flynn, K., 2015. Financial fraud in the private health insurance sector in Australia: Perspectives from the industry. *Journal of Financial Crime*, 23(1), pp. 143–158. https://doi.org/10.1108/JFC-06-2014-0032
32. Faux, M., Wardle, J. and Adams, J., 2019. Medicare billing, law and practice: complex, incomprehensible and beginning to unravel. *Journal of Law and Medicine*. Oct; 27(1), 66–93. PMID: 31682343.
33. Roman-Belmonte, J.M., De la Corte-Rodriguez, H. and Rodriguez-Merchan, E.C., 2018. How blockchain technology can change medicine. *Postgraduate Medicine*, 130(4), pp. 420–427.
34. Attaran, M., 2022. Blockchain technology in healthcare: Challenges and opportunities. *International Journal of Healthcare Management*, 15(1), pp. 70–83.
35. Nguyen, D.C., Pham, Q.V., Pathirana, P.N., Ding, M., Seneviratne, A., Lin, Z., Dobre, O. and Hwang, W.J., 2022. Federated learning for smart healthcare: A survey. *ACM Computing Surveys (CSUR)*, 55(3), pp. 1–37.
36. Taheri, R., Shojafar, M., Alazab, M. and Tafazolli, R., 2020. *FED-IIoT: A Robust Federated Malware Detection Architecture in Industrial IoT*. IEEE Transactions on Industrial Informatics. Vol. 17, no. 12, pp. 8442–8452, Dec. 2021, doi: 10.1109/TII.2020.3043458.
37. Pham, Q.-V., Dev, K., Maddikunta, P. K. R., Gadekallu, T. R. and Huynh-The, T., 2021. Fusion of federated learning and industrial internet of things: A survey. arXiv preprint arXiv:2101.00798.

38. Lian, Z., Wang, W. and Su, C., 2021. COFEL: Communication-efficient and optimized federated learning with local differential privacy. In *ICC 2021-IEEE International Conference on Communications*, pp. 1–6.
39. Liu, Yining and Wang, Weizheng, 2022. EPPDA: An efficient privacy-preserving data aggregation federated learning scheme. *IEEE Transactions on Network Science and Engineering*. PP. 10.1109/TNSE.2022.3153519. available at: https://www.researchgate.net/publication/358740281_EPPDA_An_Efficient_Privacy-Preserving_Data_Aggregation_Federated_Learning_Scheme#fullTextFileContent
40. Zhang, C., Xie, Y., Bai, H., Yu, B., Li, W. and Gao, Y., 2021. A survey on federated learning. *Knowledge-Based Systems*, 216, p. 106775.
41. Alamleh, A., Albahri, O.S., Zaidan, A.A., Albahri, A.S., Alamoodi, A.H., Zaidan, B.B., Qahtan, S., Alsatar, H.A., Al-Samarraay, M.S. and Jasim, A.N., 2022. Federated learning for IoMT applications: A standardisation and benchmarking framework of intrusion detection systems. *IEEE Journal of Biomedical and Health Informatics*, 216, pp. 1–16.

APPENDIX A

SWOT Analysis Results—Strengths

TABLE 14.3 Strengths of Blockchain

References	Strengths	Text Description
IBM https://www.ibm.com/au-en/topics/benefits-of-blockchain	Enhanced security	"By creating a record that can't be altered and is encrypted end-to-end, blockchain helps prevent fraud and unauthorized activity." [24]
	Greater transparency	"Without blockchain, each organization has to keep a separate database. Because blockchain uses a distributed ledger, transactions and data are recorded identically in multiple locations." [24]
	Instant traceability	"Blockchain creates an audit trail that documents the provenance of an asset at every step on its journey." [24]
	Increased efficiency and speed	"Traditional paper-heavy processes are time-consuming, prone to human error, and often require third-party mediation. By streamlining these processes with blockchain, transactions can be completed faster and more efficiently." [24]
	Automation	"Transactions can even be automated with "smart contracts," which increase your efficiency and speed the process even further." [24]

APPENDIX B

SWOT Analysis Results—Weaknesses

TABLE 14.4 Weaknesses of Blockchain

References	Weaknesses	Text Description
101blockchains: https://101blockchains.com/disadvantages-of-blockchain/	Node dependent	"Quality of the blockchain is determined by the quality of the nodes" [35]

(*Continued*)

TABLE 14.4 (Continued) Weaknesses of Blockchain

References	Weaknesses	Text Description
	Scalability challenges	Blockchains can become inefficient when the network grows too much, i.e., when there are too many nodes [35]
	Interoperability Issues	If there are legacy systems in use, integration to the network can be challenging [35]
	Energy consumption	Some blockchains consume too much energy [35]
	Immutability of data	Blockchain cannot go back, changes get recorded in a ledger [35]
	Not Completely Secure	Still vulnerable to certain cyber threats and employee hacks. Also "51% attacks" are also possible if one gains majority control over a blockchain and intends to manipulate it [35]
	Responsibility for the users	Users are their own bank and use their private keys [35]
	Cost and Implementation Struggle	It can require computer hardware and software updates and training of employees. Also, will require some expert knowledge [35]
	Lack of maturity	Blockchains are still quite new, therefore, there is limited experience to gauge their successes and failures [35]
[9] Schulz, et al., 2021	Require antitrust laws Require special corporate models	"In addition to the antitrust issues, the German automotive industry's AI efforts show that, beyond the technical realization of AI platforms, cooperation models are needed to enable collaboration and data exchange permanently." [9]

APPENDIX C

SWOT Analysis Results—Opportunities

TABLE 14.5 Opportunities with Blockchain (Catena-X)

References	Opportunities	Text Extract
[9]	Increased efficiency Environmental friendliness Enhanced collaboration	"The interests pursued with establishing the Catena-X Automotive Network platform are different because production is to become more efficient and environmentally friendly through networking between vehicle manufacturers and suppliers." [9]
	Smart factories Team robotics Transparent value chain Optimized production	"Furthermore, these activities represent a first step in the direction of smart factories and team robotics because Catena-X offers the opportunity for a transparent value chain so that production can be optimized." [9]
	Increased average productivity Increased marginal productivity	"If Catena-X is successfully initialized, both the average productivity and the marginal productivities of the logistics and intralogistics production functions increase for the participating companies." [9]
	Increased national product	"The increase in marginal productivity resulting from Catena-X generates a leverage effect, which leads to an improvement in operating results for companies and is reflected in the national economy in the form of an increased national product." [9]
[10]	Environmental friendliness	"This collaborative effort will support business climate action with a comprehensive technical infrastructure for sharing granular, consistent and verified product-level data on primary emissions among manufacturers of automotive parts." [10]
[11]	Enhanced collaboration Increased trust	"Initiatives like the International Data Spaces Association (IDSA), GAIA-X or the automotive-related Catena-X aim to enable cross-company collaboration in a shared environment of trust. This work takes place

(*Continued*)

TABLE 14.5 (Continued) Opportunities with Blockchain (Catena-X)

References	Opportunities	Text Extract
		in the context of the Catena-X project." [11]
[12]	Enhanced collaboration Digital twins	"Now all participants have pledged to cooperate and collaborate jointly in an open network to advance and accelerate cross-company data exchange throughout the entire automotive value chain. Specific examples include continuously connected data chains to create digital twins of automobiles" [12]
[13]	Increased transparency Increased security Increased autonomy Increased efficiency Enhanced collaboration	"Modeling a trust chain using SSI can help in resolving these interdependencies between fragmented authorities in a way that is transparent, secure, and intermediary-independent. Most importantly, it provides a framework to digitize and automate these governmental functions while reducing obstacles such as manual steps. While modelling these trust chains between governmental and private authorities, it is important that there is a joint approach between public policy expertise and technical expertise, which is why it could make sense to push for this in initiatives such as Gaia-X or Catena-X." [13]
[14]	Enhanced collaboration	"Decisionmakers in governments and businesses have recognized the economic potential of data markets and hence recently supported significant projects that provide a shared digital infrastructure for data-sharing initiatives such as GAIA-X [5] or the automotive-related Catena-X, which promote the collaboration of large enterprises in data markets." [14]
	Enhanced autonomy Enhanced interoperability Enhanced sustainability	"As Figure 14.9 illustrates, all of these measures are interrelated and represent important building blocks for realizing the shared vision of digital ecosystems for sustainable production. In the lighthouse project CATENA-X, all of these building blocks are brought together in order to realize a

(*Continued*)

TABLE 14.5 (Continued) Opportunities with Blockchain (Catena-X)

References	Opportunities	Text Extract
		continuous data exchange for all contributors along the automotive value chain and to implement sustainability and Circular Economy or Manufacturing-as-a-Service use cases." [14]
[16]	Smart factory	"The automotive industry is about to take up and drive this ambition in their Catena-X Automotive Network initiative (https://catena-x.net/en/, accessed on 15 July 2021). The Smart Factory Web architecture is brought in as a validated approach and background to this initiative." [16]
[17]	Increased environmental friendliness	"The business-to-business (B2B)-network Catena-X, involving a group of German companies in the automobile sector, is developing a digital tool that will bundle all CO2 data in the supply chain." [17]
	Enhanced collaboration	Based on the new cloud standard Gaia-X, companies such as BASF, BMW, Bosch, Fraunhofer, Mercedes-Benz, Siemens, VW, Trumpf and several small and medium-sized enterprises are building a platform for sovereign data exchange to make their ecosystem more efficient and controllable." [17]
	Increased efficiency	
[18]	Improved infrastructure	"Reliable and secure infrastructure for data storage and processing that preserves the sovereignty of users" [18]
	Improved guidelines	"Clear guidelines, fair rules, and trustworthy governance for differentiated data access and use according to the respective roles of stakeholder" [18]
	Improved scalability	"Standards and interfaces that enable efficient and flexible scaling in different use cases, as well as the expansion of the application field through interoperability with other systems" [18]

APPENDIX D

SWOT Analysis Results—Threats

TABLE 14.6 Threats with Blockchain (Catena-X)

Paper	Threats	Text Extract
[15]	Lack of collaborative thinking	"To elaborate these use cases, several barriers for broad implementation of collaborative data-driven business models in Industry 4.0 Ecosystems can be identified [30], summarized as follows: • Lack of collaborative thinking and mutual digital trust: bilateral market relations are prevalent, combined with a fear of losing data sovereignty and competitiveness. • Lack of sustainable and scalable business models: clear value propositions with a fair share of overall benefit for all market actors in the long term are often not yet seen. • Lack of financial resources and skills: smaller manufacturing companies in particular struggle with the necessary investments and knowledge for transformation. • Lack of reliable technical and legal foundations: secure digital infrastructure with clear standards for sharing data and a supportive legal framework are seen as prerequisites. " [15]
	Lack of digital trust	
	Lack of financial resources	
	Lack of skills	
	L ack of reliable technical foundations	
	Lack of reliable legal foundations	
	Lack of suitable business models	
[18]	Requirement of new infrastructure	"Reliable and secure infrastructure for data storage and processing that preserves the sovereignty of users" [18] "Standards and interfaces that enable efficient and flexible scaling in different use cases, as well as the expansion of the application field through interoperability with other systems" [18] "Clear guidelines, fair rules, and trustworthy governance for differentiated data access and use according to the respective roles of stakeholders" [18]
	Requirement of new rules and guidelines	

(*Continued*)

TABLE 14.6 (Continued) Threats with Blockchain (Catena-X)

Paper	Threats	Text Extract
[19]	Requirement of IP protection, trade secrets	"With regard to the need for a new data culture, owners at present often do not want to share their data because of strategic considerations, such as intellectual property (IP) protection. According to the interviewed experts, this phenomenon is currently seen as a major challenge in the car and automotive industry. This was mentioned to be the case in the Catena-X project (International Data Spaces Association, 2021), which aims to enable cross-company data exchange between all involved actors in the automotive value chain." [19]

IV

Human Factors

Nilmini Wickramasinghe, Freimut Bodendorf, and Mathias Kraus

The most essential aspect of healthcare is the human side. In essence, digital health is socio-technical primarily because ultimately it is the human condition or malady that must be addressed. Human beings are individual and unique and thus, several issues must be considered in order to ensure we offer personalised, precise healthcare delivery so that every life receives the best possible care.

The final section of our book, therefore, focuses on a few significant aspects regarding human factors and how and why advances in machine learning, analytics and artificial intelligence can now enable us to address unique human factors more precisely. These areas include enabling the healthcare workforce to be more familiar with the language of machine learning and artificial intelligence and thereby be best positioned to navigate the best treatment decisions for a presenting patient as well as identifying the implications and considerations for the healthcare workforce because of advances in technology and analytics solutions. In addition, this section highlights advances that have made it possible to develop digital twins to provide precise and tailored clinical decision-making with the aim of addressing the unique and specific priorities of the presenting patient in their treatment journey.

The four chapters which make up this section include

DOI: 10.1201/9781032699745-18

Chapter 15: Implications and Considerations of AI for the Healthcare Workforce: A Theoretical Perspective, by Nevin, M., highlights the need for changes in the health workforce given the introduction of artificial intelligence, analytics, and machine learning.

Chapter 16: Unplanned Readmission Risks for Comorbid Patients of Diabetes: An Action Design Research Paradigm Data-Driven Decision Support, by Nilmini Wickramasinghe, applies an action research methodology to highlight critical issues around unplanned readmission with diabetes comorbid patients.

Chapter 17: Establishing a Digital Twin Architecture for Superior Falls Risk Prediction Using a Bayesian Network Model, by Nilmini Wickramasinghe, discusses how deriving a digital twin of a patient can be of assistance in preventing falls during an acute care visit.

Chapter 18: Facilitating a Shared Meaning of AI/ML Findings amongst Key Healthcare Stakeholders: The Role of Analytic Translators, by Wendy D. Lynch et al., highlights a current key void in healthcare given the introduction of analytics, artificial intelligence and machine learning; namely the need for all healthcare stakeholders to be equally comfortable around terminology and far-reaching implications.

The human factor in healthcare delivery will always remain the most challenging and perplexing since we humans are all individuals and present with unique nuances that must be considered in order to truly provide high-quality, high-value care. The chapters that make up this section then represent only the tip of the iceberg in this regard. It is the intention of this section to build awareness of the complex human factors rather than necessarily cover all key areas. Once there is awareness, we are confident that this will then permeate the design, development, and eventual deployment of technology solutions; and thereby, it is hoped that responsibly designed solutions will ensue.

CHAPTER 15

Implications and Considerations of AI for the Healthcare Workforce

A Theoretical Perspective

Mark Nevin

INTRODUCTION

The onset of AI in clinical care heralds a range of complex matters for the health workforce to consider and respond to. In the short to medium term, many health professionals will need to become accustomed to working safely alongside AI technologies, using it ethically and supporting patients in their decision-making. In the longer term, their roles could change drastically as the technical capabilities of AI continue to advance.

This chapter considers the emerging implications for the health workforce from the onset of AI technologies in clinical care. It starts by outlining models of entry to health professions and how they are regulated, with a specific emphasis on duties to maintain their professional skills throughout their careers. The role of professional standards and pre-existing requirements to practise healthcare ethically will then be established, before analysing how professional bodies expect these

DOI: 10.1201/9781032699745-19

requirements to apply to the emerging field of AI in healthcare. The chapter will also explore the initial attitudes of health workers to medical imaging, which is at the forefront of the deployment of AI in medicine, before considering the role of health workers in the deployment of AI in this area.

This chapter will thereby establish:

- general duties for skills to remain current through continuing professional development and to practice ethically etc;
- expectation regarding workforce responsibilities and clinical oversight of AI; and
- desire to upskill to work alongside AI.

Having laid out duties, expectations and a desire to become educated in new AI technologies, the chapter will present a two-level framework for upskilling the health workforce in professions which will utilise AI in clinical care. Some signs of the manifestation of this framework are then presented. The chapter concludes by exploring foreseeable challenges from the adoption of this framework and provides some thoughts on the broader implications of AI for the health workforce.

This chapter will regularly reference medical imaging as one of the domains of healthcare at the forefront of the deployment of AI and where the implications for health workers have been widely considered and are already being acted upon. AI has thrived in medical imaging due to the existence of several important building blocks. Firstly, the availability of enormous volumes of data from hundreds of millions of scans undertaken annually around the world.[1,2] Secondly, these datasets are relatively well structured and interoperable (based on DICOM standards[3]), with an accompanying clinical interpretation in the form of a diagnostic report. Thirdly, medical imaging services are also high-value and relatively well reimbursed.[4] Fourthly, imaging equipment suppliers tend to be large multinational companies with substantial research and development budgets. These factors, in addition to rapidly advancing computational capabilities, have positioned medical imaging as a target for AI entrepreneurs and investors.

Due to this potential for AI being adopted at scale, West et al. demonstrate that substantial volumes of research have been published on the implications of these new technologies for medical imaging, often with specific consideration of the radiologist workforce.[5] Indeed, this potential is being realised, with Muehlematter et al. observing that the majority of US Food and Drug Administration (FDA) and European CE approvals of AI technologies under medical device legislation are in medical imaging.[6]

Due to the availability of suitable literature, this chapter also focuses predominantly on:

- doctors due to their greater predominance in the delivery of healthcare and the availability of academic publications and other materials focusing on medicine; and
- international bodies and specific countries due to the nuances of sub-national regulation in some major jurisdictions and the availability of materials in the English language.

Before going into the specific implications of AI for the health workforce, it is important to revisit some fundamentals regarding how the health workforce is regulated and related expectations.

REGULATION OF THE HEALTH WORKFORCE

The health workforce includes a broad range of regulated professions including medicine, nursing, dentistry, pharmacy, optometry, allied health and others. While the methods and scope of regulation of health professions varies across (and within some) countries, several common features are apparent including accreditation of training pathways, requirements for registration or licensing as a health professional, protection of titles, codes of professional conduct and requirements for continuing professional development.[7,8,9] These features set an important context to:

- ensure uniform attainment of healthcare knowledge and skills;
- protect the public when they attend health services; and
- set expectations for the health workforce to maintain the skills necessary to practise safely as new techniques and technologies emerge, such as artificial intelligence.

In order to practise as a health professional, regulation in most countries requires registration. There are two typical types of registrable qualifications for health professionals. Firstly, a university degree confers graduates the ability to register as a generalist health professional, although in some instances additional college or professional body examinations are required. A second (and subsequent) pathway exists to enter vocational training programs after initially qualifying as a generalist health professional, such as that which typically exists for specialisation within a field of medicine. [Ref vii, viii, ix] This latter pathway is frequently profession-led via colleges or boards, however, routes also exist to subspecialise via universities.[10]

As was indicated above, the level of government which regulates health professions also differs between nations. Some countries have national regulations for health professionals, including the UK, the Republic of Ireland and New Zealand, while others have state-level regulations, including the USA and Canada.[11] Notably, Australia moved from state-based regulation of health professionals to national registration and accreditation in 2010.[12] This chapter will refer more frequently to international standards and national regulatory models since their requirements are uniform within that country, therefore facilitating international comparisons.

PROFESSIONAL STANDARDS AND EXPECTATIONS

Healthcare is a dynamic industry with ongoing research into disease processes and innovations in technologies and techniques used in the delivery of healthcare. This dynamism necessitates that the expected knowledge base of health practitioners must evolve over time.

The World Federation of Medical Educators (WFME) sets global standards for quality improvement in medical education. WFME (p.8) specified that:

> In order to practise appropriately throughout their professional life, doctors must remain up-to-date, which entails engaging in some form of continuing learning and education. In fact, the role of continuing professional development (CPD) in quality assurance and quality development of the health care delivery systems is increasingly significant.[13]

The same WFME standards also require doctors to be competent in relation to the use of information and communication technology including accessing relevant patient data and healthcare information systems, and doing so ethically while maintaining patient privacy and confidentiality as technology advances.[ibid.]

Regulators also expect health professionals to maintain their base knowledge and understanding of their designated field of healthcare. To provide an example, the International Association of Medical Regulatory Authorities (IAMRA) has a membership spanning over 50 countries including medical and some other health profession regulators.[14] IAMRA (p.2) sets a clear expectation for regulators to embed continued professional competency and therefore quality improvement through career-long learning and integration of acquired knowledge into daily practice:

> Career-long learning is more important than at any time in the past; medical practice is rapidly evolving and growing more complex. The benefits of medicine have never been greater, but the risks of harm from poor practice should not be underestimated. Unless doctors keep up to date with advances in clinical knowledge, technology, innovation, and working within complex, safety-critical systems, they risk compromising the care and well-being of their patients.[15]

Several countries have made this requirement for ongoing professional development mandatory for health professionals, including within the IAMRA membership, US states and 21 countries of the European Union.[7,9]

REQUIREMENTS TO PRACTICE HEALTHCARE ETHICALLY

Ethics is integral to the disciplines of healthcare, establishing norms of conduct and behaviour for health professionals. The origins of ethics in healthcare date back to the time of Hippocrates and have evolved since into contemporary principles and codes of practice. Simply put, frameworks of healthcare ethics rest on four principles:

- respect for patient's autonomy (their ability to make decisions);
- beneficence (to act in the patient's best interest);
- non-maleficence (to do no harm);
- and justice (to treat people equitably).[16]

These principles have been further developed and contextualised by regulators and professional bodies into codes of practice that set professional standards that clinicians must adhere to for registration and maintenance of registration as a healthcare professional.[17,18,19,20,21] Notably, the onus is placed on the individual health professional to uphold ethical standards, including when using new technologies in clinical care. Should they fail to do so, provisions exist to sanction them by removing their professional registration, and therefore right to practise. [Ref vii Kreutzberg]

Other chapters of this book will also delve into ethical frameworks in relation to the use of AI in healthcare. How these apply, and to whom exactly, is pertinent to the health workforce. Health professionals have long-established duties to practise ethically and must therefore play a critical role in the ethical deployment of AI into patient care. Indeed, trusting clinician-patient relationships have long been central to the delivery of healthcare care [Ref if needed xv-ixx] and clinicians will hold the responsibility to deem the AI (or for that matter any technique or technology) suitable for that patient's presentation.

RESPONSIBILITIES FOR ETHICAL AI AND CLINICAL OVERSIGHT BY MEDICAL PRACTITIONERS

Since at least 2017, international professional bodies have been exploring and seeking means to address ethical, professional practice and governance issues relating to the adoption of AI into clinical care and the resultant implications for the health workforce. Professional bodies have an important role in healthcare as they influence the standard of care expected of practitioners via their membership.

The Academy of Medical Royal Colleges (AoMRC) convened focus groups in 2018 from a broad panel of experts across medicine, nursing, public health, AI and public institutions to explore clinical, ethical and practical considerations across a series of domains and focus predominantly on the implications for doctors and patients.[22] AoMRC (p.14) anticipated changes in behaviours and a rethink in many aspects of doctors' education and career paths:

> As AI systems become more autonomous with a greater degree of direct-to-patient advice, a significant need arises to establish the role of clinicians in maintaining quality, safety, patient education and holistic support.[ibid.]

AoMRC (p.25) foresaw inevitable implications for the training and education of clinicians, with shifting fundamental learning needs to keep pace with changing professional working practices. The same paper drew parallels with how doctors interact with the pharmaceutical industry:

> Medical students are educated to interpret and critique the output of clinical trials and strict marketing regulations are in place. As doctors seek the evidence behind pharmaceuticals, perhaps they should similarly be trained to appraise new healthcare technologies for safety and efficacy and understand their technical limitations and risks.[ibid.]

Analysis and recommendations from global radiology bodies delved deeper into the implications for their profession. The European and North American radiology leadership came together to produce a declaration that established a common understanding of the issues and ultimate goals of utilising AI in radiology.[23] The resultant Multisociety Statement comprehensively explored ethical issues relating to data, algorithms and training models, medical practice, and anticipated disruption to the radiologist workforce.

Many of the key conclusions in Multisociety Statement relate directly to the workforce, in summary:

- AI has the potential to improve radiology, help patients and deliver more cost-effective medical imaging.
- People involved with AI development, deployment in health and monitoring must understand it deeply.
- Users of AI have a duty to understand risks, alert patients and stakeholders to those pitfalls and monitor AI to guard against harm.
- Accountability for AI must be shared between its human designers and operators.
- Regulation, standards, and codes of conduct need to balance technical, clinical, population health and commercial motivations with moral concerns.
- Codes of conduct on AI will need a continual emphasis on transparency, protection of patients and vigorous control of versions and uses.[ibid.,24]

In the accompanying academic summary paper, Geis et al. (p.437) concluded that:

> Radiologists will remain ultimately responsible for patient care and will need to acquire new skills to do their best for patients in the new AI ecosystem.[ibid. [i.e. xxiv]]

Contemporaneously, in the southern hemisphere, The Royal Australian and New Zealand College of Radiologists (RANZCR) responded to the onset of AI with four major streams of work covering ethics and appropriate use of AI in medicine, standards of practice, workforce upskilling, and advocacy for a robust approach to regulating AI.[25]

RANZCR published the first global set of ethical principles for the use of AI in medicine, intended inter alia to guide the upskilling of medical practitioners using machine learning or AI in health.[26] These principles require a discerning medical practitioner to be capable of explaining a finding or recommendation from AI, applying humanitarian values and individual patient preferences and values to clinical decision-making. Regarding accountability for patient care when using AI, RANZCR held that while responsibility would primarily rest with the medical practitioner, there may be instances where responsibility is shared between the medical practitioner caring for the patient, the hospital or practice that made a decision to deploy the AI and the manufacturer developing the AI.[ibid.]

These international professional bodies express recurring themes of addressing ethical issues such as transparency, equity and explainability via human oversight, joint responsibilities (between those designing and subsequent health worker operators of AI) and expectations that medical practitioners will need to upskill to practise safely alongside AI. Moreover, expectations have been set for clinicians to be capable of explaining findings from AI to patients under their care and supporting them to make subsequent decisions about care or treatment options.

INITIAL ATTITUDES AND EXPECTATIONS OF WORKFORCE IMPLICATIONS FROM AI

Consideration of the workforce implications of AI would be incomplete without revisiting the initial hype, specifically the technology's potential to replace human workers who undertake highly skilled tasks and specialist analyses.

Earlier in this chapter, the significant potential for AI in medical imaging was illustrated. High-profile commentary from technology experts generated significant hype that AI technologies would replace radiologists in the interpretation of medical images. In 2016, Hinton proposed that "we should stop training radiologists now", implying that they would soon be redundant, a comment that was relayed across media outlets and to radiologists around the world.[27]

This was a shock to the radiology community as it foretold of radiologists becoming structurally unemployed, meaning their skills would become outdated due to advances in technology, resulting in that profession being replaced by AI. Chockley and Emanuel proposed that within a few years, there may be no speciality called radiology.[28] With the benefit of hindsight, these perspectives bought too much into the hype and were at best premature. Analyses shortly afterwards by Harvey recognised that limitations in AI technology, complexities in radiology workflows and the need for human interactions meant there would be an enduring role for radiologists.[29] Moreover, Langlotz recollected how radiologists had previously mastered MRI technology, learning to recognise its shortcomings and leverage its strengths, predicting that they would do likewise for AI and dismissed suggestions that they would be replaced.[30] Langlotz (p.2) foresaw a greater likelihood that "radiologists who use AI will replace those who don't".[ibid.]

Evidence of how the attitudes of frontline clinicians were impacted by this debate is provided by a large two-part survey of 1,000 radiologists and radiology trainees across 54 countries which was undertaken contemporaneously in early 2019. This survey by Huisman et al. (p.7059) found that:

- 48% of radiologists and residents have an open and proactive attitude towards artificial intelligence (AI), while 38% fear replacement by AI;
- Intermediate and advanced understanding of AI may enhance the adoption of AI in clinical practice, while rudimentary knowledge appears inhibitive; and
- AI should be incorporated in radiology training curricula.[31]

The same paper found a correlation between limited AI-specific knowledge and fear of replacement.[ibid.] The second part of the survey by

Huisman et al. (p.8798) focused on barriers clinicians anticipated for the implementation of AI into healthcare settings, and found:

- Demand from the radiology community to incorporate AI into residency programs, but less support to recognise imaging informatics as a radiology subspecialty.
- Ethical and legal issues and lack of knowledge are recognised as major barriers to AI implementation in radiology, while the shortage of labelled data and IT infrastructure issues are seen as less problematic.
- AI education in radiology curricula should include technical aspects of data management, risk of bias, and ethical and legal issues to aid adoption of AI in radiology.[32]

These surveys demonstrated lingering fears of replacement coupled with a desire to understand how to apply the technology to patient care. Interesting preferences are expressed for education about AI technology, and ethical and legal considerations to be incorporated into training programs, yet apparent resistance to the emergence of a formal subspecialty of radiology informatics. Other surveys of attitudes amongst radiologists, medical students and trainees in specialties which utilise medical imaging have found similarly positive attitudes towards the potential of AI and disagreement with the notion that medical specialists would be replaced by AI technology.[33,34,35]

Various publications have anticipated similar challenges from the development and use of AI in healthcare, namely the black box nature of systems, the need for large volumes of accurately labelled training data and the risks of conscious and unconscious bias in automated decision-making. [Ref xxii AoMRC, xxiii Multisociety, xxv Kenny,] [36,37,38] These challenges feed directly into ethical concerns and require a judicious approach to its adoption and oversight in patient care.

ROLE OF HEALTH WORKERS WHEN DEPLOYING AI TECHNOLOGY INTO CLINICAL CARE

This chapter has established that there are foundational duties and expectations for the health workforce to have a role in the safe deployment of new technologies, including AI, in clinical settings. It is also anticipated that clinicians and AI machines will need to work together in partnership for the foreseeable future. This section will contextualise what the adoption of AI is expected to require of health workers in real-world clinical settings.

Clinicians have responsibilities to anticipate and manage shortcomings of AI technologies, as part of overall duties for quality care. [Ref xxii AoMRC (2019), xxiii Multisociety, xxv Kenny, xxvi RANZCR,],[39] AoMRC (2019) also saw a distinct role for clinicians in educating patients, fostering public acceptance and trust in new technologies and supporting patients to consent for AI tools to be used in the delivery of care to them. [Ref xxii AoMRC] This should also extend to advocacy regarding the ethical application and protection of sensitive data generated about patients, including the secondary use of such data.

Given the complexity of new technologies, consumers will need to be supported to contextualise findings from AI and assist them in subsequent decision-making on care or treatment.

In order to fulfil these roles, all clinicians using AI will need to understand how AI technologies work, the validity of findings in relation to other clinical investigations, and how to manage shortcomings. [reference xxii AoMRC, xxiii Multisociety, xxv Kenny, xxvi RANZCR]

The importance of educating practitioners has also been raised when considering how to govern the adoption of AI in health. Reddy et al. propose a governance model with four domains (fairness, transparency, trustworthiness and accountability) to oversee the deployment of AI in health, including making specific reference to educating clinicians and patients about AI.[40]

In time, these expectations will become the de facto standard of care for health workers practising alongside AI. This chapter illustrated earlier that there are duties for health professionals to maintain the currency of their professional knowledge and understanding. If a health worker fails to do so, their registration could be called into question and their right to practice removed. Health professionals could also face malpractice allegations and be held to be professionally and financially liable for adverse incidents involving AI for patients who attended for care.

Whereas a general understanding of AI will be required of all practitioners using it, a subset of clinicians will need to develop specialist knowledge to lead and oversee the selection of AI tools and oversee their implementation via clinical governance responsibilities, including determining suitability for patient cohorts, establishing risk tolerances, managing change and training other health workers alongside adoption of specific technology, trouble-shooting of complex clinical matters relating to use of AI, overseeing periodic audits of AI performance, reporting to overarching organisational governance, and engaging with technology suppliers and vendors. In order to effectively perform these higher-order tasks, a subset of clinicians will need to possess in-depth knowledge of digital technologies and/or AI.

While management of the application of AI technologies is still in its relative infancy, an example of published bi-national standards that guide hospitals and practices in the adoption of AI in medical imaging is available from RANZCR, which we will return to in the next section.[41]

How can health workers be best prepared for these roles at the clinical coalface? Having established that requirements exist and indicated how they might apply in practice, the next section of this chapter presents a two-level framework of clinical competence: competent user of AI technologies and subspecialist AI expert.

TWO-LEVEL CLINICAL COMPETENCE FRAMEWORK: COMPETENT USER AND AI EXPERT

Having evaluated how the workforce is regulated, analysed expectations from professional bodies and attitudes from areas of medicine where AI is most advanced, we have seen that the health workforce will have duties, expectations and a desire to upskill to practice safely alongside AI.

We have seen how clinical disciplines practising with or alongside AI will have distinct responsibilities to understand the technology, its limitations and how to contextualise findings in line with patient preferences, history and symptoms, test results and other clinical findings.

This framework argues that a two-level upskilling framework will be required for disciplines of health that embed AI into clinical areas.

At the first level, a general understanding of the technologies of AI and knowledge of how that would apply in clinical care will be required of those practitioners to become competent users of AI. Clinicians using AI in their practice or hospital need to have a solid baseline understanding of AI including machine learning, neural networks and algorithms, and how large and complex volumes of data are analysed by AI tools to produce a finding or recommendation for patients under their care. Fundamentally, they will need to be capable of interrogating what data an AI tool was trained and tested on, applying it ethically, determining its suitability or otherwise for patient cohorts, and explaining its findings to patients.

At the second level, a subset of clinicians will need to develop deep subject matter expertise, layering AI expertise on top of their existing clinical skillset, and guiding the application of AI within their discipline. These AI experts are necessary due to the complexity of the technology and the need for clinical input and oversight of all aspects of AI in health care (from its design, testing, approval for use, deployment, oversight and audit and associated troubleshooting).

We will now explore further the rationale for this framework and early signs of it manifesting.

Level 1: Competent User of AI

We have seen that clinicians are expected by their regulators to continue their professional development through their careers to become abreast of new technologies. Over time, expectations to practise safely with any new technology or treatment become embedded. In relation to AI, professional bodies have set expectations that clinicians will be responsible for the ethical application of AI into patient care [Ref xxii AoMRC, xxiii Multisociety Statement, xxv Kenny, xxvi RANZCR].

Others have argued for the need for an overhaul of medical education to incorporate AI. Wartman and Combs argue for a shift in medical education from knowledge acquisition (which risks information overload) to knowledge management, equipping doctors to be effective users of AI, highly skilled to explain treatment options empathetically to patients.[42] Shortly afterwards, Sapci and Sapci undertook a systematic review of publications recommending the incorporation of AI into both medical education and health informatics training.[43] They propose a framework to equip these disciplines to understand AI technologies, minimise bias, assess problematic results, and take precautions where needed.

Building further on how these expectations might apply, the extensive Topol Review of innovative health technologies for Health Education England proposed that the UK launch a nationwide training program for health and social care professionals within the NHS to position it to capitalise on genomics, digital medicine, artificial intelligence and robotics with a goal of improving health services.[44] The Topol Review (p.15) recommended that:

> Educational resources should be developed to educate and train all healthcare professionals in: health data provenance, curation, integration and governance; the ethics of AI and autonomous systems/tools; critical appraisal and interpretation of AI and robotics technologies.[ibid.]

Furthermore, the Topol Review (p.17) specified that:

> Professional, Statutory and Regulatory Bodies (PSRBs) and practitioners need to identify the knowledge, skills, professional attributes and behaviours needed for healthcare graduates to work in a technologically enabled service, and then work with educators to redesign the curricula for this purpose.[ibid.]

Reddy and Cooper (2020) propose components of an educational package to train the health workforce in AI: covering proficiency in understanding fundamentals of the technology; how and where to apply it; and governance of AI systems. [Ref xxxix Reddy and Cooper]

An early manifestation that the required bar (i.e. professional standard to attain registration) has been raised to incorporate AI for two professions that rely on medical imaging is provided by the revisions made by RANZCR to its training curricula for clinical radiologists and radiation oncologists, which came into effect in early 2021. The learning outcomes articulated in RANZCR (2021a) and RANZCR (2021b) set expectations that clinical radiologists and radiation oncologists respectively will need to understand AI technologies, apply them ethically and take responsibility for their use in patient care.[45,46] This inaugural revision to incorporate AI is noteworthy because RANZCR's training curricula are the de facto professional standards that a clinical radiologist or radiation oncologist must meet in order to register to practise and therefore also maintain registration in Australia or New Zealand. Later the same year, the Royal College of Radiologists (2021) followed suit, adding requirements for UK trainees in clinical radiology to keep up to understand the fundamentals of emerging new technologies such as AI, including their pitfalls, and to be prepared to adopt these tools into clinical practice once the technology is validated.[47]

It will be interesting to observe how and when other health professions and jurisdictions follow suit as AI becomes more commonplace and clinicians are expected to safeguard its adoption into clinical care and support patients in related decision-making.

Level 2: Subspecialist AI Expert

There are numerous models of subspecialism in healthcare, ranging from formally recognised (and registrable) qualifications, becoming dual qualified (e.g. in another discipline which might be informatics or data science) to credentialing by payers or employers through to "special interests" whereby someone chooses to deepen their knowledge beyond a generalist understanding in a particular area. There are also various routes into subspecialist practice, for example by gaining exposure by working in a high-volume centre; through research, CPD or via attending conferences; through informal supervised training or apprenticeships; or potentially through a combination of learning, gaining exposure and building experience over time.

This framework proposes that the complexity of the technology and the need for clinical input and oversight of all aspects of AI necessitates the emergence of subspecialist experts in AI.

The closely related field of health informatics also encompasses many of the specialist skills required to assess digital health technologies and oversee their deployment into clinical care. The field of health informatics has also been displaying signs of the emergence of a formal subspecialty for clinicians. Gundlapalli et al. undertook a study to determine the extent of formal regulator-approved certification of health informatics for doctors (physicians), and found two countries (Germany and Belgium) in addition to the USA that have regulator-approved training pathways leading to formal certification, with some others planning to do so.[48] Furthermore, nursing informatics has been certified in the USA by the Accreditation Board for Nursing Certification since 1992, although this is not apparent in other countries.[49]

In the UK, the Topol Review (2019) resulted in a new subspecialist training program called the Topol Fellowship which supports a select number of health professionals (anticipated to be 50 in 2023) to develop specialist expertise in the adoption of innovative new technologies (including AI). [Ref xliv Topol] Although admittedly broader than just AI, the Topol Review (2019, p.11) anticipated the need for new specialist skills and individuals who would champion the adoption of new technologies:

> NHS organisations should invest in their existing workforce to develop specialist skills, including the assessment and commissioning of genomics and digital technologies. With all new technologies, it is essential to identify future champions early and create networks to enable collaborative learning. [Ref xliv Topol]

The clinical roles of these health practitioners subspecialising in AI will evolve accordingly, akin to the emergence of health informaticians in the USA and elsewhere who hold roles such as chief clinical informatics officers and oversee the deployment of complex digital health technologies into clinical care.

As was noted for level 1: competent user, we are still at the outset of deployment of AI into clinical care. There is however some evidence of subspecialist expert AI roles taking shape, again from Australia and New Zealand. RANZCR published standards of practice to support the deployment of AI in radiology practices and hospitals. [ref xli RANCZR] RANZCR (2020, p.17) craft a chief radiologist information officer (CRIO) role, articulating a series of higher-order responsibilities which will require deep subspecialist knowledge of AI:

> 4.4 The Practice will appoint a CRIO with direct access to senior management. The CRIO will have defined responsibility and authority for implementing and maintaining ML and AI tools within the Practice.[ibid.]

A series of indicators, or evidence of the standard being met, are also provided, including

i. The CRIO will have a broad understanding of standards frameworks relating to digital health, including enterprise IT governance, information security, knowledge and data management, risk management, business analysis, change management and how to resolve issues that may arise through implementation.

ii. The CRIO will work with the implementing governing body to recognise the preferences, cultural values and other values of the Practice's patients, and how they may affect the use of ML and AI tools in the Practice.

iii. The CRIO and radiology team at the Practice will identify tasks or decisions that should not be delegated to technology.

iv. The CRIO and governance body will consider how to guard against (contain and manage) automation bias.

v. The CRIO will oversee ongoing monitoring of ML and AI software to ensure optimal performance.[ibid.]

Another example of a subspecialist training route for medical specialists is the professional diploma in digital health provided by the Royal College of Surgeons Ireland (RCSI), the professional training body for surgeons and other medical specialties in Ireland. According to RCSI (n.d.), this training course is intended to provide the skills and confidence to lead digital transformation in the attendee's healthcare setting.[50] Numerous other training programs for artificial intelligence have come into existence including MSc programs and informal training fellowships which would support the development of subspecialist skills in AI. A holistic consideration of these is unfortunately beyond the scope of this chapter.

At this stage, and recalling the lack of support expressed by survey respondents in Huisman et al. (2021b), it is unclear whether there will be formalised recognition of subspecialist AI expertise, at least for the foreseeable future. [Ref xxii Huisman et al. 2021b] There is also potential for AI subspecialist expertise to be encompassed within the broader domain of health informatics, avoiding the need for parallel recognition.

More likely in the foreseeable future is that individual health practitioners will determine their own subspecialist upskilling journey through a mix of formal learning, CPD at conferences, exposure to AI and experience resolving complex problems which arise.

New professional standards and regulations for health workers can take some years to become a reality, following extensive analysis, consultation, and in some cases, revisions to government legislation. Whether and how this two-level framework is adopted will need to be revisited periodically to ascertain the extent to which it is shaping up across and within jurisdictions.

CHALLENGES REGARDING THE ADOPTION OF A TWO-LEVEL FRAMEWORK AND AREAS FOR FUTURE CONSIDERATION AND RESEARCH

As was flagged by Topol Review (2019), consideration is needed of what technologies such as AI would mean for training institutions that provide education services for the two entry pathways into health professions (i.e. university and postgraduate apprenticeship style training). [ref xliv Topol] They will need to take responsibility for embedding AI into training pathways and therefore ensure new entrants to the health workforce have the requisite knowledge and skills to practice safely alongside AI.

There are also implications for the accrediting bodies which oversee these training institutions as they accredit their governance and procedures covering the development of training curricula.

There are also significant questions for those already registered and practising as health workers in professions where AI is being adopted. Regulators of these professions will need to apply requirements for them to upskill via professional standards in order for those clinicians to practise safely alongside AI and support patients as needed. This has in fact been publicly recognised by the General Medical Council (GMC) in the UK. In response to a government consultation on standards in public life relating to AI, the GMC stated that regulators should consider and respond to the impact of AI in the fields they regulate.[51]

Numerous complexities remain to be worked through, including unforeseeable implications for patient care from the adoption of AI. Should a series of adverse incidents result, further consideration must be given to the merits of formally recognising subspecialist roles of AI experts and how that could be built upon existing training pathways for the health workforce.

THOUGHTS ON FUTURE BROADER IMPLICATIONS OF AI FOR THE HEALTH WORKFORCE

Numerous papers referenced in this chapter have discussed the potential for the delivery of more and better care when health workers work in partnership with AI. But what are the precise implications for workforce productivity and how can this be measured? Whereas there are claims from AI suppliers of productivity improvements, indeed these are expected, they are yet to be demonstrated at scale in academic studies.[52] Furthermore, in order to demonstrate the improvements, a sound baseline of current productivity rates first needs to be established within varied and complex health environments. Such research into the productivity implications of adopting AI would be welcome.

More broadly, consideration should also be given to the macroeconomic implications of AI for workforce demand and supply. While fair to say that there will be productivity dividends from adopting AI, the timing and the precise nature of these are uncertain, and analysis will be further complicated by evolving roles and responsibilities for health professionals. Research into the productivity implications of AI (initially working alongside health professionals) would help determine what that means for future workforce demand, numbers, mix and distribution of health workers needed to deliver services safely, and the resultant implications for training program content and numbers.

CONCLUSION

This chapter began by considering models of entry to health professions and how they are regulated, emphasising duties to maintain their professional skills throughout their careers. It also explored how professional bodies expect these requirements to apply to the emerging field of AI in healthcare, and the initial attitudes of health workers in medical imaging which expressed a desire to upskill to understand AI technologies.

This chapter established:

- general duties for health practitioners to maintain and advance their skills through continuing professional development and to practice ethically etc;
- expectations regarding workforce responsibilities and clinical oversight of AI; and
- desire to upskill to work alongside AI,

The chapter then introduced a two-level framework for upskilling the health workforce in professions which will utilise AI in clinical care, and presented early signs of this framework being introduced. The chapter concludes with some foreseeable challenges from the adoption of this framework and provides some thoughts on the broader implications of AI for the health workforce.

The implications of AI technologies for the health workforce are substantial. This chapter has covered the anticipated impacts on health professionals' roles, responsibilities and the skills they will require to continue to practice safely alongside AI. Whether and how these manifest will continue to be of great interest to the numerous health professions that AI will impact.

NOTES

1. United Nations Scientific Committee on the Effects of Atomic Radiation (UNSCEAR) (2008) *Sources and Effects of Ionizing Radiation Access, Report to General Assembly*, viewed 18 December 2022, <https://www.unscear.org/docs/reports/2008/09-86753_Report_2008_Annex_A.pdf>
2. Organisation for Economic Cooperation and Development (OECD) (2019) Health Care Utilisation Statistics, viewed 18 December 2022, <https://stats.oecd.org/index.aspx?queryid=30160>
3. Integrating the Health Enterprise (IHE) (2022) *Radiology*, IHE, viewed 18 December 2022, <https://www.ihe.net/ihe_domains/radiology/>
4. Squires D and Anderson C (2015) *Spending, Use of Services, Prices, and Health in 13 Countries*, The Commonwealth Fund, viewed 18 December 2022, <https://www.commonwealthfund.org/publications/issue-briefs/2015/oct/us-health-care-global-perspective>
5. West et al. (2019) '*Global Trend in Artificial Intelligence–Based Publications in Radiology From 2000 to 2018*', *American Journal of Roentgenology* vol.213, no.6, pp.1204–1206, https://doi.org/10.2214/AJR.19.21346
6. Muehlematter et al. (2021) '*Approval of Artificial Intelligence and Machine Learning-based Medical Devices in the USA and Europe (2015–20): A Comparative Analysis*', *The Lancet Digital Health* vol.3, no.3, pp.195–203, https://doi.org/10.1016/S2589-7500(20)30292-2
7. Kreutzberg A, Reichebner C, Maier CB, et al. (2019) '*Regulating the input: health professions*', in: Busse R, Klazinga N, Panteli D, et al, editors (2019) '*Improving healthcare quality in Europe: Characteristics, effectiveness and implementation of different strategies*', European Observatory on Health Systems and Policies 2019 Health Policy Series, vol.53, no.5, viewed 17 December 2022, <https://www.ncbi.nlm.nih.gov/books/NBK549267/>
8. Moore J. (2018) '*Professions Regulation in the United States*', *Journal of Health Law (Revista de Direito Sanitario)*, vol.19, no.2, pp.131–155, https://doi.org/10.11606/issn.2316-9044.v19i2p131-155
9. Greiner AC, Knebel E and editors (2003) '*Health Professions Education: A Bridge to Quality*', in Institute of Medicine (US) (2003), '*Health Professions Oversight Processes: What They Do and Do Not Do, and What They Could Do, Committee on the Health Professions Education Summit*', National Academies Press, Washington (DC), viewed 18 December 2022, <https://www.ncbi.nlm.nih.gov/books/NBK221526/>
10. International Association of Medical Regulatory Authorities (IAMRA) (n.d.), '*Statement on Accreditation of Postgraduate (Specialist) Medical Education Programs*', IAMRA, viewed 11 December 2022, <https://www.iamra.com/resources/Documents/IAMRA%20Stmt%20on%20Accred%20of%20PG%20Spec%20%20Med%20Ed.pdf>
11. Leslie K, et al. (2021) '*Regulating Health Professional Scopes of Practice: Comparing Institutional Arrangements and Approaches in the US, Canada,*

Australia and the UK', *Human Resources Health* vol.19, no.15, https://doi.org/10.1186/s12960-020-00550-3

12. Australian Government Department of Health and Aged Care, Canberra (n.d.) '*National Registration and Accreditation Scheme*', Department of Health and Aged Care, viewed 17 December 2022, <https://www.health.gov.au/our-work/national-registration-and-accreditation-scheme>
13. WFME (2015) '*Standards for Quality Improvement*', WFME, viewed 11 December 2022, <https://wfme.org/download/wfme-global-standards-cpd-english/>
14. IAMRA (n.d.) '*Membership Listing*', IAMRA, viewed 11 December 2022, <https://www.iamra.com/membership-listing>
15. IAMRA (2021) '*Statement on Continuing Competency*', IAMRA, viewed 11 December 2022, <https://www.iamra.com/resources/Documents/IAMRA%20Statement%20on%20Continued%20Competency.pdf>
16. Varkey B (2021), '*Principles of Clinical Ethics and Their Application to Practice*', *Medical Principles and Practice*, vol.30 no.1, pp.17–28, https://doi.org/10.1159/000509119
17. General Medical Council (2019) '*Good Medical Practice*', General Medical Council, viewed 14 December 2022, <https://www.gmc-uk.org/ethical-guidance/ethical-guidance-for-doctors/good-medical-practice>
18. Australian Medical Council (2016) '*Good Medical Practice: Professionalism Ethics and Law, 4th Edition*', Australian Medical Council, viewed 14 December 2022, <https://www.amc.org.au/amc-good-medical-practice/>
19. Irish Medical Council (2019) '*Medical Council - Professional Conduct & Ethics 8th Edition*', Irish Medical Council, viewed 14 December 2022, <https://www.medicalcouncil.ie/public-information/professional-conduct-ethics/>
20. Medical Council of New Zealand (2021) '*Good Medical Practice*', Medical Council of New Zealand, viewed 14 December 2022, <https://www.mcnz.org.nz/assets/standards/b3ad8bfba4/Good-Medical-Practice.pdf>
21. International Council for Nurses (2021) '*The ICN Code of Ethics for Nurses*', International Council for Nurses, viewed 29 December 2022, <https://www.icn.ch/sites/default/files/inline-files/ICN_Code-of-Ethics_EN_Web.pdf>
22. AoMRC (2019) '*Artificial Intelligent in Healthcare*', AoMRC, viewed 18 December 2022, <https://www.aomrc.org.uk/wp-content/uploads/2019/01/Artificial_intelligence_in_healthcare_0119.pdf>
23. European and North American Multisociety Statement (2019) '*Ethics of AI in Radiology*', *Radiology*, vol.293 no.2, ACR, viewed 18 December 2022, <https://www.acr.org/-/media/ACR/Files/Informatics/Ethics-of-AI-in-Radiology-European-and-North-American-Multisociety-Statement--6-13-2019.pdf>
24. Geis et al. (2019) '*Ethics of Artificial Intelligence in Radiology: Summary of the Joint European and North American Multisociety Statement*', *Radiology*, vol.293, no.2, pp.436–440, https://doi.org/10.1148/radiol.2019191586

25. Kenny L, Nevin M and Fitzpatrick K (2021) '*Ethics and Standards in the Use of Artificial Intelligence in Medicine on behalf of the Royal Australian and New Zealand College of Radiologists*', *Journal of Medical Imaging and Radiation Oncology, vol.*65, no.5, pp.486–494, https://doi.org/10.1111/1754-9485.13289
26. RANZCR (2019) '*Ethical Principles for AI in Medicine*', RANZCR, viewed 19 December 2022, <https://www.ranzcr.com/documents/4952-ethical-principles-for-ai-in-medicine/file>
27. Hinton G (2016) '*Comments on radiology and deep learning at the 2016 Machine Learning and Market for Intelligence Conference*', You Tube, viewed 18 December 2022, <https://youtu.be/2HMPRXstSvQ>
28. Chockley and Emanuel (2016) '*The End of Radiology? Three Threats to the Future Practice of Radiology*', *Journal of the American College of Radiology, vol.*13, no.12, pp.1415–1420, https://doi.org/10.1016/j.jacr.2016.07.010
29. Harvey H (2018) '*Why AI will not Replace Radiologists*', Towards Data Science, viewed 18 December 2022, <https://towardsdatascience.com/why-ai-will-not-replace-radiologists-c7736f2c7d80>
30. Langlotz C (2019) '*Will Artificial Intelligence Replace Radiologists?*', *Radiology: Artificial Intelligence* vol.1, no.3, pp.1–3, https://pubs.rsna.org/doi/10.1148/ryai.2019190058
31. Huisman et al. (2021) '*An International Survey on AI in Radiology in 1,041 Radiologists and Radiology Residents Part 1: Fear of Replacement, Knowledge, and Attitude*', *European Radiology*, vol.31, pp.7058–7066, https://doi.org/10.1007/s00330-021-07781-5
32. Huisman et al. (2021) '*An International Survey on AI in Radiology in 1041 Radiologists and Radiology Residents part 2: Expectations, Hurdles to Implementation, and Education*', *European Radiology*, vol.31, pp. 8797–8806, https://doi.org/10.1007/s00330-021-07782-4
33. Pinto dos Santos D, et al. (2018) '*Medical Students' Attitude towards Artificial Intelligence: A Multicentre Survey*', *European Radiology*, vol.29, pp.1640–1646, https://doi.org/10.1007/s00330-018-5601-1
34. European Society of Radiology (ESR) (2019) '*Impact of Artificial Intelligence on Radiology: a EuroAIM Survey Among Members of the European Society of Radiology*', *Imaging Insights*, vol.10, no.1, p.105, https://doi.org/10.1186/s13244-019-0798-3
35. Scheetz J, Rothschild P, McGuinness M, et al. (2021) '*A Survey of Clinicians on the Use of Artificial Intelligence in Ophthalmology, Dermatology, Radiology and Radiation Oncology*',*Scientific Reports*, vol.11, p.5193, https://doi.org/10.1038/s41598-021-84698-5
36. Chartrand G, et al. (2017) '*Deep Learning: A Primer for Radiologists*', *RadioGraphics*, vol.37, no.7, https://doi.org/10.1148/rg.2017170077
37. Wong et al. (2018) '*Artificial Intelligence in Radiology: How will we be Affected?*', European Radiology, vol.29, pp.141–143, https://doi.org/10.1007/s00330-018-5644-3

38. Castiglioni I, et al. (2021) '*AI Applications to Medical Images: From Machine Learning to Deep Learning*', *Physica Medica*, vol.83, pp.9–24, https://doi.org/10.1016/j.ejmp.2021.02.006
39. Reddy S, and Cooper P (2021) '*Health workforce learning in response to artificial intelligence*', in: Butler-Henderson K, Day K, Gray K, editors '*The health informatician workforce*', Springer Cham. https://doi.org/10.1007/978-3-030-81850-0_8
40. Reddy S, et al. (2020) '*A Governance Model for the Application of AI in Health Care*', *Journal of the American Medical Informatics Association*, vol.27, no.3, pp.491–497, https://doi.org/10.1093/jamia/ocz192
41. RANZCR (2020) '*Standards of Practice for Artificial Intelligence*', RANZCR, viewed date 18 December 2022, <https://www.ranzcr.com/search/standards-of-practice-for-artificial-intelligence>
42. Wartman SA and Combs CD (2019) '*Reimagining Medical Education in the Age of AI*', *AMA Journal of Ethics*, vol.21, no.2, pp.146–152, https://doi.org/10.1001/amajethics.2019.146.
43. Sapci AH and Sapci HA (2020) '*Artificial Intelligence Education and Tools for Medical and Health Informatics Students: Systematic Review*', *JMIR Medical Education*, vol.6, no.1, p.19285, https://doi.org/10.2196/19285. PMID: 32602844; PMCID: PMC7367541.
44. Topol et al. (2019) *Topol Review, Preparing the Health Workforce to Deliver the Digital Future* for Health Education England, Health Education England, viewed 18 December 2022, <https://topol.hee.nhs.uk/wp-content/uploads/HEE-Topol-Review-2019.pdf>
45. RANZCR (2021) '*Clinical Radiology Curriculum Learning Outcomes*' (see *Section Three AI*, p.25) RANZCR, viewed 3 January 2023, <https://www.ranzcr.com/documents/5399-ranzcr-clinical-radiology-learning-outcomes/file>
46. RANZCR (2021) '*Radiation Oncology Learning Outcomes and Handbook*' (see Leader (and Manager), p.129) RANZCR, viewed 3 January 2023, <https://www.ranzcr.com/trainees/radiation-oncology-training-program/learning-outcomes-and-handbook>
47. RCR (2021) 'Clinical Radiology Specialty Training Curriculum' RCR viewed 3 January 2023, <https://www.rcr.ac.uk/sites/default/files/clinical_radiology_curriculum_2020.pdf>
48. Gundlapalli et al. (2015)'*Clinical Informatics Board Specialty Certification for Physicians: A Global View*', *Studies in Health Technology and Informatics*, vol.216, pp.501–505.
49. Cummins et al. (2016) '*Nursing Informatics Certification Worldwide: History, Pathway, Roles, and Motivation*', *Yearbook Medical Informatics 2016*, vol.10, no.1, pp.264–271, https://doi.org/10.15265/IY-2016-039
50. RCSI (n.d.) '*Study digital health*', Royal College of Surgeons in Ireland viewed 3 January 2023 <https://www.rcsi.com/online/study-digital-health?Campaign=RCSIOnline-March+2022+Campaign&Provider=Facebook>

51. General Medical Council (2020) '*GMC Response to Committee on Standards in Public Life on Artificial Intelligence*', GMC viewed 3 February 2022, <https://www.gmc-uk.org/-/media/documents/gmc-response-to-committee-on-standards-in-public-life-on-artificial-intelligence-and-public-85283035.pdf>
52. Hazarika I (2020) '*Artificial Intelligence: Opportunities and Implications for the Health Workforce*', *International Health*, vol.12, no.4, pp.241–245, https://doi.org/10.1093/inthealth/ihaa007

CHAPTER 16

Unplanned Readmission Risks for Comorbid Patients of Diabetes

An Action Design Research Paradigm Data-Driven Decision Support

Nilmini Wickramasinghe

INTRODUCTION

Facilitating better judgement in decision-making entails the use of data, statistical analysis, and machine learning to guide humans through a systematic approach that identifies hidden insights that will proffer solutions via the identification of trends, visualization, and correlation of events (Bohanec et al. 2017; Sarker 2021). This means that principles, processes, and frameworks that will analyse data through feature engineering, and predictive analytics will be needed to identify the probable solutions to problems (Fayyad et al. 1996), which can only be meaningful to decision-makers after the interpretation of results. As a result of this capability, the surge in Information Technology (IT) through the Internet of Things (IoT) and other smart devices has augmented decision-making in healthcare (Chatterjee et al. 2020) paving the way for improved caregiving that enhances patients' outcomes. To this end, numerous studies on data-driven decision support for healthcare applications have been

DOI: 10.1201/9781032699745-20

carried out. Lejarza et al. (2021) used a data-driven technique that hinges on discrete state space for capturing the physiological state of Intensive Care Unit (ICU) patients to recommend the optimal time for their discharge. Todd et al. (2022) used survival analysis to propose applications for managing readmission in public hospitals to identify high-risk patients who may need more attention to forestall URA.

Unfortunately, most of the studies in this area have focused on descriptive and explanatory studies without the consideration and inclusion of the design principles for solving the data-driven problem in a complex healthcare context. As a result, this chapter follows a holistic approach to identifying the risk factors by using the Action Design Research (ADR) paradigm to construct and implement IT artifacts for data-driven decision support aimed at identifying the risk factors of 30-day URA for patients of diverse cultural backgrounds. This will help to identify the patients that are at a high risk of 30-day URA and enable a better characterization of comorbid patients with diabetes on admission, hence, giving the clinicians the opportunity of effective and tailored caregiving that will help to forestall the early URA.

BACKGROUND

Despite the chances of reducing 30-day Unplanned Readmission (URA) of patients with diabetes through self-management and reduction of preventable causes (Fluitman et al. 2016; Soh et al. 2020), 14–21% of patients still have URA (Budnitz et al. 2011; Friedman et al. 2008). Many factors such as age, gender, race, cardiovascular conditions, renal disease, chronic kidney disease, cancer, depression, dementia, respiratory illnesses, insulin therapy, and insurance status (Gould et al. 2020; Soh et al. 2020) have been identified as risks of URA of diabetes patients. Png et al. (2018) relied on Electronic Medical Records (EMR) to analyse 30-day URA, which showed illness burden and diabetes medication as risk factors of early URA whereas Rubin and Shah (2021) showed that socioeconomics, comorbidities, Length of hospital Stay (LOS), history of readmission are the determinants of 30-day URA. Even though numerous risk factors of 30-day URA have been identified by researchers, there is still the need to understand how the risk factors influence patients from diverse cultural backgrounds by considering medication therapies. Other researchers such as Shang et al. (2021), Collin et al. (2017), and Rie et al. (2015) have also identified the risk factors of early URA of patients with diabetes to include race, sex, age, admission type, admission location, length of stay, and drug use.

The rest of the chapter will include methodology, which describes the Action Design Research (ADR), data acquisition, feature engineering and statistical analysis techniques. The results and the implication of the study are captured in the discussion section while highlighting the limitations and the direction for future research.

METHODOLOGY

Action Design Research

The need for solving Information System (IS) problems that make both theoretical and practical contributions is vital in research if there will be any abstraction that will benefit practitioners. ADR is an offshoot of the action and design research concept that provides theoretical contributions to IS problems by collecting, analyzing, building, and evaluating IT artifacts in an organizational context to solve these problems (Sein et al. 2011). This helps to solve current and future problems by providing a framework that facilitates quick and better decisions for the numerous IS problems while enabling practitioners to work smarter in a more productive manner. ADR relies on the theoretical knowledge gained about a problem to develop a design architecture for solving the problem via a stepwise approach that evaluates the IT artifacts following problem formulation, building, intervention, evaluation, reflection and learning, and formulation of learning. Despite this robust approach used by ADR, some researchers have argued that the effectiveness of ADR rests in the practical translation of problems into solutions that are endorsed by stakeholders. This ensures that the solutions are shaped within practical IT artifacts that will involve end-users of the project early while balancing the political, economic, and societal values of the ensuing results of such projects (Keijzer-Broers and de Reuver 2016).

Problem Formulation

Even though design science research projects can be diverse, the fundamental step in a design project is the identification of a problem that needs solutions, thus allowing researchers to construct IT artifacts for defining the problem before creating specific artifacts for some specific contexts. In this study, the need to understand the risk factors of 30-day URA and their severities for comorbid patients of diabetes from diverse cultural backgrounds treated with numerous medications forms the basis. Since the reliance on theories for designing the IT artifacts cannot be

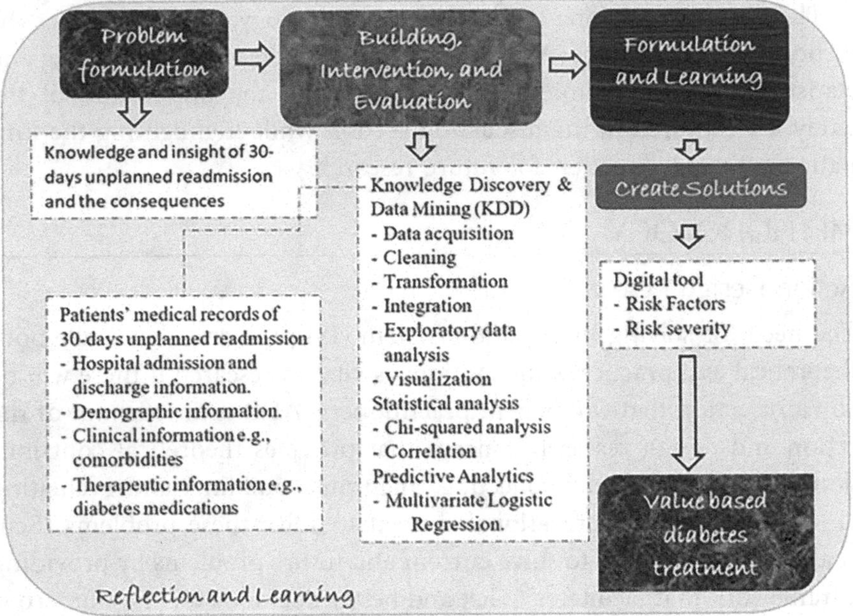

FIGURE 16.1 Action design research (ADR) architecture for data-driven decision support for 30-day unplanned readmission risk estimation of culturally diverse patients with diabetes.

overlooked, the study depends on the data-driven theory of KDD (Fayyad et al. 1996) for crafting the steps for analyzing data, obtaining the artifacts, and sub-artifacts for managing 30-day URA following Figure 16.1. The conceptualization of this project was informed by the challenges posed by the 30-day URA of comorbid patients with diabetes whose experiences after admission are not good due to the diminished quality of life after discharge and the subsequent 30-day URA. Furthermore, 30-day URA results in financial penalties on hospitals from health insurance, casts the stigma of poor-quality care services on the hospitals, deprives future patients of the opportunity of bed space, and increases the financial burden on the populace through increased cost of managing healthcare (AIHW 2017; Clement et al. 2014; Shebeshi et al. 2020).

Building, Intervention and Evaluation

Since the 30-day URA of comorbid diabetes patients is not economic and impacts the overall quality of life of patients, it becomes imperative to understand the risk factors, their severities, and how they apply to a culturally diverse society. This understanding and the implementation of requisite adjustments for patients affected by the risks will make room for improved caregiving at the hospitals since optimal care engagement can potentially reduce 30-day URA (Bianco et al. 2012; Considine et al. 2020; van der Does et al. 2020). This stage of ADR involves the implementation of the various steps in KDD through the analysis of patients' medical records to compute the probability, and risk factors (and their severities) using Multivariate Logistic Regression (MLR). There is also data engineering to facilitate high-quality information that will produce a better result following the transformation of some of the predictors of 30-day URA. The implementation of statistical analysis helps to establish the nature of the artifacts (risk factors) at a 95% significant level. The implementation of exploratory data analysis helps to identify the trends and patterns of the 30-day URA rate amongst the various cultural backgrounds and comorbidities. With this systematic implementation of KDD on the historic patients' records, the artifacts, which form the basis for decision support in managing patients are identified. More details about the building, intervention and evaluation steps are discussed in the next 3 sub-sections.

Data Acquisition

De-identified data obtained from the Health Facts database (Cerner Corporation, Kansas City, MO), which collects comprehensive clinical records across hospitals in the United States (Strack et al. 2014) is used for the KDD analysis. Over 74 million records from more than 130 hospitals' unique records of patients treated for diabetes and other health conditions provided hospital-specific records such as admission and discharge categories, demographic, and clinical information for this study that relied on information such as emergency, outpatient, and inpatients visits, diagnosed comorbidities following ICD-9-CM codes. From the preliminary analysis, a total of 101,766 records related to comorbid diabetes patients were identified with over 55 features that included medication types and HbA1C levels.

Feature Engineering

Further analysis of the 10,766 records to identify patients treated with at least one diabetes medication who stayed at least 1 day on hospital admission resulted in 17,933 records used for this study. After dropping the features with more than 10% of missing values and eliminating features that have no direct relevance to 30-day URA, the following features were left for the analysis:- race, gender, age, admission type (ADT), admission source

(ADM), discharge disposition (DSC), time in hospital (TIH), number of labs (NLB), number of procedures (NPR), number of medications (NMD), number of outpatient visits (NOU), number of inpatient visits (NIP), primary diagnosis (PDGN), number of diagnoses (NDG), A1C test result (HbA1C), diabetes medications used (MED). The "race" is classified into 3 categories in recognition of the minorities by using the acronym black, Indigenous and people of colour (BIPOC), hence, non-BIPOC are Caucasians, BIPOC is Asians, Hispanics, and other races while AA-BIPOC represents African Americans. Age is grouped into < 40 years, 40–50 years, 50–60 years, 60–70 years, 70–80 years, and >80 years. The sub-classes of the remaining features are ADM: 4, PDGN: 9, DSC: 3, HbA1C: 3, gender: 2, therapy: 2, and MED: 39. The data also identified mono and combo therapies for diabetes medications that include metformin (MET), glipizide (GLP), Insulin (INS), glimepiride (GLI), glyburide (GLY), rosiglitazone (ROS), pioglitazone (PIO) and their combinations.

Statistical Analysis

The association between the features used for the analysis was determined with Chi-squared analysis while using Multivariate Logistic Regression (MLR) to compute risk factors and their severities by computing the relative risks (RR) at a 95% confidence level. The probability of 30-day URA was determined from the MLR following Eq. (16.1). Thus, for the 30-day URA (η) (that has predictor values denoted by x_1, x_2, .., x_n) with a dichotomous representation of 1 and 0 (1: 30-day URA, 0: no URA), if the probability of 30-day URA $Pr = Pr(\eta = 1)$, and there is an assumption of a linear relationship, then the probability Pr, log-odd l and RR of 30-day URA at η =1 is expressed in Eq. (16.1).

$$\begin{cases} P_r &= \dfrac{1}{1 + e^{-l}} \\ l &= log_{10}\dfrac{P_r}{1 - P_r} = \alpha_0 + \alpha_1 x_1 + \ldots + \alpha_k x_n \\ RR &= e^{-l} \end{cases} \tag{16.1}$$

where α_0, α_1, … , α_n are the coefficient of the intercept, and the coefficient of predictors 1, …, n.

The benchmark described by Ayatollahi et al. (2017) for estimating the risk severities in hospitals as low, moderate, and high was adopted for understanding the trends of 30-day URA risk for the various cultures considered. The computation of the RR based on Eq. (16.1) provided information about the influences of the various artifacts and sub-artifacts relating to the risk of 30-day URA. The accuracy, brier score loss, and AUC of the 30-day URA were determined by using the ground truth and predicted 30-day URA status.

Reflection, Learning, and Formalization of Design Principles

The reflection and learning are paralleled stages that are continuous in the entire process of designing and formulating the requisite digital solution for the risk factors and their severities for 30-day URA of patients with diabetes. Hence, minimizing 30-day URA involves understanding the artifacts (contributing risk factors and their severities) to facilitate quick and efficient management of patients to improve their hospitalization experience as well as improve their quality of life after discharge. The interaction of the ADR processes in the architecture shown in Figure 16.1 leads to the building of digital intervention tools that will also provide healthcare practitioners with a medium for both learning and reflective practices to forestall 30-day URA vis-à-vis providing value-based treatment for comorbid patients with diabetes. Imperatively, the learning and reflective process during problem formulation; building, intervention, and evaluation, and the formulation of learning into a creative solution in the form of a digital tool helped to maximize the benefits of effective digital tool development. The benefit of this reflection and learning is maximized via a cost-effective and practical strategy utilization to facilitate meaningful actions (Anseel et al. 2009) that help clinicians minimize 30-day URA. This can result in an improvement in patients' experience of diabetes and comorbid diabetes treatment, seeing that therapeutic misconception, healthcare workers' levity, comorbidity burden, and poor diagnosis (Bianco et al. 2012; van der Does et al. 2020; Considine et al. 2020) can hamper recovery post-discharge and result in 30-day URA.

RESULTS

Overview of 30-Day Unplanned Readmission of Comorbid Patients with Diabetes

Of the 17,933 patients identified for this study, 10.71% had 30-day URA with 10.93% females and 10.47% males returning to the hospital after discharge within 30 days. Patients who are described as non-BIPOC have the highest 30-day URA of 10.98%, followed by AA-BIPOC with 9.94%, while BIPOC patients have the least 30-day URA at 9.63%. The 30-day

URA for the age groups varied from 9.28 to 10.95%, PDGN is from 8.62 to 12.22% with patients in the age group of 60–70 years having the highest rate. For medication therapy and types, those on combo therapy have 9.44% of 30-day URA, monotherapy-treated patients have 11.59%, whereas patients treated with GLY-PIO have a 17.31% rate, which is the highest. The remainder of the baseline characteristics of the cohorts are shown in Table 16.1.

Table 16.2 shows the cumulative rate of 30-day URA for the various cultural backgrounds and primary comorbidity diagnosis of the patients treated with the various diabetes medications. Patients diagnosed with circulatory system conditions (CIR) are most prone to 30-day URA with non-BIPOC patients having the most likelihood at 3.69%, compared to the BIPOC and AA-BIPOC which have 3.18% and 3.3%, respectively. Apart from those who were diagnosed with DIA, RES, and OTH disease conditions as their primary diagnosis, the 30-day URA rates of the remaining comorbidities are < 1%.

According to Figure 16.2, the patients at high risk of 30-day URA are <1% of the population prone to URA despite their cultural group, while BIPOC patients have the highest rate of patients at low risk of 30-day URA followed by AA-BIPOC, but non-BIPOC patients constituted the most moderate risk-prone patients. The number of BIPOC patients exposed to high risk of 30-day URA is 238%, 177%, and 780% respectively more than all the patients, non-BIPOC, and AA-BIPOC patients at high risk.

Risk Factors of 30-Day Unplanned Readmission

The risk factors for 30-day URA and their severities measured as the *RR* for all the patients and the various cultural groups are shown in Table 16.3. At 95% significant level, the risk factors are as follows: all patients {ADM(TRF), ADT (ELE, UGT, EMG), ages, PDGN (DIG, INJ, MUS, OTH, RES), DSC (FAC, HOSP, OTH), HbA1C (7–8, >8), MED (GLY), NDG, NEM, NIP, NOU, NLB, race (AA-BIPOC)}. So, compared to non-BIPOC patients, AA-BIPOC patients are prone to 30-day URA after discharge, but not BIPOC patients. The most pronounced risk factors for all the patients are DSC (FAC) – 1.41(1.25–1.59), P: <0.0001; DSC (HOSP) – 1.41(1.06–1.86), P: 0.0165; DSC(OTH) – 1.27(1.08–1.51), P: 0.0047; and NIP – 1.23(1.19–1.28), P: <0.0001. Table 16.3 highlights the 30-day URA risk factors for culturally diverse patients and shows that DSC (FAC, HOSP, OTH) are the only risk factor for 30-day URA for non-BIPOC patients. For AA-BIPOC patients, NIP – 1.23(1.12–1.36), P:

TABLE 16.1 Baseline Characteristics of the Study Population Showing the Cohorts That Have 30-Day Unplanned Readmission (NB: *mean ± std)

Features	No (n, %)	Yes (n, %)	Features	No (n, %)	Yes (n, %)
Samples	16013(89.29%)	1920(10.71%)	MED		
Race			GLI	189(90.43%)	20(9.57%)
AA-BIPOC	3370(90.06%)	372(9.94%)	GLI-INS	276(89.9%)	31(10.1%)
BIPOC	713(90.37%)	76(9.63%)	GLI-PIO-INS	53(89.83%)	6(10.17%)
non-BIPOC	11930(89.02%)	1472(10.98%)	GLP	637(87.14%)	94(12.86%)
Gender			GLP-INS	728(89.88%)	82(10.12%)
Female	8275(89.07%)	1015(10.93%)	GLP-PIO	76(95%)	4(5%)
Male	7738(89.53%)	905(10.47%)	GLP-PIO-INS	81(89.01%)	10(10.99%)
Age			GLP-ROS	67(93.06%)	5(6.94%)
40–50 years	1917(89.2%)	232(10.8%)	GLP-ROS-INS	80(87.91%)	11(12.09%)
50–60 years	3006(90.41%)	319(9.59%)	GLY	570(90.19%)	62(9.81%)
60–70 years	3269(89.05%)	402(10.95%)	GLY-INS	483(91.13%)	47(8.87%)
70–80 years	3579(88.11%)	483(11.89%)	GLY-PIO	43(82.69%)	9(17.31%)
<40 years	1584(90.72%)	162(9.28%)	GLY-PIO-INS	58(90.63%)	6(9.38%)
>80 years	2658(89.19%)	322(10.81%)	GLY-ROS	47(94%)	3(6%)
HbA1C			GLY-ROS-INS	65(90.28%)	7(9.72%)
<7	4775(89.12%)	583(10.88%)	INS	6761(88.34%)	892(11.66%)
7–8	3761(89.04%)	463(10.96%)	MET	770(88.4%)	101(11.6%)
>8	7477(89.53%)	874(10.47%)	MET-GLI	71(95.95%)	3(4.05%)
PDGN			MET-GLI-INS	159(89.33%)	19(10.67%)
CIR	4663(87.93%)	640(12.07%)	MET-GLP	226(89.68%)	26(10.32%)
DIA	2561(89.99%)	285(10.01%)	MET-GLP-INS	372(93%)	28(7%)
DIG	1073(87.95%)	147(12.05%)	MET-GLP-PIO-INS	52(92.86%)	4(7.14%)
GEN	672(88.42%)	88(11.58%)	MET-GLP-ROS	105(88.24%)	14(11.76%)
INJ	403(91.38%)	38(8.62%)	MET-GLY	306(92.45%)	25(7.55%)

(Continued)

TABLE 16.1 (Continued) Baseline Characteristics of the Study Population Showing the Cohorts That Have 30-Day Unplanned Readmission (NB: *mean ± std)

Features	No (n, %)	Yes (n, %)	Features	No (n, %)	Yes (n, %)
MUS	489(90.22%)	53(9.78%)	MET-GLY-INS	290(92.95%)	22(7.05%)
NEO	309(87.78%)	43(12.22%)	MET-GLY-ROS	51(92.73%)	4(7.27%)
OTH	3272(89.45%)	386(10.55%)	MET-GLY-ROS-INS	52(88.14%)	7(11.86%)
RES	2571(91.46%)	240(8.54%)	MET-INS	980(91.33%)	93(8.67%)
Therapy			MET-PIO	65(97.01%)	2(2.99%)
combo	6686(90.56%)	697(9.44%)	MET-PIO-INS	136(90.07%)	15(9.93%)
mono	9327(88.41%)	1223(11.59%)	MET-ROS	81(84.38%)	15(15.63%)
ADM			MET-ROS-INS	135(88.24%)	18(11.76%)
EMG	8879(89.33%)	1061(10.67%)	OTH	831(91.12%)	81(8.88%)
OTH	3113(88.11%)	420(11.89%)	PIO	182(87.08%)	27(12.92%)
REF	3229(89.77%)	368(10.23%)	PIO-INS	327(86.74%)	50(13.26%)
TRA	792(91.77%)	71(8.23%)	REP	44(88%)	6(12%)
ADT			REP-INS	129(88.36%)	17(11.64%)
ELE	1522(90.76%)	155(9.24%)	ROS	149(88.17%)	20(11.83%)
EMG	8180(89.65%)	944(10.35%)	ROS-INS	286(89.38%)	34(10.63%)
OTH	3719(87.63%)	525(12.37%)	NDG*	7.31(±2.03)	7.62(±1.82)
UGT	2592(89.75%)	296(10.25%)	NEM*	0.2(±0.75)	0.42(±1.38)
DSC			NIP*	0.47(±1.04)	1.02(±1.96)
FAC	4783(86.74%)	731(13.26%)	NLB*	48.59(±20.09)	48.47(±20.61)
HOME	9409(91.15%)	913(8.85%)	NMD*	16.77(±8.27)	17.8(±8.37)
HOSP	411(86.16%)	66(13.84%)	NOU*	0.39(±1.33)	0.43(±1.15)
OTH	1410(87.04%)	210(12.96%)	NPR*	1.18(±1.69)	1.24(±1.7)
			TIH*	4.81(±3.09)	5.17(±3.11)

TABLE 16.2 Cumulative Rate of 30-Day Unplanned Readmission for Different Cultural Diversities and Patients' Primary Diagnosis

Features	All Patients (n = 1920, 10.71%)	Non-BIPOC (n = 1472, 10.98%)	AA-BIPOC (n = 372, 9.94%)	BIPOC (n = 76, 9.63%)
CIR	640(3.57%)	495(3.69%)	119(3.18%)	26(3.3%)
DIA	285(1.59%)	203(1.51%)	70(1.87%)	12(1.52%)
DIG	147(0.82%)	115(0.86%)	25(0.67%)	7(0.89%)
GEN	88(0.49%)	69(0.51%)	17(0.45%)	2(0.25%)
INJ	38(0.21%)	30(0.22%)	6(0.16%)	2(0.25%)
MUS	53(0.3%)	41(0.31%)	11(0.29%)	1(0.13%)
NEO	43(0.24%)	31(0.23%)	9(0.24%)	3(0.38%)
OTH	386(2.15%)	288(2.15%)	83(2.22%)	15(1.9%)
RES	240(1.34%)	200(1.49%)	32(0.86%)	8(1.01%)

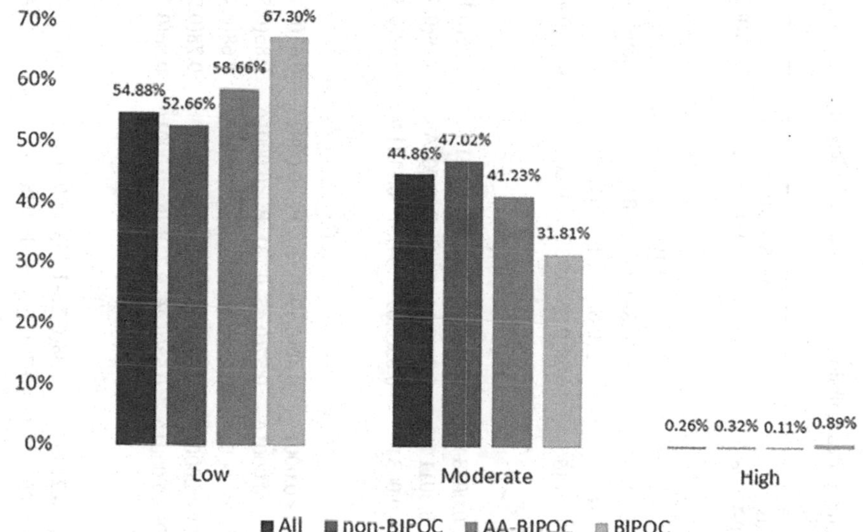

FIGURE 16.2 30-Day unplanned readmission risk of the patients arranged according to risk severity and cultural diversity.

<0.0001; NEM – 1.15(1.04–1.28), P: 0.0087; and NPR – 1.09(1.01–1.17), P: 0.0338 are risk factors of concern whereas NIP – 1.31(1.03–1.65), P: 0.0251 remains the risk factor of concern for BIPOC patients.

The accuracy of prediction of the probability of the 30-day URA for the various cultural groups has been captured in Figure 16.3 which showed patients with BIPOC backgrounds were predicted with the highest accuracy {acc: 90.75%, AUC: 76%, BSL: 7.57%} while non-BIPOC patients have the least accuracy {acc: 89.07%, AUC: 64%, BSL: 9.47%}.

TABLE 16.3 Predictors of 30-Day Unplanned Readmission for Patients of Different Cultural Backgrounds (^, Significant at 95% Confidence Level; CI, Confidence Interval)

Parameters	All Patients RR (95% CI), P-Value	Non-BIPOC RR (95% CI), P-Value	AA-BIPOC RR (95% CI), P-Value	BIPOC RR (95% CI), P-Value
ADM				
OTH	ref	ref	ref	ref
EMG	0.97(0.8–1.17), P: 0.7163	0.99(0.8–1.23), P: 0.9338	0.69(0.42–1.13), P: 0.1423	1.04(0.4–2.75), P: 0.9316
REF	0.9(0.73–1.1), P: 0.3136	0.79(0.62–1), P: 0.0495^	1.08(0.64–1.83), P: 0.7709	1.72(0.65–4.57), P: 0.274
TRA	0.68(0.5–0.93), P: 0.0146^	0.49(0.33–0.73), P: 0.0004^	0.86(0.46–1.62), P: 0.6454	2.11(0.5–8.86), P: 0.3088
ADT				
OTH	ref	ref	ref	ref
ELE	0.7(0.55–0.88), P: 0.0028^	0.94(0.72–1.22), P: 0.6216	0.26(0.13–0.49), P: <0.0001^	0.18(0.05–0.7), P: 0.0134^
EMG	0.77(0.66–0.9), P: 0.0011^	0.79(0.66–0.94), P: 0.007^	0.79(0.51–1.2), P: 0.264	0.5(0.23–1.08), P: 0.0777
UGT	0.76(0.64–0.91), P: 0.0034^	0.85(0.69–1.04), P: 0.1121	0.49(0.3–0.79), P: 0.0039^	0.72(0.32–1.61), P: 0.4198
AGE				
<40 years	ref	ref	ref	ref
>80 years	0.53(0.43–0.65), P: <0.0001^	0.49(0.39–0.62), P: <0.0001^	0.67(0.4–1.13), P: 0.1347	0.78(0.24–2.51), P: 0.6718
40–50 years	0.67(0.55–0.81), P: <0.0001^	0.57(0.45–0.73), P: <0.0001^	0.85(0.58–1.22), P: 0.3723	1.32(0.48–3.67), P: 0.5919
50–60 years	0.59(0.49–0.71), P: <0.0001^	0.55(0.44–0.7), P: <0.0001^	0.68(0.47–0.99), P: 0.0433^	0.46(0.15–1.4), P: 0.1699
60–70 years	0.67(0.56–0.81), P: <0.0001^	0.62(0.5–0.78), P: <0.0001^	0.78(0.53–1.15), P: 0.2063	0.92(0.33–2.57), P: 0.871
70–80 years	0.64(0.53–0.78), P: <0.0001^	0.58(0.46–0.72), P: <0.0001^	0.86(0.57–1.28), P: 0.4506	1.21(0.43–3.43), P: 0.7165
PDGN				
DIA	ref	ref	ref	ref
CIR	0.91(0.78–1.06), P: 0.2185	0.88(0.73–1.05), P: 0.1632	1.07(0.77–1.5), P: 0.6877	0.62(0.27–1.43), P: 0.2615
DIG	0.7(0.57–0.87), P: 0.0012^	0.7(0.55–0.9), P: 0.0053^	0.76(0.47–1.24), P: 0.2791	0.37(0.13–1.04), P: 0.0597

GEN	0.79(0.61–1.02), P: 0.0725	0.77(0.57–1.03), P: 0.0765	1.13(0.63–2.01), P: 0.6866	0.25(0.05–1.29), P: 0.0978
INJ	0.53(0.37–0.76), P: 0.0005^	0.47(0.31–0.71), P: 0.0003^	1.09(0.43–2.76), P: 0.8567	0.23(0.04–1.31), P: 0.0983
MUS	0.57(0.41–0.78), P: 0.0005^	0.5(0.35–0.72), P: 0.0002^	1.33(0.65–2.75), P: 0.4335	0.13(0.01–1.23), P: 0.0753
NEO	0.85(0.6–1.21), P: 0.374	0.75(0.5–1.14), P: 0.1778	1.34(0.6–2.97), P: 0.4748	0.91(0.18–4.7), P: 0.911
OTH	0.65(0.55–0.76), P: <0.0001^	0.6(0.5–0.72), P: <0.0001^	0.89(0.64–1.24), P: 0.5022	0.3(0.13–0.69), P: 0.0042^
RES	0.54(0.45–0.65), P: <0.0001^	0.56(0.46–0.69), P: <0.0001^	0.52(0.33–0.8), P: 0.0034^	0.23(0.08–0.65), P: 0.0051^
DSC				
HOME	ref	ref	ref	ref
FAC	1.41(1.25–1.59), P: <0.0001^	1.48(1.29–1.7), P: <0.0001^	1.12(0.84–1.5), P: 0.4488	1.86(0.97–3.57), P: 0.0627
HOSP	1.41(1.06–1.86), P: 0.0165^	1.47(1.08–2), P: 0.0132^	1.31(0.59–2.9), P: 0.51	1.46(0.3–7.1), P: 0.6383
OTH	1.27(1.08–1.51), P: 0.0047^	1.36(1.12–1.65), P: 0.002^	1.16(0.8–1.7), P: 0.4273	1.27(0.39–4.11), P: 0.6896
Gender				
Female	ref	ref	ref	ref
Male	0.83(0.75–0.91), P: <0.0001^	0.82(0.73–0.91), P: 0.0003^	0.85(0.69–1.06), P: 0.1506	1.18(0.69–1.99), P: 0.5467
HbA1C				
<7	ref	ref	ref	ref
7–8	0.78(0.69–0.88), P: <0.0001^	0.73(0.63–0.84), P: <0.0001^	1.03(0.76–1.4), P: 0.8319	1.01(0.51–2.02), P: 0.9695
>8	0.67(0.6–0.75), P: <0.0001^	0.69(0.6–0.78), P: <0.0001^	0.69(0.54–0.87), P: 0.002^	0.42(0.22–0.8), P: 0.0081^
MED				
INS	ref	ref	ref	ref
GLI	0.8(0.5–1.29), P: 0.3615	0.84(0.49–1.43), P: 0.5185	0.63(0.19–2.14), P: 0.4635	0.57(0.06–5.23), P: 0.6215
GLI-INS	0.35(0.05–2.78), P: 0.3238	0.47(0.06–3.86), P: 0.4833	-	0(0–0), P: 0.9998
GLI-PIO-INS	0.41(0.05–3.67), P: 0.4241	0.7(0.07–6.74), P: 0.7599	-	0(0–0), P: 0.9997
GLP	0.96(0.76–1.22), P: 0.7599	1.01(0.78–1.32), P: 0.9224	0.78(0.43–1.43), P: 0.423	0.75(0.23–2.47), P: 0.6304
GLP-INS	0.32(0.04–2.47), P: 0.2755	0.53(0.07–4.2), P: 0.547	-	-
GLP-PIO	0.12(0.01–1.18), P: 0.0694	0.11(0.01–1.37), P: 0.0864	-	-

(Continued)

TABLE 16.3 (Continued) Predictors of 30-Day Unplanned Readmission for Patients of Different Cultural Backgrounds (^, Significant at 95% Confidence Level; CI, Confidence Interval)

Parameters	All Patients RR (95% CI), P-Value	Non-BIPOC RR (95% CI), P-Value	AA-BIPOC RR (95% CI), P-Value	BIPOC RR (95% CI), P-Value
GLP-PIO-INS	0.37(0.04–3.14), P: 0.3651	0.65(0.07–5.67), P: 0.6933	-	-
GLP-ROS	0.19(0.02–1.79), P: 0.1486	0.39(0.04–3.69), P: 0.4096	-	-
GLP-ROS-INS	0.35(0.04–2.95), P: 0.3373	0.61(0.07–5.32), P: 0.6556	-	-
GLY	0.73(0.55–0.96), P: 0.027^	0.76(0.56–1.04), P: 0.0849	0.71(0.36–1.43), P: 0.3434	0.5(0.06–4.48), P: 0.5365
GLY-INS	0.27(0.03–2.06), P: 0.2055	0.43(0.05–3.43), P: 0.4236	-	-
GLY-PIO	0.52(0.06–4.5), P: 0.5527	0.92(0.1–8.21), P: 0.9397	-	-
GLY-PIO-INS	0.34(0.04–3.03), P: 0.3313	0.62(0.07–5.72), P: 0.6705	-	-
GLY-ROS	0.19(0.02–2.01), P: 0.1694	0.25(0.02–3.11), P: 0.2834	-	-
GLY-ROS-INS	0.33(0.04–2.89), P: 0.3163	0.37(0.04–3.65), P: 0.3928	-	-
MET	0.9(0.72–1.13), P: 0.3551	0.96(0.74–1.24), P: 0.7429	0.67(0.39–1.16), P: 0.1526	1.31(0.44–3.95), P: 0.6256
MET-GLI	0.14(0.01–1.41), P: 0.0941	0.28(0.03–2.97), P: 0.2905	-	-
MET-GLI-INS	0.41(0.05–3.3), P: 0.4038	0.61(0.07–5.11), P: 0.6463	-	-
MET-GLP	0.33(0.04–2.57), P: 0.2877	0.56(0.07–4.6), P: 0.5905	-	-
MET-GLP-INS	0.23(0.03–1.8), P: 0.1617	0.38(0.05–3.15), P: 0.372	-	-
MET-GLP-PIO-INS	0.24(0.02–2.32), P: 0.2168	0.23(0.02–2.81), P: 0.249	-	-
MET-GLP-ROS	0.48(0.06–3.93), P: 0.4952	0.88(0.1–7.53), P: 0.9082	-	-
MET-GLY	0.23(0.03–1.78), P: 0.1571	0.37(0.05–3.07), P: 0.3599	-	-
MET-GLY-INS	0.22(0.03–1.76), P: 0.154	0.43(0.05–3.55), P: 0.4335	-	-
MET-GLY-ROS	0.2(0.02–1.96), P: 0.1675	0.3(0.03–3.21), P: 0.3201	-	-
MET-GLY-ROS-INS	0.41(0.05–3.59), P: 0.4193	0.77(0.08–7.21), P: 0.8212	-	-
MET-INS	0.27(0.04–2.09), P: 0.2122	0.4(0.05–3.14), P: 0.3811	-	-

MET-PIO	0.09(0.01–1.09), P: 0.0585	0.19(0.02–2.33), P: 0.1947	-	-
MET-PIO-INS	0.36(0.04–2.88), P: 0.3328	0.61(0.07–5.24), P: 0.6528	-	-
MET-ROS	0.46(0.06–3.78), P: 0.4721	0.97(0.11–8.22), P: 0.9791	-	-
MET-ROS-INS	0.42(0.05–3.36), P: 0.4121	0.64(0.08–5.43), P: 0.683	-	-
OTH	0.32(0.04–2.4), P: 0.2682	0.5(0.07–3.85), P: 0.5067	-	-
PIO	1.02(0.67–1.55), P: 0.9371	0.94(0.57–1.57), P: 0.8251	1.02(0.43–2.42), P: 0.9704	1.23(0.16–9.2), P: 0.8393
PIO-INS	0.4(0.05–3.06), P: 0.3748	0.61(0.08–4.88), P: 0.6383	-	-
REP	0.99(0.41–2.38), P: 0.986	0.81(0.28–2.33), P: 0.6941	0.86(0.1–7.23), P: 0.8879	6.66(0.52–85.05), P: 0.1445
REP-INS	0.4(0.05–3.2), P: 0.3859	0.6(0.07–5.1), P: 0.6435	-	-
ROS	0.93(0.58–1.5), P: 0.7674	1.13(0.67–1.92), P: 0.648	0.48(0.14–1.67), P: 0.2487	-
ROS-INS	0.31(0.04–2.45), P: 0.2693	0.47(0.06–3.81), P: 0.4781	-	-
NDG	0.91(0.89–0.94), P: <0.0001^	0.91(0.89–0.94), P: <0.0001^	0.92(0.87–0.97), P: 0.0021^	0.92(0.8–1.06), P: 0.2383
NEM	1.09(1.04–1.14), P: 0.0006^	1.07(1.02–1.13), P: 0.0102^	1.15(1.04–1.28), P: 0.0087^	1.05(0.76–1.45), P: 0.7672
NIP	1.23(1.19–1.28), P: <0.0001^	1.23(1.19–1.28), P: <0.0001^	1.23(1.12–1.36), P: <0.0001^	1.31(1.03–1.65), P: 0.0251^
NLB	0.99(0.99–1), P: 0.0002^	1(0.99–1), P: 0.0138^	0.99(0.98–1), P: 0.0012^	0.99(0.97–1), P: 0.0942
NMD	1(0.99–1.01), P: 0.7948	1(0.99–1.01), P: 0.7067	1.01(0.99–1.03), P: 0.57	1.01(0.96–1.06), P: 0.7926
NOU	0.94(0.9–0.98), P: 0.0075^	0.95(0.91–1), P: 0.0323^	0.89(0.77–1.04), P: 0.1491	0.9(0.68–1.21), P: 0.4959
NPR	1.03(0.99–1.06), P: 0.1047	1.01(0.97–1.05), P: 0.6192	1.09(1.01–1.17), P: 0.0338^	1.21(1–1.46), P: 0.0554
TIH	1.01(0.99–1.03), P: 0.5364	1.01(0.98–1.03), P: 0.5545	1(0.96–1.04), P: 0.9309	0.98(0.88–1.1), P: 0.7457
Therapy				
mono	ref	ref		
combo	2.63(0.35–19.84), P: 0.3488	1.73(0.22–13.49), P: 0.6002	-	-
RACE				
non-BIPOC	ref			-
AA-BIPOC	0.78(0.69–0.89), P: 0.0001^	-	-	-
BIPOC	0.78(0.61–1), P: 0.0507	-	-	-

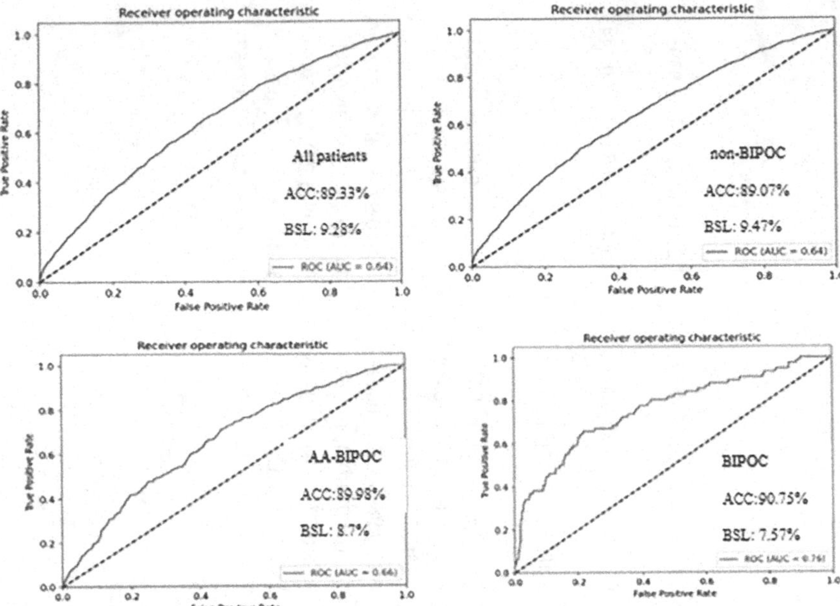

FIGURE 16.3 Prediction accuracy of multivariate Logistic regression model used for predicting the risk factors of 30-day unplanned readmission of all the patients and the cultural diversity. BSL, Brier score loss; acc, accuracy; AUC, area under the curve.

DISCUSSION

This study relies on the ADR paradigm to identify the artifacts that relate to 30-day URA of comorbid patients with diabetes treated with either mono or combo therapy that includes INS, MET, GLY, GLI, GLP, ROS, ROS, PIO, MET-GLY, and the combinations of the various medications. By gaining insights from the secondary data of patients from different cultural backgrounds treated for primary diagnosis based on ICD-9 coding using KDD, the risk factors and their severities were identified. The risk factors such as age, comorbidities (DIG, INJ, MUS, NEO), DSC, HbA1C, and race (AA-BIPOC) are similar to some of the findings by previous researchers (Collin et al. 2017; Rie et al. 2015). However, medications (except GLY- 0.73(0.55–0.96), P: 0.027) are not risk factors at 95% confidence level since the P-values are >0.05. Even at this, other researchers such as Png et al. (2018) attributed diabetes-related medication adherence to late URA, which occurs between 31 and 180 days.

The significance of this study on diabetes management cannot be overemphasized seeing that the knowledge of the risk factors has a far-reaching implication for effective clinical practice, which can reduce the practice variation that is inherent across many healthcare settings (Atsma et al. 2020). Even though the ability of clinicians to draw inferences from previous experiences and that of others in managing health conditions is vital for reflective practice (Mantzourani et al. 2019), the combination of this approach with the pre-knowledge of the risk factors will enhance patients' outcomes.

The patients who have African American background are shown to be at risk of 30-day URA. Unfortunately, African Americans also have a very high rate of diabetes-related morbidity (Cunningham et al. 2018), which is one of the risk attributes of patients who have 30-day URA (Bianco et al. 2012; van der Does et al. 2020). Again, the HbA1C of patients with a reading of <7% is not very different from those whose readings are 7–8% and >8%. Previous studies have also linked the increased mortality of patients with diabetes to the increasing levels of HbA1C (Forbes et al. 2018). HbA1C abnormality is also linked to comorbidities such as microvascular diseases, peripheral arterial disease, cardiovascular diseases, and chronic kidney disease (Kang et al. 2015; Li et al. 2020; Muntner et al. 2005; Saba et al. 2013; Yang et al. 2020). Thus, despite the low-risk level (as indicated by the RR) of HbA1C for all the patients {7–8%: 0.78(0.69–0.88), P: <0.0001; >8%: 0.67(0.6–0.75), P: <0.0001}, it is important that intensive glycaemic normalization and glucose variability controls are targeted in diabetes treatment to ensure optimal clinical outcome (Yang et al. 2020) that will forestall 30-day URA.

Some of the limitations of this study are the small populations of some of the sub-classes of the predictors used. This caused the MLR not to have results for the risk severity of some of the predictors because of the infinite values obtained following the few or no 30-day URA associated with such features. This calls for bigger data that will be able to capture the 30-day URA status of patients in a reasonable size for the various classes of predictors considered. It may also be necessary to reduce some of the sub-classes to a more manageable size to make it easier to interpret the results obtained from the analysis, an approach that may be suitable for the medications considered in this study. The need for considering late URA for patients who were readmitted after 30 days of discharge would have complimented this study, seeing that understanding the risk factors of long-term URA will help to reduce the cost of healthcare despite the cogent need for minimizing early URA before 30 days of discharge. Finally, lumping the comorbidities in broader classes such as

CIR conditions makes it difficult to figure out the real impacts of most comorbidities on 30-day URA. This makes it imperative to narrow the study down to unique comorbidities such as stroke, hypertension, heart failure, dementia, etc.

CONCLUSIONS

This study relied on ADR to develop a strategy for identifying the artifacts associated with the risk of 30-day URA for comorbid patients of diabetes treated with mono and combo therapies that include INS, MET, GLY, GLI, GLP, ROS, ROS, PIO, MET-GLY, MET-PIO-INS, and their combinations. Hence, the formulation of a strategy that hinged on the KDD for identifying the risk factors and their severities for patients from diverse cultural backgrounds such as non-BIPOC, BIPOC, and AA-BIPOC to understand how the various predictors considered in the study contribute to an early URA 30 days after hospital discharge. Following the reflection and learning obtained from the problem formulation stage of the ADR, and the building, intervention, and evaluation of the secondary data from patients' records, it was possible to formulate a creative solution that identified the risk factors and their severities for all the patients and those from the Caucasian background (non-BIPOC), African American race (AA-BIPOC) and other races that are neither Caucasians nor African Americans (BIPOC).

It was found that patients from AA-BIPOC backgrounds are most prone to 30-day URA when compared to other cultural backgrounds even though the rate of 30-day URA for all races is within a 2% difference from 9.63–10.98%. The risk of 30-day URA for all patients is highest with patients who are discharged to other facilities (DSC-FAC) and hospitals (DSC-HOSP). For non-BIPOC patients, the highest risk factor is associated with DSC-FAC while NIP is the highest risk factor for patients of AA-BIPOC and BIPOC backgrounds. The risk associated with HbA1C levels is low (RR of <1), however, the potential of uncontrollable blood sugar levels triggering a major health crisis for patients with diabetes cannot be overemphasized, thus the need for intensive glycaemic normalization and glucose variability controls to ensure optimal clinical outcomes for comorbid patients with diabetes.

ACKNOWLEDGEMENTS

This chapter is from a project around risk mitigation and readmission that was made possible from funding received by the author from

Epworth Medical Foundation. The author acknowledges with gratitude the work of the key research assistant Dr Chinedu Ossai who was responsible for all the technical aspects of the project.

REFERENCES

Anseel, F., Lievens, F. and Schollaert, E., 2009. "Reflection as a strategy to enhance task performance after feedback". *Organizational Behavior and Human Decision Processes*, 110(1), pp.23–35.

Atsma, F., Elwyn, G. and Westert, G., 2020. "Understanding unwarranted variation in clinical practice: A focus on network effects, reflective medicine and learning health systems". *International Journal for Quality in Health Care*, 32(4), pp.271–274.

Australian Institute of Health and Welfare (AIHW). 2017. Australia's Hospitals 2016–17 at a Glance; Australian Institute of Health and Welfare: Canberra, Australia.

Avison, D.E., Lau, F., Myers, M.D. and Nielsen, P.A., 1999. "Action research". *Communications of the ACM*, 42(1), pp.94–97.

Ayatollahi, H. and Shagerdi, G., 2017. "Information security risk assessment in hospitals". *The Open Medical Informatics Journal*, 11, p.37.

Bianco, A., Molè, A., Nobile, C.G., Di Giuseppe, G., Pileggi, C. and Angelillo, I.F., 2012. "Hospital readmission prevalence and analysis of those potentially avoidable in southern Italy". *PloS One*, 7(11), p.e48263.

Bohanec, M., Robnik-Šikonja, M. and Borštnar, M.K., 2017. "Decision-making framework with double-loop learning through interpretable black-box machine learning models". *Industrial Management & Data Systems*. Vol. 117, No. 7, pp. 1389–1406. https://doi.org/10.1108/IMDS-09-2016-0409

Budnitz, D.S., Lovegrove, M.C., Shehab, N. and Richards, C.L., 2011. "Emergency hospitalizations for adverse drug events in older Americans". *New England Journal of Medicine*, 365(21), pp.2002–2012.

Chatterjee, P., Tesis, A., Cymberknop, L.J. and Armentano, R.L., 2020. "Internet of things and artificial intelligence in healthcare during COVID-19 pandemic—A South American perspective". *Frontiers in Public Health*. Dec 16; 8: 600213. doi: 10.3389/fpubh.2020.600213. PMID: 33392139; PMCID: PMC7772467.

Clement, R.C., Kheir, M.M., Derman, P.B., Flynn, D.N., Speck, R.M., Levin, L.S. and Fleisher, L.A., 2014. "What are the economic consequences of unplanned readmissions after TKA?". *Clinical Orthopaedics and Related Research®*, 472(10), pp.3134–3141.

Collins, J., Abbass, I.M., Harvey, R., Suehs, B., Uribe, C., Bouchard, J., Prewitt, T., DeLuzio, T. and Allen, E., 2017. "Predictors of all-cause 30 day readmission among Medicare patients with type 2 diabetes". *Current Medical Research and Opinion*, 33(8), pp.1517–1523.

Considine, J., Berry, D., Sprogis, S.K., Newnham, E., Fox, K., Darzins, P., Rawson, H. and Street, M., 2020. "Understanding the patient experience of early unplanned hospital readmission following acute care discharge: A qualitative descriptive study". *BMJ Open*, 10(5), p.e034728.

Considine, J., Fox, K., Plunkett, D., Mecner, M., O'Reilly, M. and Darzins, P., 2017. "Factors associated with unplanned readmissions in a major Australian health service". *Australian Health Review*, 43(1), pp.1–9.

Cunningham, A.T., Crittendon, D.R., White, N., Mills, G.D., Diaz, V. and LaNoue, M.D., 2018. "The effect of diabetes self-management education on HbA1c and quality of life in African-Americans: A systematic review and meta-analysis". *BMC Health Services Research*, 18(1), pp.1–13.

Fayyad, U.M., Piatetsky-Shapiro, G. and Smyth, P., 1996, August. "Knowledge discovery and data mining: Towards a unifying framework". In *KDD*. Vol. 17, Issue 3, pp. 37–54.

Fluitman, K.S., Van Galen, L.S., Merten, H., Rombach, S.M., Brabrand, M., Cooksley, T., Nickel, C.H., Subbe, C.P., Kramer, M.H.H. and Nanayakkara, P.W.B., 2016. "Exploring the preventable causes of unplanned readmissions using root cause analysis: Coordination of care is the weakest link". *European Journal of Internal Medicine*, 30, pp.18–24.

Forbes, A., Murrells, T., Mulnier, H. and Sinclair, A.J., 2018. "Mean HbA1c, HbA1c variability, and mortality in people with diabetes aged 70 years and older: A retrospective cohort study". *The Lancet Diabetes & Endocrinology*, 6(6), pp.476–486.

Friedman, B., Jiang, H.J. and Elixhauser, A., 2008. "Costly hospital readmissions and complex chronic illness". *Inquiry: The Journal of Health Care Organization, Provision, and Financing*, 45(4), pp.408–421.

Gould, D., Dowsey, M., Jo, I. and Choong, P., 2020. "Patient-related risk factors for unplanned 30-day readmission following total knee arthroplasty: A narrative literature review". *ANZ Journal of Surgery*, 90(7–8), pp.1253–1258.

Kang, S.H., Jung, D.J., Choi, E.W., Cho, K.H., Park, J.W. and Do, J.Y., 2015. "HbA1c levels are associated with chronic kidney disease in a non-diabetic adult population: A Nationwide survey (KNHANES 2011–2013)". *PLoS One*, 10(12), p.e0145827.

Keijzer-Broers, W. and de Reuver, M., 2016. "Action design research for social innovation: Lessons from designing a health and wellbeing platform". Thirty Seventh International Conference on Information Systems, Dublin 2016.

Lejarza, F., Calvert, J., Attwood, M.M., Evans, D. and Mao, Q., 2021. "Optimal discharge of patients from intensive care via a data-driven policy learning framework". arXiv preprint arXiv:2112.09315.

Li, S., Nemeth, I., Donnelly, L., Hapca, S., Zhou, K. and Pearson, E.R., 2020. "Visit-to-visit HbA1c variability is associated with cardiovascular disease and microvascular complications in patients with newly diagnosed type 2 diabetes". *Diabetes Care*, 43(2), pp.426–432.

Mantzourani, E., Desselle, S., Le, J., Lonie, J.M. and Lucas, C., 2019. "The role of reflective practice in healthcare professions: Next steps for pharmacy education and practice". *Research in Social and Administrative Pharmacy*, 15(12), pp.1476–1479.

Muntner, P., Wildman, R.P., Reynolds, K., DeSalvo, K.B., Chen, J. and Fonseca, V., 2005. "Relationship between HbA1c level and peripheral arterial disease". *Diabetes Care*, 28(8), pp.1981–1987.

Png, M.E., Yoong, J., Chen, C., Tan, C.S., Tai, E.S., Khoo, E.Y. and Wee, H.L., 2018. "Risk factors and direct medical cost of early versus late unplanned readmissions among diabetes patients at a tertiary hospital in Singapore". *Current Medical Research and Opinion*, 34(6), pp.1071–1080.

Ries, Z., Rungprai, C., Harpole, B., Phruetthiphat, O.A., Gao, Y., Pugely, A. and Phisitkul, P., 2015. "Incidence, risk factors, and causes for thirty-day unplanned readmissions following primary lower-extremity amputation in patients with diabetes". *JBJS*, 97(21), pp.1774–1780.

Rubin, D.J. and Shah, A.A., 2021. "Predicting and preventing acute care re-utilization by patients with diabetes". *Current Diabetes Reports*, 21(9), pp.1–13.

Saba, L., Ikeda, N., Deidda, M., Araki, T., Molinari, F., Meiburger, K.M., Acharya, U.R., Nagashima, Y., Mercuro, G., Nakano, M. and Nicolaides, A., 2013. "Association of automated carotid IMT measurement and HbA1c in Japanese patients with coronary artery disease". *Diabetes Research and Clinical Practice*, 100(3), pp.348–353.

Sarker, I.H., 2021. "Data science and analytics: An overview from data-driven smart computing, decision-making and applications perspective". *SN Computer Science*, 2(5), pp.1–22.

Sein, M.K., Henfridsson, O., Purao, S., Rossi, M. and Lindgren, R., 2011. "Action design research". *MIS Quarterly*, pp.37–56.

Shang, Y., Jiang, K., Wang, L., Zhang, Z., Zhou, S., Liu, Y., Dong, J. and Wu, H., 2021. "The 30-days hospital readmission risk in diabetic patients: Predictive modeling with machine learning classifiers". *BMC Medical Informatics and Decision Making*, 21(2), pp.1–11.

Shebeshi, D.S., Dolja-Gore, X. and Byles, J., 2020. "Unplanned readmission within 28 days of hospital discharge in a longitudinal population-based cohort of older Australian women". *International Journal of Environmental Research and Public Health*, 17(9), p.3136.

Soh, J.G.S., Wong, W.P., Mukhopadhyay, A., Quek, S.C. and Tai, B.C., 2020. "Predictors of 30-day unplanned hospital readmission among adult patients with diabetes mellitus: A systematic review with meta-analysis". *BMJ Open Diabetes Research and Care*, 8(1), p.e001227.

Strack, B., DeShazo, J.P., Gennings, C., Olmo, J.L., Ventura, S., Cios, K.J. and Clore, J.N., 2014. "Impact of HbA1c measurement on hospital readmission rates: Analysis of 70,000 clinical database patient records". *BioMed Research International*, 2014.

Todd, J., Gepp, A., Stern, S. and Vanstone, B.J., 2022. "Improving decision making in the management of hospital readmissions using modern survival analysis techniques". *Decision Support Systems*, p.113747.

van der Does, A.M., Kneepkens, E.L., Uitvlugt, E.B., Jansen, S.L., Schilder, L., Tokmaji, G., Wijers, S.C., Radersma, M., Heijnen, J.N.M., Teunissen, P.F. and Hulshof, P.B., 2020. "Preventability of unplanned readmissions within

30 days of discharge. A cross-sectional, single-center study". *PLoS One*, 15(4), p.e0229940.

Yang, C.Y., Su, P.F., Hung, J.Y., Ou, H.T. and Kuo, S., 2020. "Comparative predictive ability of visit-to-visit HbA1c variability measures for microvascular disease risk in type 2 diabetes". *Cardiovascular Diabetology*, 19(1), pp.1–10.

ACRONYMS

ADM-EMG	admission source (emergency)
ADM-OTH	admission source (planned)
ADM-REF	admission source (referrals)
ADM-TRA	admission source (transferred from other facilities)
ADR	action design research
ADT-ELE	admission type (elective)
ADT-EMG	admission type (emergency)
ADT-OTH	admission type (planned)
ADT-UGT	admission type (urgent)
AUC	area under the curve
BIPOC	Black, Indigenous, and people of colour
BSL	Brier score loss
CMB-CIR	comorbidity (circulatory system)
CMB-DIA	comorbidity (diabetes)
CMB-DIG	comorbidity (digestive)
CMB-GEN	comorbidity (genitourinary)
CMB-INJ	comorbidity (injury and poisoning)
CMB-MUS	comorbidity (musculoskeletal system and connective tissue)
CMB-NEO	comorbidity (neoplasms)
CMB-OTH	comorbidity (others)
CMB-RES	comorbidity (respiratory system)
DSC-FAC	discharge source (care facility)
DSC-HOME	discharge source (home)
DSC-HOSP	discharge source (hospital)
DSC-OTH	discharge source (others)
GLI	Glimepiride
GLI	glimepiride and insulin
GLP	glipizide
GLP-INS	glipizide and insulin
GLY	glyburide

GLY-INS	glyburide-insulin
GLY-MET	glyburide-metformin
GLY-MET-INS	glyburide-metformin-insulin
GLY-ROS	glyburide-rosiglitazone
GLY-ROS-INS	glyburide-rosiglitazone-insulin
HbA1C (<7)	HbA1C less than 7%
HbA1C (>8)	HbA1C greater than 8%
HbA1C (7–8)	HbA1C 7–8%
ICD	International classification of diseases
INS	insulin
IS	information system
IT	information technology
KDD	knowledge discovery and data mining
MED	medication
MET	metformin
MET-GLI-INS	metformin, glimepiride, and insulin
MET-GLP	metformin and glipizide
MET-GLP-INS	metformin, glipizide, and insulin
MET-INS	metformin and insulin
MLR	multivariate logistic regression
NDG	number of diagnoses
NEM	number of emergency visits
NIP	number of inpatient visits
NLB	number of labs
NMD	number of medications
NOU	number of outpatient visits
NPR	number of procedures
NTF	The number of trees in the forest
PDGN	primary diagnosis
PIO	pioglitazone
PIO-INS	pioglitazone, and insulin
ROS-INS	rosiglitazone, and insulin
RR	relative risk
SFT	standard deviation of fit time
STS	standard deviation of test score
THM	monotherapy
TIH	time in hospital
URA	unplanned readmission

CHAPTER 17

Establishing a Digital Twin Architecture for Superior Falls Risk Prediction Using a Bayesian Network Model

Nilmini Wickramasinghe

INTRODUCTION

Falls are most common among the frail and elderly; recent studies show that 70% of inpatients have experienced one form of fall or another in the last 12 months (Coussement et al. 2008) with 2%–15% of those in acute care hospitals experiencing the same feat (Salgado et al. 2004; Nakai et al. 2006). Falls risk assessment using different risk factors such as gait instability, agitated confusion, urinary incontinence, falls history and use of some medications, especially, sedatives/hypnotics have been done by many researchers in different contexts (Woolcott et al. 2009; Seppala et al. 2019; Eglseer et al. 2020), but the need for an effective falls intervention requires enhanced assessment tools; this will make it possible for patients with reversible and manageable risk factors to be given adequate priority to forestall falls on admission and the catastrophic consequences. Some of these consequences such as death, injury, reduced confidence

DOI: 10.1201/9781032699745-21

and performance of functions of daily living, increased length of stay, anxiety and guilt for staff and relatives, and complaint and litigation (Oliver 2008; Ahmad et al. 2012) contribute significantly to the increased cost of healthcare.

To manage fall risk, a recommended strategy of using a fall risk assessment tool has been a standard practice. Some of these tools include Tyndall Bailey Falls Risk Assessment Tool (Tyndall et al. 2020), ONTARIO Modified Stratify (Oliver et al. 1997), environmental risk assessment for Falls (Lai et al. 2011), Falls Risk Assessment Scale for the Elderly (Jester et al. 2005), Morse falls scale (Morse et al. 1989; Kim et al. 2007) and the falls risk assessment Tool (Nandy et al. 2004). Despite the authenticity of these tools in different hospital contexts with respect to the validity of results (Narayanan et al. 2016), the possibility of considering the intrinsic effects of different demographic, clinical and psychosocial conditions is not possible. Again, most of the tools are specific for the elderly (Tyndall et al. 2020) and the use context has been shown to be quite effective for managing falls associated with some characteristic age-dependent factors.

In the context of these challenges, the research question we are asking is *"How can't the chances of an effective interfacing of a digital twin inpatient, the historic falls risk database, and Bayesian network facilitate a flawless prediction of falls risk acuity?"* Considering the importance of fall risk assessment to patients' safety on admission and the need to have an approach that will be able to consider a combination of psychosocial, clinical, demographic, and intrinsic factors associated with the patients, in making decisions about the risk acuity, digital twin becomes a viable alternative. From the agent perspective, the digital twin provides a valuable blueprint for conceiving and designing virtual environments for mirroring the physical world, providing models to replicate trends and outcomes, and supporting decision-making with human users (via an assistance system), it provides a viable alternative (Angelo et al. 2020) for effective falls risk replication framework. For this purpose, we believe that the adoption of a framework that provides an assistance system, which incorporates the Bayesian network model-based falls risk assessment of a digital twin of inpatients, will be vital. This will enhance the quick definition of the clinical, demographic, and psychosocial attributes of inpatients, in a model that highlights the expected fall risk vulnerabilities for specific condition combinations. This structure will also provide personalized information, that will be adopted by the assistance system in making recommendations about the fall risk predisposition of patients on admission.

A SYNOPSIS OF THE DIGITAL TWIN CONCEPT

The concept of digital twins has evolved from NASA in 2002 as a strategy for virtual representation of physical phenomena using simulation and physical models to enhance a seamless understanding of the physical system (Glaessgen et al. 2012; Fuller et al. 2019). The technique has found applications in manufacturing (Josifovska et al. 2019; Zhou et al. 2020), supply chain management (Park et al. 2020), smart cities (Ruohomaki et al. 2018) and healthcare (Rivera et al. 2019; Angelo et al. 2020; Liu et al. 2020) by a combination of physical, mathematical models and artificial intelligence to allows for pure virtual renderings with amazing precision to make it easier to design and enhance physical systems in real-time (Tao et al. 2018). The importance of digital twins in healthcare, especially, in precision medicine is making it possible for healthcare professionals to make pathway planning, medical resource allocation, medical activity prediction, and prognostic and diagnostic medicine (Liu et al. 2019; Rivera et al. 2019). Liu et al. (2019) showed that digital twins can effectively help in personal health management for the elderly by designing a cloud-based digital twin for monitoring, diagnosing, and predicting their health conditions following the analysis of wearable medical devices. According to Rivera et al. (2019), digital twin provides a way to better monitor chronic diseases and their ways of treatment, to minimize the risk to patients while improving their quality of life. The tendency to enhance the decision process for healthcare professionals using digital twins cannot be overemphasized seeing that autonomous computing assistance can be obtained for planning and decision-making processes in treatment, especially, complex conditions (Rivera et al. 2019). Angelo et al. (2020) integrated digital twins and multi-agent systems in trauma management by considering when a patient is helped by a physician at an accident scene before transferring to the hospital emergency department and the trauma management process.

STUDY DESIGN AND METHODOLOGY

Design Science Research Methodology

We have applied the Design Science Research Methodology (DSRM) that involves the development and study of artifacts that use identifiable genres described as computational, optimization, representation and information systems (IS) economic (Elragal and Haddara 2019) to solve practical IS problems (Hevner 2007). The framework follows activities, which can include problem explanation, artifact and requirement definition, artifact design and development, artifact demonstration and artifact evaluation (Martin et al. 2018). To ensure that the fall risk predisposition of inpatients on admission is known with a Bayesian network model-based digital twin, the patient's clinical, demographic, and psychosocial data predisposed to different fall risk levels (low and high) is required. The virtual platform artifact that will be developed uses a system assistance containing secondary data that are modelled with a mathematical formulation, thus, enabling seamless estimation of fall risk. The use of a Bayesian network to identify the hidden patterns in inpatient digital twins considering the characteristic features of the secondary data obtained from hospitals, aligns with the computational and optimization genre of DSRM (Elragal and Haddara 2019). Since the mathematical basis for the evaluation of the artifact involves optimization and simulation, the design artifact used in this study will allow for the implementation of the qualitative evaluation (Von Alan 2004) of inpatients' digital twin to facilitate the estimation of fall risk predisposition. The potential of using the Bayesian network to establish the probability of occurrence of events based on the causal relationships (Sesen et al. 2013; Masegosa and Moral 2013), makes it a good strategy for determining the fall risk vulnerabilities based on the clinical, demographic, and psychosocial parameters. Since it is a probabilistic tool for interactive relationship estimation, it is vital for intelligent clinical decision support following the optimal computation of trends and events (Flores et al. 2011), thus providing a good framework for fall risk vulnerability estimation of inpatients.

Digital Twin-Based Bayesian Network Falls Risk Framework

The traditional techniques for fall risk assessment consist of numerous shortfalls that have been previously elaborated (Jester et al. 2005; Tyndall et al. 2020); unfortunately, these challenges make it difficult to have a holistic consideration of patients' conditions in fall risk assessment. If we consider the two health scenarios of inpatients with different clinical, demographic, and psychosocial conditions shown in Figure 17.1, the challenges faced by healthcare professionals using the known falls risk assessment tools can be summarized as follows:

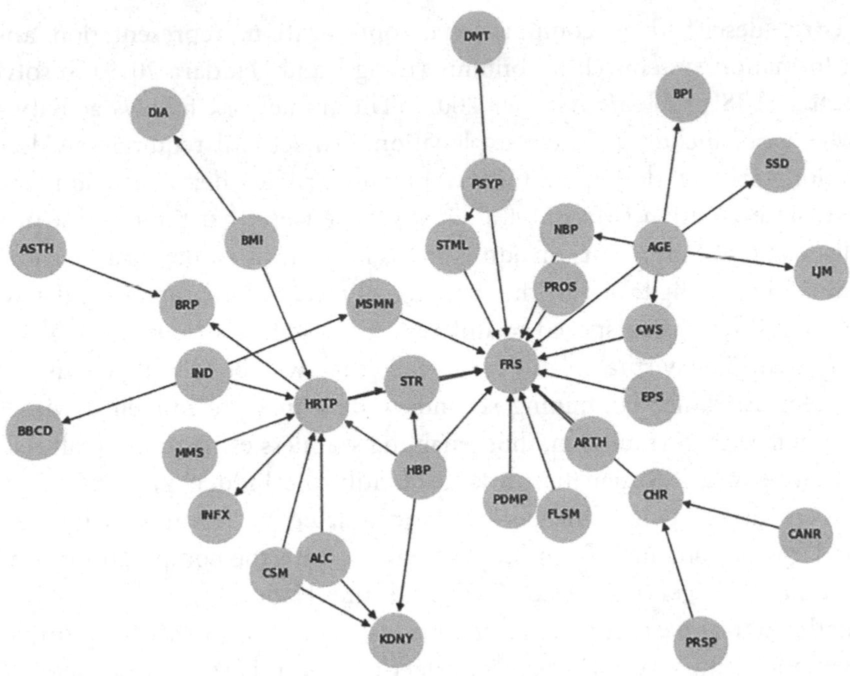

FIGURE 17.1 Illustration of the challenges of using the traditional falls risk assessment tools for estimating patient's proneness to falls on hospital admission.

- Correlating the influence of the clinical, demographic, and psychosocial parameters on fall risk susceptibility of the patients because of the causal-effect relationships of the parameters.
- Effective utilization of these variable patients' characteristics and their influences in falls risk estimation when they are not part of the considered parameters in the assessment model.
- Monitoring the varying patients' characteristics and the use of established patterns of acquired data for effective estimation of fall risk.

To tackle these challenges, we design a digital twin framework to serve as an assistance system in the context of fall risk assessment in acute care hospitalization (Figure 17.2). This solution relies on three main components – the database or Electronic Medical Record (EMR), the Digital twin platform and the assistance system. This close-loop system enables the assistance system that provides the state of inpatients (digital twin of

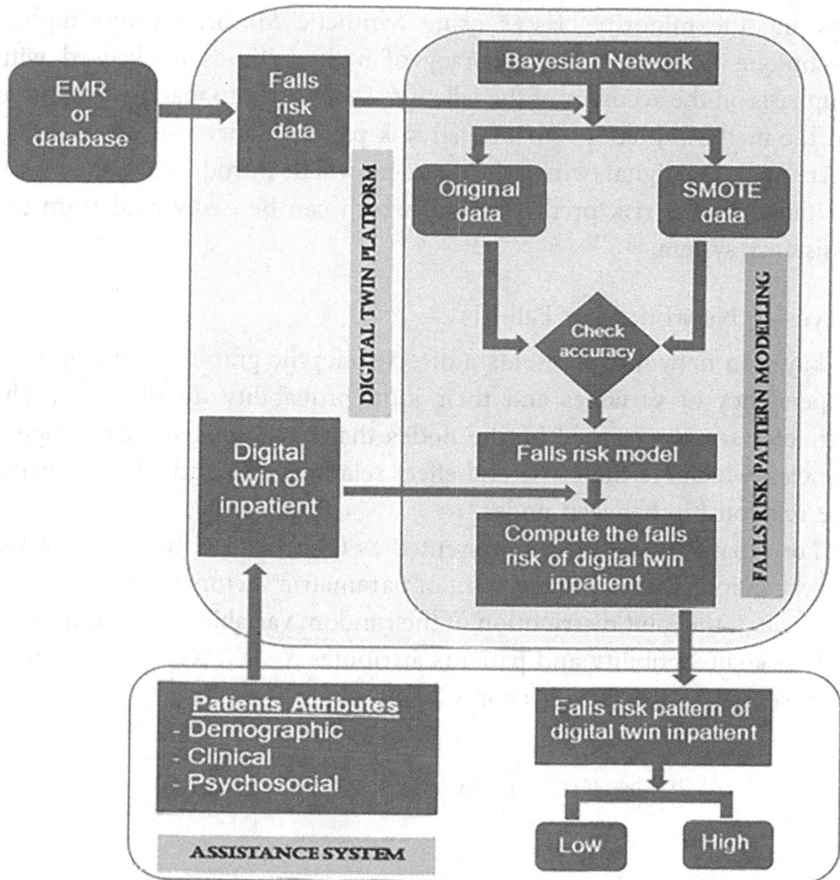

FIGURE 17.2 The framework for digital-twin-based Bayesian network falls risk acuity estimation. SMOTE, Synthetic Minority Oversampling Technique; EMR, Electronic Medical Records.

inpatient attributes) to interact with the fall risk records from the cloud using a mathematical model (Bayesian network) to facilitate seamless prediction of patient's falls risk susceptibility. The digital twin platform contains the historical data of patients' fall risk predisposition levels and their attributes (clinical, demographic and psychosocial conditions); the digital twin of inpatient that will be tested and the architecture for falls risk pattern modelling with Bayesian network. The Bayesian network initially models the historic secondary data to determine the pattern of the fall risk levels (low and high). To ensure that the pattern is dependable, the modelling relies on the original data that has the fall risk predisposition of patients for their various attributes for the classification, and later by upsizing the minority classes using Synthetic Minority Oversampling Technique (SMOTE). The accuracy of both methods is checked with emphasis on the accuracy of the fall risk classes prior to making a decision on the method to adopt for the fall risk pattern. Once this decision has been made, the digital twin of the inpatient will be introduced to the model to know the fall risk predisposition, which can be easily read from the assistance system.

Bayesian Network Mfor Fall Risk

A Bayesian network represents a directed acyclic graph for showing the dependency of variables and their joint probability distributions. The variables are represented by the nodes that have links showing dependencies, which are the cause and effect relationships, and edges showing the relationship between nodes.

For a Bayesian network represented as (G,α) with G being a directed acyclic graph (DAG) and α is a set of parametric vectors given by $\alpha = \{\alpha_1, \alpha_2, \ldots, \alpha_n\}$, the joint distribution of the random variables representing the falls risk susceptibility and patients attributes $X = \{X_1, X_2, \ldots, X_n\}$ can be represented by Eq. (17.1) (Lauria 2008).

$$P(x|\alpha, G) = \prod_{i=1}^{n} P(x_i|\pi(x_i), \alpha, G) = \prod_{i=1}^{n} \alpha_{i,k}(j) \qquad (17.1)$$

where $P(x|\alpha,G)$ is the probability of the conjunction of a given task $x_1, x_2, \ldots, x_n$ to the falls risk variables $X_i \in X$, $\pi(x_i)$ identifies the list of parents that are directly linked to X_i in the DAG G and n is the number of discrete variables.

The conditional probability at the nodes $X_i \in X$ are depicted by Eq. (17.2) (Lauria 2008).

$$\alpha = \{\alpha_1, \alpha_2, \ldots, \alpha_n\} = \left\{ [\alpha_{i,k}(j)]_{k=1}^{r_i} \right\}_{j=1, i=1,2,\ldots n}^{q_i} \qquad (17.2)$$

where r_i represents the state of the variables $X_i \in X$, q_i is the valid configuration values of $X_i \in X$ $(\pi(x_i))$.

If the random variables of the fall risk X has one target variable θ representing the fall risk levels of the patients and (n-1) feature variables representing the patient's attributes $\lambda = \{\lambda_1, \lambda_2, \ldots, \lambda_{n-1}\}$ such that $X = \{\theta, \lambda\}$, we can therefore classify new attribute feature vector $\alpha = \{\alpha_1, \alpha_2, \ldots, \alpha_{n-1}\}$

into θ* if $D = \{D_1, D_2, \ldots, D_n\}$ set of data has been trained, following optimization of the objective function in Eq. (17.3).

$$\theta* = \underset{\theta}{\text{argmax}}\{P(\theta|\alpha, D)\} \tag{17.3}$$

Since the solution of the maximum likelihood estimation shown in Eq. (17.3) is difficult to find analytically, the Expectation-Maximization (*EM*) algorithm (Dempster et al. 1977) can be employed to find the optimal local solution through *M* iterations. Suppose the classification accuracy of the original fall risk data is ACC(θ|α,D). The accuracy of the SMOTE data obtained by upsizing the minority class of the falls risk class of the original dataset is ACC(θ|Ǧ, ά). In that case, the *EM* algorithm for determining the Bayesian network (G, α) for estimating the fall risk class of digital twin inpatient is shown in Algorithm 17.1.

ALGORITHM 17.1 EM{X,D,G,A,M}

Required: X is a set of random variables representing the fall risk parameters (patients attributes and the fall risk classes), *G* is the Bayesian network structure for representing the fall risk, patients attribute relationship, *α* is the initial parametric values and *M* is the number of iterations and *D* is the training dataset.

Ensure: A Bayesian network of the structural representation of the relationship.

Compute the accuracy of the original fall risk data
for i = 1 to M do
$\theta^* = \underset{\theta}{\text{argmax}}\{P(\theta|\alpha, D)\}$
Compute $Acc(\theta \mid \alpha, D)$
end for
Compute the accuracy of SMOTE updated fall risk data
for i = 1 to *M* do
$\theta^{**} = \underset{\theta}{\text{argmax}}\{P(\theta|\check{G}, ά)\}$
Compute $Acc(\theta \mid \check{G}, ά)$
end for

Compare: Compare the accuracies of the original data and SMOTE data Bayesian networks
if $Acc(\theta \mid \alpha, D) < Acc(\theta \mid \check{G}, ά)$
return $Acc(\theta \mid \check{G}, ά)$
else:
return $Acc(\theta \mid \alpha, D)$

CASE STUDY

We decided to apply the concept of Bayesian network-based digital twin of inpatients to determine the risk predisposition of patients with different clinical, psychosocial, and demographic characteristics to establish the fall risk on admission. The artifact we developed with the DSRM relied on secondary data from a not-for-profit healthcare organization in Australia to demonstrate the feasibility of the technique. To this end, de-identified data of 1014 inpatients with more than 40 demographic, clinical and psychosocial conditions and fall risk susceptibilities were randomly selected for the study. The patient records that were obtained between February 2017 and June 2018 included clinical conditions such as heart failure, chronic obstructive pulmonary disease, diabetes, dementia, stroke, epilepsy, cancer, prostate, arthritis, asthma, high blood pressure, *etc.* The demographic and psychosocial conditions considered include age, Body Mass Index (BMI), history of previous falls, smoking habit, alcohol consumption, fall in the last six months, impaired vision and hearing loss, use of prosthesis, wound and skin break, hospitalization in the past 12 months, and the history of infectious diseases.

The Bayesian network shown in Figure 17.3 is used to model the fall risk considering the patient's attributes represented as the nodes. The link between the various patients' clinical, psychosocial, and demographic conditions and the fall risk has been shown.

The summary of the patient's characteristics, showing the proportions that have the various psychosocial and clinical conditions used for this study and the various classes of demographic conditions such as age and BMI is shown in Table 17.1.

By using a 10-fold cross-validation ensemble with 80% of the dataset for training and 20% for testing, we confirmed the difference in accuracy of the Bayesian network model of the original falls risk data and SMOTE upsizing of the original dataset. The estimation results showing the precision, recall, f1-score, accuracy, and area under the curve (AUC) are shown in Table 17.2. Although the accuracy and the AUC of the original data are slightly higher than those of the SMOTE upsized dataset for the cross-validation of the training dataset, the very low precision of the high-risk class of the falls risk of the original dataset makes it imperative to use the SMOTE upsized model. The SMOTE upsized Bayesian network model estimated the precision of the high-risk class to 110% higher accuracy than that with the original data from 34.72% to 72.81%.

Scenario A

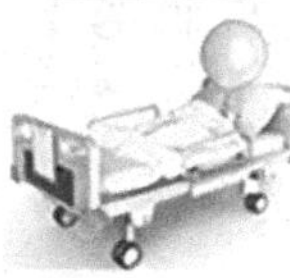

- Primary diagnosis: *heart problem*
- Age: 55
- BMI: 28
- Smoker: yes
- Comorbidities: diabetes, arthritis, asthma, dementia
- Fall in last 12 months: no
- Others: prosthesis, history of infectious disease

Scenario B

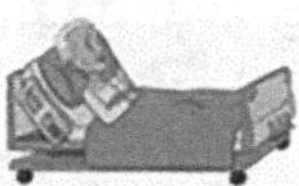

- Primary diagnosis: *stroke*
- Age: 85
- BMI: 38
- Alcohol consumption: yes
- Smoker: no
- Comorbidities: heart problems, cancer, asthma, kidney disease
- Fall in last 12 months: no
- Others: limited jaw movement, neck, and back problems

FIGURE 17.3 Bayesian network Model for Falls risk acuity of patients considering clinical and psychosocial parameters. Alcohol (ALC), arthritis (ARTH), bowel bleeding, constipation, diarrhoea (BBCD), blood clotting problems (BCP), bladder problems, incontinence (BPI), cancer (CANR), chemotherapy, radiation (CHR), Current Smoker (CSM), current wounds, skin breaks (CWS), Diabetes (DIA), Dementia (DMT), epilepsy/seizures (EPS), fallen in last 6 months (FLSM), Falls risk (FRS), H/L blood pressure (HBP), heart problems (HRTP), infectious diseases (IND), indigestion, reflux (INFX), impaired vision, hearing(IVH), kidney disease (KDNY), limited jaw movement (LJM), migraines/motion sickness (MMS), Multi sclerosis/Motor Neuron disease (MSMN), neck/back problems (NBP), physical disability, mobility problems (PDMP), prosthesis (PROS), prostate problems (PRSP), psychiatric problems (PSYP), Speech, swallowing difficulties (SSD), short term memory loss (STML), Stroke (STR), body mass index (BMI).

Furthermore, the higher accuracy of the SMOTE upsized model (78.87% and AUC 92.91%) compared to the model that relied on the original dataset (accuracy:74.38% and AUC: 91.57%) makes it imperative to rely on the SMOTE-based Bayesian network model for the falls risk estimation of the digital twin of inpatients.

Illustrative Case of a Digital Twin of a Cancer Inpatient

For a digital twin inpatient suffering from cancer and other comorbidities such as heart problems, stroke, dementia, and has a history of falls per the patient attributes shown in Table 17.3, the digital twin platform via the SMOTE-based Bayesian network model shows that this patient is predisposed to high-risk of falls on admission. Following the attributes and fall risk diagnosis of this digital inpatient, the triage nurse can be in the position to use the clinical, demographic, and psychosocial attributes to facilitate a fall mitigation plan that is suitable for inpatients of similar

TABLE 17.1 Clinical, Demographic, and Psychosocial Parameters of the Patients Used for the Study

Parameter	Class	Percent	Parameter	Class	Percent
Age (AGE)	<18	4.64%	Fallen in last 6 months (FLSM)	No	84.01%
	18–39	73.22%		Yes	15.99%
	40–65	34.65%	Falls risk (FRS)	Low	82.72%
	>65	23.49%		High	12.78%
Alcohol (ALC)	No	97.14%	High and Light blood pressure (HBP)	No	71.08%
	Yes	2.86%		Yes	28.92%
Arthritis (ARTH)	No	81.54%	Heart problems (HRTP)	No	87.66%
	Yes	18.46%		Yes	12.34%
Asthma(ASTH)	No	81.34%	History of infectious diseases (IND)	No	96.84%
	Yes	18.66%		Yes	3.16%
Bowel bleeding, constipation, diarrhoea (BBCD)	No	80.16%	indigestion, reflux (INFX)	No	77.00%
	Yes	19.84%		Yes	23.00%
Blood clotting problems (BCP)	No	92.40%	Impaired vision, hearing (IVH)	No	72.46%
	Yes	7.60%		Yes	27.54%
BMI	<20	9.77%	Kidney disease (KDNY)	No	93.48%
	21–25	29.91%		Yes	6.52%
	26–30	29.81%	Limited jaw movement (LJM)	No	96.25%
	>30	30.50%		Yes	3.75%
Bladder problems, incontinence (BPI)	No	87.27%	Migraines/motion sickness (MMS)	No	81.05%
	Yes	12.73%		Yes	18.95%
Breathing problems (BRP)	No	82.53%	Multi sclerosis/motor neuron disease (MSMN)	No	98.22%
	Yes	17.47%		Yes	1.78%

Cancer (CANR)	No	75.12%	Neck/back problems (NBP)	No	73.35%
	Yes	24.88%		Yes	26.65%
Chemotherapy, radiation (CHR)	No	84.90%	Physical disability, mobility problems (PDMP)	No	81.84%
	Yes	15.10%		Yes	18.16%
Current Smoker (CSM)	No	75.02%	Prosthesis (PROS)	No	87.46%
	Yes	24.98%		Yes	12.54%
Current wounds, skin breaks (CWS)	No	85.09%	Prostate problems (PRSP)	No	93.78%
	Yes	14.91%		Yes	6.22%
Diabetes (DIA)	No	90.42%	Psychiatric problems (PSYP)	No	78.58%
	Yes	9.58%		Yes	21.42%
Dementia (DMT)	No	53.11%	Speech, swallowing difficulties (SSD)	No	95.26%
	Yes	46.89%		Yes	4.74%
Epilepsy/seizures (EPS)	No	95.46%	Short-term memory loss (STML)	No	92.99%
	Yes	4.54%		Yes	7.01%
			Stroke(STR)	No	95.66%
				Yes	4.34%

TABLE 17.2 Summary of Accuracy of the Cross-Validation of the Training Dataset and Testing Dataset Accuracy for Bayesian Network Classification of Falls Risk of the Original Dataset and SMOTE (of the Original) Dataset

		Original Dataset			
		10-Fold Cross-Validation of the Training Dataset			
k-Folds	Precision	Recall	f1 Score	Accuracy	AUC
1	0.9260	0.9232	0.9243	0.9232	0.9660
2	0.9369	0.9369	0.9369	0.9369	0.9683
3	0.9412	0.9410	0.9411	0.9410	0.9685
4	0.9296	0.9287	0.9291	0.9287	0.9653
5	0.9439	0.9451	0.9441	0.9451	0.9685
6	0.9381	0.9383	0.9382	0.9383	0.9665
7	0.9242	0.9218	0.9228	0.9218	0.9673
8	0.9405	0.9396	0.9400	0.9396	0.9744
9	0.9357	0.9355	0.9356	0.9355	0.9688
10	0.9350	0.9355	0.9353	0.9355	0.9662
		Test Data Accuracy			
Risk class	Precision	Recall	f1-Score	Accuracy	AUC
High risk	0.3472	0.8333	0.4902	0.7438	0.9157
Low risk	0.9618	0.7283	0.8289		
All	0.8710	0.7438	0.7788		
		SMOTE of Original Dataset			
		10-Fold Cross-Validation of the Training Dataset			
k-Folds	Precision	Recall	f1 Score	Accuracy	AUC
1	0.9173	0.9171	0.9171	0.9171	0.9585
2	0.9138	0.9138	0.9138	0.9138	0.9589
3	0.9206	0.9204	0.9204	0.9204	0.9596
4	0.9155	0.9154	0.9154	0.9154	0.9541
5	0.9188	0.9187	0.9187	0.9187	0.9554
6	0.9173	0.9171	0.9171	0.9171	0.9572
7	0.9187	0.9187	0.9187	0.9187	0.9611
8	0.9180	0.9179	0.9179	0.9179	0.9527
9	0.9181	0.9179	0.9179	0.9179	0.9629
10	0.9150	0.9146	0.9146	0.9146	0.9591
		Test Data Accuracy			
Risk class	Precision	Recall	f1 Score	Accuracy	AUC
High risk	0.7281	0.9294	0.8165	0.7887	0.9291
Low risk	0.8992	0.6446	0.7509		
All	0.8126	0.7887	0.7840		

TABLE 17.3 Characteristics of Digital Twin Inpatient Used for Illustrative Case Study

AGE	95	MMS	No	BBCD	Yes	PROS	No
BMI	25	MSMN	No	BPI	Yes	CWS	Yes
DIA	No	EPS	No	KDNY	No	IND	No
HBP	Yes	STML	Yes	CANR	Yes	FLSM	Yes
SSD	No	PSYP	No	CHR	No	CSM	No
DMT	Yes	HRTP	Yes	PRSP	No	ALC	No
STR	Yes	BCP	No	PDMP	Yes	NBP	Yes
LJM	No	BRP	No	ARTH	Yes	IVH	No
INFX	No	ASTH	No	Falls risk level: High			

characteristics. In situations where a multi-disciplinary team is needed for strategic fall mitigation actions, the seamless acquisition of the fall risk predisposition will enhance the timeliness of developing such plans.

Implications for Theory and Practice

Precision medicine involves an enhanced and more detailed data analysis, as well as the ability of computers to evaluate, integrate, and exploit these data, and ultimately construct the 'digital twin' of a patient (Joyner et al. 2019; Khoury 2019). Since digital twin in the healthcare context can denote the vision of a comprehensive, virtual tool that integrates the clinical data acquired over time as determined with mechanistic and statistical models (Alber et al., 2019), our integration of the inpatients attributes in the form of clinical, demographic, lifestyle and circumstances data is inevitable for proffering a better control of falls risk. By implementing a Bayesian network, which is synonymous with the mechanistic and statistical model in a digital twin architecture of inpatients subjected to different clinical, psychosocial, and demographic characteristics, it is possible to have a smart falls risk management strategy through the optimization and control of some risk factors of falls on admission. This is because the digital twin inpatients helps to provide a mirror world that augments the real state of inpatients visiting acute care hospitals, hence, providing a cognitive, social and temporal reinforcement (Ricci et al. 2019) that will facilitate patient management in real-time. Imperatively, the advantage of our study in effective patient care interventions cannot be overemphasised since the understanding of how different comorbidities and other patient attributes can impact the entire patient experience is guaranteed, thus, helping in the strategic planning and care intervention (Angelo et al. 2020). Moreover, the proffered approach enables a personalised and more individually tailored fall risk assessment to ensue.

Considering the tendency to minimize fall risk by relying on fall risk predictions, the quality of life of patients will increase (Rivera et al. 2019). This is because falls on hospital admissions, which have been attributed mostly to high-risk patients can be minimized (Blain et al. 2019). There is also the high possibility of managing those patients through person-tailored fall mitigation plans where clinical conditions predispose them to a high fall risk. Implementing the digital twin model will also ensure that fall risk is not superficially determined by neglecting the causal relationships between different patients' attributes, which are intrinsic parameters contributing to falls, unfortunately, some of these intrinsic factors and their interactions have been overlooked in many fall risk models.

CONCLUSIONS

The importance of precision medicine facilitated by digital twins in the superior management of patients at all levels of hospital care via a well-integrated analysis of available data cannot be ignored in ensuring improved patient well-being and minimized cost of healthcare. This study relied on the clinical, psychosocial, and demographic information from inpatients in acute care hospitals to develop a Bayesian network-based digital twin framework for predicting the fall risk of patients on admission. By using secondary data of historic fall risk of inpatients from the database or the Electronic Medical Record (EMR), it was possible to develop this virtual environment to provide an assistance system for seamless management of falls and the associated risks via real-time estimation of patients' vulnerabilities. To ensure that the Bayesian network that acted as a mathematical model in the digital twin platform predicts the fall risk level with higher accuracy, we relied on the Synthetic Minority Oversampling Technique (SMOTE) to upsize the minority class of the fall risk levels in the historic data. This helped to ensure that the healthcare professionals managing falls-related risk in the hospital will have the estimated fall risk levels to an acceptable level of accuracy, thereby, helping to mitigate against falls on admissions and the associated consequences.

The demonstration of the technique we developed in this study with data from a non-profit healthcare organization in Australia went a long way to cement the viability of the framework developed and represents one of the first studies of this kind. Despite this feat, this study has some limitations; namely, the need to include a fall risk mitigation strategy to the digital twin architecture to enhance the quick implementation of fall risk level findings at triage. Our future work will expand this study from this pilot phase to incorporate more data for a robust and generalisable outcome.

ACKNOWLEDGEMENTS

This work is as a result of an Epworth Medical Fund research grant awarded to the author. The author is indebted to the work of the research assistant Dr Chinedu Ossai for performing the necessary technical aspects of this project.

REFERENCES

Ahmad, B.S., Hill, K.D., O'Brien, T.J., Gorelik, A., Habib, N. and Wark, J.D., 2012. Falls and fractures in patients chronically treated with antiepileptic drugs. *Neurology*, 79(2), pp.145–151.

Alber, M., Tepole, A.B., Cannon, W.R., De, S., Dura-Bernal, S., Garikipati, K., Karniadakis, G., Lytton, W.W., Perdikaris, P., Petzold, L. and Kuhl, E., 2019. Integrating machine learning and multiscale modeling—Perspectives, challenges, and opportunities in the biological, biomedical, and behavioral sciences. *NPJ Digital Medicine*, 2(1), pp.1–11.

Angelo, C., Matteo, G., Montagna, S. and Ricci, A., 2020. On the integration of agents and digital twins in healthcare. *Journal of Medical Systems*, 44(9).

Blain, H., Dabas, F., Mekhinini, S., Picot, M.C., Miot, S., Bousquet, J., Boubakri, C., Jaussent, A. and Bernard, P.L., 2019. Effectiveness of a programme delivered in a falls clinic in preventing serious injuries in high-risk older adults: A pre-and post-intervention study. *Maturitas*, 122, pp.80–86.

Coussement, J., De Paepe, L., Schwendimann, R., Denhaerynck, K., Dejaeger, E. and Milisen, K., 2008. Interventions for preventing falls in acute-and chronic-care hospitals: A systematic review and meta-analysis. *Journal of the American Geriatrics society*, 56(1), pp.29–36.

Dempster, A., Laird, N. and Rubin, D., 1977. Maximum likelihood from incomplete data via the EM algorithm. *Journal of the Royal Statistical Society, Series B* 39, pp.1–38.

Eglseer, D., Hoedl, M. and Schoberer, D., 2020. Malnutrition risk and hospital-acquired falls in older adults: A cross-sectional, multicenter study. *Geriatrics & Gerontology International*, 20(4), pp.348–353.

Elragal, A. and Haddara, M., 2019. Design science research: Evaluation in the lens of big data analytics. *Systems*, 7(2), p.27.

Flores, M.J., Nicholson, A.E., Brunskill, A., Korb, K.B. and Mascaro, S., 2011. Incorporating expert knowledge when learning Bayesian network structure: A medical case study. *Artificial Intelligence in Medicine*, 53(3), pp.181–204.

Fuller, A., Fan, Z. and Day, C., 2019. Digital twin: enabling technology, challenges and open research. *arXiv preprint arXiv:1911.01276.*

Glaessgen, E. and Stargel, D., 2012, April. The digital twin paradigm for future NASA and US Air Force vehicles. In *53rd AIAA/ASME/ASCE/AHS/ASC structures, structural dynamics and materials conference 20th AIAA/ASME/AHS adaptive structures conference 14th AIAA* (p. 1818).

Hevner, A.R., 2007. A three cycle view of design science research. *Scandinavian Journal of Information Systems*, 19(2), p.4.

Jester, R., Wade, S. and Henderson, K., 2005. A pilot investigation of the efficacy of falls risk assessment tools and prevention strategies in an elderly hip fracture population. *Journal of Orthopaedic Nursing*, 9(1), pp.27–34.

Josifovska, K., Yigitbas, E. and Engels, G., 2019, July. A digital twin-based multimodal ui adaptation framework for assistance systems in industry 4.0. In International Conference on Human-Computer Interaction (pp. 398–409). Springer, Cham.

Joyner, M.J. and Paneth, N., 2019. Promises, promises, and precision medicine. *The Journal of Clinical Investigation*, 129(3), pp.946–948.

Kim, E.A.N., Mordiffi, S.Z., Bee, W.H., Devi, K. and Evans, D., 2007. Evaluation of three fall-risk assessment tools in an acute care setting. *Journal of Advanced Nursing*, 60(4), pp.427–435.

Khoury, M.J., 2019. Precision medicine vs preventive medicine. *JAMA*, 321(4), pp.406–406.

Lai, P.C., Wong, W.C., Low, C.T., Wong, M. and Chan, M.H., 2011. A small-area study of environmental risk assessment of outdoor falls. *Journal of Medical Systems*, 35(6), pp.1543–1552.

Lauría, E.J., 2008. An information-geometric approach to learning Bayesian network topologies from data. In Innovations in Bayesian Networks (pp. 187–217). Springer, Berlin, Heidelberg.

Liu, Y., Zhang, L., Yang, Y., Zhou, L., Ren, L., Wang, F., Liu, R., Pang, Z. and Deen, M.J., 2019. A novel cloud-based framework for the elderly healthcare services using digital twin. *IEEE Access*, 7, pp.49088–49101.

Martin, N., Bergs, J., Eerdekens, D., Depaire, B. and Verelst, S., 2018. Developing an emergency department crowding dashboard: A design science approach. *International Emergency Nursing*, 39, pp.68–76.

Masegosa, A.R. and Moral, S., 2013. An interactive approach for Bayesian network learning using domain/expert knowledge. *International Journal of Approximate Reasoning*, 54(8), pp.1168–1181.

Morse, J.M., Morse, R.M. and Tylko, S.J., 1989. Development of a scale to identify the fall-prone patient. *Canadian Journal on Aging/La Revue Canadienne du Vieillissement*, 8(4), pp.366–377.

Nakai, A., Akeda, M. and Kawabata, I. (2006). Incidence and risk factors for inpatient falls in an academic acute-care hospital. *Journal of Nippon Medical School*, 73(5), pp.265–270.

Nandy, S., Parsons, S., Cryer, C., Underwood, M., Rashbrook, E., Carter, Y., Eldridge, S., Close, J., Skelton, D., Taylor, S. and Feder, G., 2004. Development and preliminary examination of the predictive validity of the Falls Risk Assessment Tool (FRAT) for use in primary care. *Journal of Public Health*, 26(2), pp.138–143.

Narayanan, V., Dickinson, A., Victor, C., Griffiths, C. and Humphrey, D., 2016. Falls screening and assessment tools used in acute mental health settings: A review of policies in England and Wales. *Physiotherapy*, 102(2), pp.178–183.

Oliver, D., 2008. Falls risk-prediction tools for hospital inpatients. Time to put them to bed? *Age and Ageing*, 37(3), pp.248–250.

Oliver, D., Britton, M., Seed, P., Martin, F.C. and Hopper, A.H., 1997. Development and evaluation of evidence based risk assessment tool (STRATIFY) to predict which elderly inpatients will fall: Case-control and cohort studies. *BMJ*, 315(7115), pp.1049–1053.

Park, K.T., Son, Y.H. and Noh, S.D., 2020. The architectural framework of a cyber physical logistics system for digital-twin-based supply chain control. *International Journal of Production Research*, pp.1–22.

Ricci, A., Tummolini, L. and Castelfranchi, C., 2019. Augmented societies with mirror worlds. *AI & Society*, 34(4), pp.745–752.

Rivera, L.F., Jiménez, M., Angara, P., Villegas, N.M., Tamura, G. and Müller, H.A., 2019, November. Towards continuous monitoring in personalized healthcare through digital twins. In *Proceedings of the 29th Annual International Conference on Computer Science and Software Engineering*; Markham, ON, Canada. 4–6 November 2019; (pp. 329–335).

Ruohomäki, T., Airaksinen, E., Huuska, P., Kesäniemi, O., Martikka, M. and Suomisto, J., 2018, September. Smart city platform enabling digital twin. In *2018 International Conference on Intelligent Systems (IS)* (pp. 155–161). IEEE.

Salgado, R.I., Lord, S.R., Ehrlich, F., Janji, N. and Rahman, A. (2004). Predictors of falling in elderly hospital patients. *Archives of Gerontology and Geriatrics*, 38(3), pp.213–219.

Seppala, L.J., Van der Velde, N., Masud, T., Blain, H., Petrovic, M., van der Cammen, T.J., Szczerbińska, K., Hartikainen, S., Kenny, R.A., Ryg, J. and Eklund, P., 2019. EuGMS task and Finish group on Fall-Risk-Increasing drugs (FRIDs): Position on knowledge Dissemination, management, and future research. *European Geriatric Medicine*, 10(2), pp.275–283.

Sesen, M.B., Nicholson, A.E., Banares-Alcantara, R., Kadir, T. and Brady, M., 2013. Bayesian networks for clinical decision support in lung cancer care. *PLoS One*, 8(12), p.e82349.

Tao, F., Cheng, J., Qi, Q., Zhang, M., Zhang, H. and Sui, F., 2018. Digital twin-driven product design, manufacturing and service with big data. *The International Journal of Advanced Manufacturing Technology*, 94(9–12), pp.3563–3576.

Tyndall, A., Bailey, R. and Elliott, R., 2020. Pragmatic development of an evidence-based intensive care unit–Specific falls risk assessment tool: The Tyndall Bailey Falls Risk Assessment Tool. *Australian Critical Care*, 33(1), pp.65–70.

Von Alan, R.H., March, S.T., Park, J. and Ram, S., 2004. Design science in information systems research. *MIS Q*, 28, pp.75–105

Woolcott, J.C., Richardson, K.J., Wiens, M.O., Patel, B., Marin, J., Khan, K.M. and Marra, C.A., 2009. Meta-analysis of the impact of 9 medication classes on falls in elderly persons. *Archives of Internal Medicine*, 169(21), pp.1952–1960.

Zhou, G., Zhang, C., Li, Z., Ding, K. and Wang, C., 2020. Knowledge-driven digital twin manufacturing cell towards intelligent manufacturing. *International Journal of Production Research*, 58(4), pp.1034–1051.

CHAPTER 18

Facilitating a Shared Meaning of AI/ML Findings amongst Key Healthcare Stakeholders

The Role of Analytic Translators

Wendy D. Lynch, John Zelcer, and Nilmini Wickramasinghe

INTRODUCTION

Today, given advances in computer technology and the Internet of Things (IoT) we are able to collect, store and analyze vast amounts of data. In fact, we are now in the Knowledge Economy or Information Age where data is a critical raw asset and input (Wickramasinghe et al., 2022). Healthcare, while historically slow to embrace technology and the potential of digital technologies, is finally catching up and a myriad of digital solutions now permeate numerous areas of healthcare such as electronic medical records (EMRs), mobile Apps and clinical decision support solutions.

However, while we are witnessing a rapid diffusion of technology into healthcare accompanied by an embracing of various analytic, machine learning and artificial intelligence algorithms to rapidly process the volumes of generated data, healthcare professionals often struggle with

DOI: 10.1201/9781032699745-22

interpreting and understanding the outputs (Wickramasinghe et al., 2022). We contend that in such a context a critical missing link is the skill of analytic translation, i.e., for clinicians to understand data science/ computer engineering terminology, and for computer scientists and engineers, in turn, to better understand the healthcare contexts in which their solutions must operate. Hence in this chapter, we answer the questions “How can analytic translation mitigate challenges of next-level analytics in healthcare?” and “How can translation demystify AI and analytics in healthcare?”

keywords: black box, translation, demystify, analytic translator, data science

BACKGROUND

Similar to other industries, healthcare is experiencing a revolution in the application of big data analytics (Khanra et al., 2020). In almost every dimension of clinical practice, from hospital capacity to personalized cancer treatment to infection control, data scientists are incorporating advanced analytics models (such as machine learning and AI) to optimize the safety, efficacy and efficiency of care (Wickramasinghe et al., 2022). In parallel to improving process outcomes, such analytic models and methods are, understandably, also increasing in complexity (2022).

Despite their associated improvements in health and delivery outcomes, the adoption of new technologies and methods comes with significant dissemination challenges (2022). Namely, frontline practitioners, their colleagues, and ultimately patients, must accept and trust the value of new information and recommendations they receive from such novel sources. The degree of acceptance will depend largely on how and by whom the information is communicated, as well as the capacity of the receiver to understand and incorporate that information into their decision-making.

As context, misunderstandings and reluctance regarding methods (such as AI) occur for a myriad of reasons. For example:

1. **Natural silos**. Few data scientists, clinicians or administrators are highly trained in each others’ fields; their expertise is narrow. This results in a lack of familiarity with priorities, principles, terminology and challenges faced by the other team. While organizations encourage cross-functional education, expert-level training in multiple areas is rare.

2. **Distrust**. Humans naturally distrust things they do not understand. In the case of AI, strong opinions have been expressed in the lay media (Pd, 2022) and academic circles (DeCamp & Tilburt, 2019) about its potential harms.

3. **Low data literacy.** Levels of data literacy vary, even among highly trained health professionals (Johnson, 2014). Statistical knowledge, the ability to discern probabilities, or interpret the relative value of options may be limited in the people who intend to receive and apply complex analytic results. Adding to the potential for misinterpretation, there is often a difference between what is statistically significant versus clinically significant (Madjarova et al., 2022).

4. **Urgency and pace.** Tight schedules in healthcare settings create time constraints, placing limits on the time allowed for thorough explanations and discussions. Further, some decisions must occur expediently to optimize outcomes. These pressures hinder extended discussions or explanations.

5. **Terminology.** Similar to silos of knowledge, specialization requires precise language by those with shared expertise. This particular terminology aids communication within members of an occupation, but simultaneously impedes understanding for those outside that group.

6. **Values.** People in different roles often have different values. While data scientists may strive to apply novel, complex models to achieve greater levels of predictive accuracy, they may not place value on comprehension by non-analysts (Sajee, 2020). Similarly, practitioners may place value on instilling trust in patients, which requires their own comfort or familiarity with a course of treatment (Epstein & Pro Publica, 2017).

7. **Interests**. Data scientists and technology developers may have strong commercial or competitive interests in their products. Conversely, clinicians' interests are predominantly directed towards the best health outcomes of their patients.

Facing these potential barriers, it follows that the proliferation of AI and machine learning methods in healthcare may not produce their intended potential advances in healthcare without some attention to natural communication barriers.

Options for Bridging the Knowledge Gap

The ever-widening gap between clinical and analytic domains manifests in several ways. Clinicians may misinterpret important information, reject new approaches, or continue outdated practices. In parallel, analysts may deliver results in complicated formats that non-analysts cannot absorb, or oversimplify results and suggest that clinicians trust an analytic finding that they, i.e., the clinicians, do not understand. This dysfunction is not limited to healthcare, but there are few industries where miscommunication has greater consequences — in missed opportunity or potential harm.

Efforts to mitigate communication challenges take many forms. For example, some organizations call for improving data literacy for everyone (Sucich, 2022). This involves widespread assessments of data-handling skills, peer-to-peer education, and intensive training. Arguments in favour of literacy education focus on the need for informed, data-driven decisions at all levels of healthcare.

While commendable, the aspiration of elevating an entire workforce to high levels of data literacy may be difficult to reach. It requires extensive time, money and effort, especially given estimates that fewer than 25% of employees currently have high numeric literacy (Sucich, 2022), and many medical professionals struggle with data as well (Berwick et al., 1981).

Another approach to implementing sophisticated solutions is to take black-box machine learning results and convert them into more digestible formats, such as decision trees (Cohen, 2021). Decision trees do give visual, logical illustrations of interdependencies that guide predictions, which can help demystify the underlying information. And, decision trees have been shown to combine diverse sets of information to accurately identify illness (Liu et al., 2022). However, full, complex models often contain too many branches to easily represent in a straightforward visual aid.

Some experts envision a future where a computerized AI assistant supports clinicians by listening to patient interactions, incorporating previous lab reports and symptoms, and providing evidence-based recommendations (Hsu, 2019). This would free the clinician to focus on the more human aspects of care, while the assistant supports diagnostics and treatment decisions. To date, information capture, transcription, and diagnostic accuracy of AI systems have advanced

(DeepScribe), but AI has not yet been adopted to bridge communication gaps. Furthermore, in cases where clinicians and patients distrust complex AI and machine learning, there may be a reluctance to accept the "voice" of artificial intelligence as the source of translation (Simonite, 2020).

Until the advent of AI assistants or universal data literacy, there is another alternative to improve communication - one that will remain relevant and valuable even as such approaches evolve. Analytic translators are interdisciplinary professionals designated to promote understanding and facilitate the appropriate application of complex analytics. The remainder of this chapter highlights the qualifications and activities of this role.

What Is an Analytic Translator?

Definition: An advisor trusted by data analysts and health care professionals to crystalize, explain, and shepherd complex analytic projects efficiently and collaboratively from initial concept to a relevant, insightful decision, or application, in ways that recognize and elevate the contribution of everyone involved (from *Become an Analytic Translator*) (Lynch, 2022).

Like language translators, analytic translators work between teams to make sure communication is clear and goals are aligned. Analytic translators are acutely aware of the potential for misunderstanding and are equipped with a combination of:

1. Working knowledge of complex analytic methods.

   The individual has enough experience in analytics to understand and assess the appropriateness of methods, interpret output, and convert statistical results into clear statements or images. If the translator will be focused on AI or machine learning, they must have sufficient comfort with those methods and outputs.

2. Solid grounding in an organization's main priorities — in this case, clinical.

   Analytic translators have a familiarity with an organization's business functions. In healthcare settings, the translator must understand the clinical or operational goals and have a sufficient grasp of what the teams want to accomplish.

3. Advanced communication and people skills.

   Analytic translators must be skilled communicators. In essence, they interact with experts, primarily discussing topics about which those experts have limited expertise (e.g., talking to doctors about machine learning, or data scientists about neurology). Done poorly, such conversations can be uncomfortable. Important skills include awareness, active listening, empathy, questioning and patience. Preferably, the translator also has credibility with both teams.

The Goals of an Analytic Translator Are To

1. **Recognize, highlight, and promote opportunities where data and analytics can explain or solve key medical challenges.**

   Clinicians may not have a deep understanding of all data sources, analytic tools, or expertise available to investigate important medical questions. Similarly, data teams may not grasp the subtleties of evolving clinical or operational priorities.

   Translators operate in between. They become familiar with both environments and stay mindful of the priorities, advantages and limitations of each. They identify opportunities others may not see.

2. **Facilitate analytic projects that meet healthcare needs efficiently and effectively by understanding both clinical and analytic domains.**

   Healthcare professionals often make rushed or cryptic requests that have not been carefully considered. What is the underlying clinical question, and how can it best be answered? Or the healthcare professional is unfamiliar with the sorts of data or methods that might be available.

   Conversely, data scientists may focus more on the technical aspects of data manipulation and modelling than the nuances of what the clinician/administrator needs to accomplish. Because clinical teams and analytic teams operate in separate silos, misunderstandings are common.

   Whether in the initial request, during technical updates, or when results get delivered, there are many instances where miscommunication is likely. While medical professionals want quick, definitive answers, analysts want to apply appropriate methods and perform data checks. Where analysts want to explain detailed limitations associated with data and models, clinicians would prefer straightforward conclusions.

Translators act as the go-between, making sure both teams follow what is happening, adjustments are understood, and results are clear. In this way, organizations avoid the rework caused by miscommunication.

3. **Deliver analytic results in optimal language and formats for the audience.**

   Expertise is a double-edged sword. The more advanced our knowledge, the more specialized and unique terminology becomes. When CFOs, pilots, endocrinologists, or data scientists speak with each other, they necessarily rely on their own unique vocabulary. Within a profession, a precise lexicon helps teams build collective understanding.

   When used between two professions, complex, technical language has the opposite impact: it divides and confuses. Clinical professionals and data scientists can find themselves lost in each other's jargon. Analytic translators are trained to extract key findings that are necessary and relevant, converting them into clear, meaningful implications for a specific audience.

4. **Build strong relationships between medical and analytic teams based on mutual respect.**

   Analytic translators understand that trust builds over time and appreciation develops from a consistent understanding of each other's contributions. As such, translators take deliberate steps to acknowledge team members' roles and achievements in a project, educating both teams.

   By facilitating clear communication, avoiding misunderstandings, and delivering clear results, translators support positive collaboration.

Healthcare professionals will be required to make critical decisions based on results they may not totally understand, created from methods they can't comprehend. To be successful, someone — trusted by both teams — will need to translate from one team to another. There is a critical need for people dedicated to useful pathways that connect data capabilities to healthcare-related problems.

THE ANALYTIC TRANSLATION PROCESS

Translators have the designated role of promoting mutual understanding at the optimal level for the stakeholder, rather than insisting that each stakeholder become more expert in another's domain. They participate in conversations or sometimes have separate conversations with analytic experts and those who will receive analytic results.

While an observer might simply notice a series of conversations where the translator listens, confirms, asks for clarification and confirms again, there are specific questions and skills they use. The translator knows they are listening for the respondent's motivation behind their request, decision criteria they will use to assess the value of an answer and signs of confidence or uncertainty. In this way, the translator assesses each team's understanding of, and comfort with, the other's work. The translator identifies clinical challenges that analytics can support and helps convert complex analytic findings into actionable clinical decisions.

The translation process is a sequence of steps where the translator uncovers the crux of an issue, and then converts it into language the other audience will best understand. The full process follows the sequence of discovering, distilling and deciphering with specific goals in each step. The next section provides an abbreviated overview of the sequence.

FROM THE CLINICAL TEAM TO THE ANALYTIC TEAM

1. **Discovery**

Translation begins with understanding the practitioners' perspective. What matters to the clinicians? What problems are they trying to solve? How do they do their job now? First, a translator listens to the clinician's priorities, concerns and challenges, taking note of their terminology. This conversation builds a context. The translator explores what clinicians wish they knew, and what decisions they need to make. How would they decide if new information is useful?

The goal is to understand *how* an analytic project might be useful to the clinician, in ways that help them do their jobs better. Practitioners are often not analytically-oriented, and will not be interested in advanced

TABLE 18.1 Digital Twin Example

Digital Twin Example
An initial conversation with the clinician focuses on their usual practices, exploring what matters to them. • *Tell me about your practice and the types of patients you see* • *Can you tell me about the patient interactions you find most rewarding* • *Tell me about the patients you find most challenging* • *How do you know when a treatment isn't working or needs to be changed?*
When a patient isn't responding well to treatment • *How do you decide which treatment to try next?* • *How do you decide if new information is useful?*
When a key question is identified • *If you had an answer to these questions, how would that be useful?*
The translator listens, discovering how the clinician perceives their role and the ways they make decisions. For example, do they focus predominantly on lab metrics? If so, which ones? Do they focus more on patient feedback? Or some combination of those? What does the practitioner find most frustrating in their role? Is it the trial-and-error aspect of treatment options? Is it patient compliance with a specific regimen? Or something else? What would be useful to know? By understanding the practitioner's values and concerns, the translator can articulate important objectives to the analytic team, while also understanding the context to better position a new solution such as Digital Twin in the future.

analytics as methods. Their acceptance of analytics will depend on how much value analytic results can provide (Table 18.1).

2. Distill and Decipher

After a dialogue with the clinician(s), the translator distils their understanding of clinician priorities, concerns and challenges into clear language that makes sense to the analytic team. Distillation means selecting the things that inform and shape what the analytic team needs to know and do. It also means leaving out extraneous details that analysts do not need.

Because translators understand the analyst role, they can then decipher the clinician's questions in terminology that guide analysis. Which processes, outcomes or metrics are most important? What question should their analysis answer? Which outcome should their models predict? What factors should be included, or at least understood? (Table 18.2).

TABLE 18.2 Digital Twin Example Cont.

Digital Twin Example
In the initial conversation with the analytic team, translators will summarize the key issues that are important to practitioners, focusing on the analytic approach and goals. For example, a practitioner might have reported that their greatest concern is achieving clinical improvement in HbA1c levels for a patient at risk of developing diabetes, that their patients receive an effective treatment with fewer side effects, or maintaining their patients' trust. They may also report that they need to hear from other clinicians that they have been successful before trying something new. Any of these concerns can be converted into an analysis within a digital twin platform (presuming the platform includes measures of HbA1c, clinical outcomes, side effects, and patient satisfaction). The translator poses specific questions to the analytic team related to these clinical priorities. Such as: 1. Compared to patients getting regular care, how much more successful are digital twin patients in achieving an HbA1c below 6.0.? 2. Compared to patients receiving the usual progression of treatments, what portion of digital twin patients have to discontinue treatment due to side effects? 3. Compared to patients getting usual care, how often do digital twin patients receive a successful treatment on the first try? How does patient satisfaction compare? 4. How many clinicians have used the digital twin platform, and of those, how many have decided not to continue? If the digital twin platform does not include some of the clinical priorities — patient satisfaction for example — this is an opportunity for analysts to explore the feasibility of adding them.

FROM THE ANALYTIC TEAM TO THE CLINICAL TEAM

1. Discover

Once analytic results have been produced, the translator reviews them and listens to what analysts have learned. This conversation allows the analytic team to describe their findings and methodologies in detail, if desired, while the translator focuses on extracting what will be important to clinicians. The goal is to gain a full understanding of the results, and their implications, and to clarify as needed. While the analytic team may focus on all the intricacies of their advanced methods, the translator will focus on what will be important to the practitioner (Table 18.3).

TABLE 18.3 Digital Twin Example with Further Elaboration

Digital Twin Example

Imagine that the analytic team was given the following question using their digital twin platforms.

1. Compared to patients getting regular care, how much more successful are digital twin patients in achieving an HbA1c below 6.0.?

Often, their results focus on platform complexity, such as an AI neural network approach, data collection through monitors connected through IoT, real-time measures and model dependencies, explaining that answers depend on multiple factors. No single measure can be determined without knowing more about the system because that is the nature of a Digital Twin.

Note: This is a common occurrence when data scientists have been immersed in complicated analytic platforms, they become reluctant to oversimplify system elegance because it minimizes their achievement. Data scientists often focus on how they have achieved an answer more than the direct answer itself. Scientists are trained to be cautious about conclusions and to focus heavily on methods and limitations, which can be confusing to non-analysts.

Listening to the explanation of how the Digital Twin informs medication, dietary and physical activity steps in response to biometrics levels, the analytic translator reinforces the value of this achievement and reiterates the value of the platform.

After confirming their understanding of how the digital twin platform works, the translator can inquire about some hypothetical modelling using the platform.

For instance, assume there are two identical patients, with similar starting HbA1c levels of 9.0, who do not follow dietary guidelines or get sufficient exercise. If one followed the usual standard of care without support from the digital twin to guide medical and lifestyle activities, how likely would they be to achieve an HbA1c below 6.0? Then, if another follows the digital twin guidelines, what might their likelihood be?

After the translator helps the analytic team define the characteristics of a hypothetical group of patients, they are able to run models that indicate that following the digital twin recommendations, 80% of patients would not only achieve reversal of diabetes, but also be taken off medication in 4–6 months. Additionally, they report on previous trials that compare outcomes for digital twin users and non-users.

Thinking ahead to other questions or objections that might come up for practitioners, the translator also explores questions about the rate of patient acceptance of digital twin guidance. In the trials, how often did patients comply or drop out? What does the information look like and how is it given?

2. Distill and Decipher

After hearing the analytic team's explanation of how and what results have been achieved, the translator extracts findings that are most relevant and meaningful to the primary issues faced by practitioners. They prepare concise statements and graphs that can illustrate the main findings, as well as brief answers to logical follow-up questions that are likely to arise.

While analytic methods are important to some audiences, not all clinicians will have an interest in understanding or learning about them. For them, it is more important that the source of information can be trusted and that any changes in their practice will not be burdensome. Their concerns are most often practical, not methodological (Table 18.4).

TABLE 18.4 Digital Twin Example with Final Elaboration

Digital Twin Example

With results in hand, the translator begins their meeting with the clinician by reviewing their previous conversation and what matters most to them.

> *Last time, we talked about your frustration that patients do not achieve clinical improvement and their low rate of compliance. While you support the idea of value-based medicine, you were concerned that clinicians were not being given sufficient support to make a significant improvement in diabetic care.*

The translator then allows the clinician to confirm that this topic remains important to them and to give an update about their thoughts.

Then, the translator introduces the topic by asking about interests relative to the clinician's own concerns.

> *Given the frustration you've had in promoting clinical improvement, I'm wondering, if there was a way to dramatically improve the likelihood that patients achieve optimal HbA1c levels using a method that other patients and doctors have found useful, would that be of interest?*

This question highlights a possible solution to one of the clinician's concerns (clinical improvement), while reducing potential objections (patient and clinician acceptance), and offering it in a non-threatening way (giving them a choice to be interested or not).

If the clinician expresses interest, the translator focuses on the benefits of the digital twin rather than the methods.

> *Our analytic team has developed an interactive system that personalizes recommendations in a simple, but sophisticated way. Patients who used it were 8 times more likely to achieve an HbA1c below 6.0 in 4–6 months. Most patients reported liking it, and doctors report it did not take more time. In fact, it reduced their time doing documentation.*

(Continued)

TABLE 18.4 (Continued) Digital Twin Example with Final Elaboration

I can provide as much detail about the advanced methods on the back end as you would like, but before I do that, would you like to see how the interface works and what it would be like for your patients?

In most cases, the clinicians are more interested in how this approach impacts their patients, followed by how it affects their team. But some do have natural concerns about unfamiliar methodologies and the use of "black boxes." To address these concerns, the translator explores the clinician's criteria for trust.

I know the analytic team would be happy to explain the methodologies used in their digital twin platform. They have extensive experience building these systems and the metrics built into the inputs and feedback were informed by the head of Endocrinology Research. So, we can set up a meeting.

Before I do that, I'm curious, how would you decide if this approach was acceptable for your patients?

This question allows the clinician to identify what would make them comfortable. They will likely not have a complete answer right away and may need to give several responses that the translator confirms. Eventually, the clinician can articulate what they require to feel comfortable. Most often it is the opinion of a trusted expert, or documentation by a trusted person or group, or a statement of validated results from a recognized group or publication.

DISCUSSION AND CONCLUSION

The rapid diffusion of advanced analytics into healthcare will inevitably create challenges as professionals struggle to interpret and understand complex outputs. While some believe that the solution is to insist that all professionals achieve a sufficient level of data and analytic literacy, our position is that the role of analytic translator can bridge the gap between data scientists and healthcare professionals.

The gap between analytic and clinical teams will only widen. Computing and analytics get increasingly complicated and specialized every year (or month, for that matter). Technologically, we are generating, collecting, storing, and processing more and more data, which require talent to digest and interpret. Machine learning and AI techniques will help us handle the complexity, but the tradeoff is less straightforward: "black box" results that are harder and harder to explain.

As described in this chapter, an analytic translator has both clinical and analytic expertise, as well as strong communication skills. Their role is to identify key opportunities where analytics can advance clinical decisions, define those opportunities in ways that facilitate effective analytic work, convert complex findings into meaningful, applicable results, and build allegiances that promote effective collaboration.

Except in cases where people unofficially assume this role, analytic translators have been missing in healthcare. As AI, machine learning and other complex Big Data analytics continue to proliferate, clinicians and their patients will benefit from incorporating trained, experienced Analytic Translators into their teams.

This chapter has served to present the case for the need for analytic translators by highlighting the current challenges that are emerging around a lack of shared meaning and suboptimal comprehension of the outputs from machine learning and AI or analytics digital health solutions. Further, it has served to answer the posed research questions; namely "How can analytic translation mitigate challenges of next-level analytics in healthcare?" and "How can translation demystify AI and analytics in healthcare?" Clearly, there is a need for more systematic research in this important area. It is our intention to progress this important area of inquiry but also hope others will join this effort. There is little doubt that analytics, AI and ML will become key differentiators in the delivery of optimal and excellent healthcare; but if we want this to be for all and not widen current disparities further, it is of vital importance to begin to address the translation aspect.

REFERENCES

Berwick, D., Fineberg, H., & Weinstein, M. (1981). When doctors meet numbers. *The American Journal of Medicine*, *71*(6), 991–998. 10.1016/0002-9343(81)90327-2

Cohen, I. (2021). Explainable AI (XAI) with a decision tree: A practical guide for XAI analysis with decision tree visualization. *Towards Data Science*. Retrieved January 18, 2023, from https://towardsdatascience.com/explainable-ai-xai-with-a-decision-tree-960d60b240bd

DeCamp, M., & Tilburt, J. C. (2019). Why we cannot trust artificial intelligence in medicine. *The Lancet. Digital Health*, *1*(8), e390–e390. 10.1016/S2589-7500(19)30197-9

DeepScribe. Retrieved Jan 18, 2023 from https://www.deepscribe.ai/

Epstein, D., & Pro Publica. (2017). When evidence says no, but doctors say yes. *The Atlantic*. Retrieved January 20, 2023, from https://www.theatlantic.com/health/archive/2017/02/when-evidence-says-no-but-doctors-say-yes/517368/

Hsu, J. (2019). Artificial intelligence could improve healthcare for all — Unless it doesn't. *Undark*. Retrieved Jan 18, 2023, from https://undark.org/2019/07/29/ai-collaboration-medicine-doctors/

Johnson, T. M., Abbasi, A., Schoenberg, E. D., Kellum, R., Speake, L. D., Spiker, C., Foust, A., Kreps, A., Ritenour, C., Brawley, & Master, V. A. (2014). Numeracy among trainees: Are we preparing physicians for evidence-based medicine? *Journal of Surgical Education*, *71*(2), 211–215. 10.1016/j.jsurg.2013.07.013

Khanra, S., Dhir, A., Islam, A. K. M. N., & Mäntymäki, M. (2020). Big data analytics in healthcare: A systematic literature review. *Enterprise Information Systems*, *14*(7), 878–912. 10.1080/17517575.2020.1812005

Liu, X., Wang, X., Wen, C., & Wan, L. (2022). Decision tree distinguish affective disorder diagnosis from psychotic disorder diagnosis with clinical and lab factors. *Heliyon*, *8*(11), e11514. 10.1016/j.heliyon.2022.e11514

Lynch, W. D. (2022). *Become an analytic translator: Make sense of data in business. Make allies of analysts and business leaders*. Triple D Press. https://www.amazon.com/Become-Analytic-Translator-Business-Analysts/dp/0578316803/ref=tmm_pap_swatch_0?_encoding=UTF8&qid=1666978415&sr=8-1

Madjarova, S. J., Williams, R. J., Nwachukwu, B. U., Martin, R. K., Karlsson, J., Ollivier, M., & Pareek, A. (2022). Picking apart p values: Common problems and points of confusion. *Knee Surgery, Sports Traumatology, Arthroscopy*, *30*(10), 3245–3248. 10.1007/s00167-022-07083-3

Pd. (2022). Elon Musk Says AI Will Take Over in 5 Years. *Neuralink*. Retrieved January 20, 2023, from https://elonmuskneuralink.com/elon-musk-says-ai-will-take-over-in-5-years-neuralink/

Sajee, A. (2020). Model Complexity, Accuracy and Interpretability. *Towards Data Science*. Retrieved January 20, 2023, from https://towardsdatascience.com/model-complexity-accuracy-and-interpretability-59888e69ab3d

Simonite, T. (2020). AI can help patients—but only if doctors understand it. *WIRED*. Retrieved January 20, 2023, from https://www.wired.com/story/ai-help-patients-doctors-understand/

Sucich, K. (2022). How to improve data literacy within healthcare organizations. *MedCity News*. Retrieved Jan 18, 2023, from https://medcitynews.com/2022/10/how-to-improve-data-literacy-within-healthcare-organizations/

Wickramasinghe, N., Chalasani, S., & Sloane, E. (Eds.). (2022). *Digital disruption in healthcare*. Springer Nature Switzerland AG. 10.1007/978-3-030-95675-2.

Epilogue

This volume has only touched the tip of the iceberg with respect to the possibilities of analytics, artificial intelligence and machine learning for enabling superior, patient-centred, high-value healthcare delivery to be realised for all. We trust that on reading this book you now have more questions than you had at the start, or as Albert Einstein once eloquently noted "The important thing is not to stop questioning." It is only through questioning and refining that we can be sure we invoke continuous improvement and through imagination that we can truly develop appropriate solutions.

We are still in the infancy of the possibilities of analytics, artificial intelligence and machine learning in the healthcare domain. The road ahead is indeed less travelled and challenging but we also believe the future is bright. What is clear is that as we move forward, analytics, artificial intelligence and machine learning will continue to play a pivotal role in enabling high-quality, high-value patient-centred healthcare delivery. We hope you are hungry to join in creating this new dawn for healthcare delivery and have enjoyed this book at least as much as we have in preparing it.

The Editors
Nilmini Wickramasinghe
Freimut Bodendorf
Mathias Kraus

Index

Printed in the United States
by Baker & Taylor Publisher Services

Printed in the United States
by Baker & Taylor Publisher Services